ONE WEEK LOAN
UNIVERSITY OF GLAMORGAN
GLYNTAFF LEARNING RESOURCES CENTRE

Renew Items on PHONE-it: 01443 654456
Help Desk: 01443 482625 Media Services Reception: 01443 482610
Items are to be returned on or before the last date below

NUTRITION AND WOUND HEALING

CRC Series in Modern Nutrition Science

Series Editor
Stacey J. Bell
Ideasphere, Inc.
Grand Rapids, Michigan

Phytopharmaceuticals in Cancer Chemoprevention
Edited by Debasis Bagchi and Harry G. Preuss

Handbook of Minerals as Nutritional Supplements
Robert A. DiSilvestro

Intestinal Failure and Rehabilitation: A Clinical Guide
Edited by Laura E. Matarese, Ezra Steiger,
and Douglas L. Seidner

Nutrition and Wound Healing
Edited by Joseph Molnar

NUTRITION AND WOUND HEALING

Edited by
Joseph Molnar
Wake Forest University School of Medicine,
Winston-Salem, North Carolina

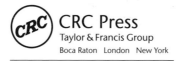

CRC Press
Taylor & Francis Group
Boca Raton   London   New York

CRC Press is an imprint of the
Taylor & Francis Group, an informa business

CRC Press
Taylor & Francis Group
6000 Broken Sound Parkway NW, Suite 300
Boca Raton, FL 33487-2742

© 2007 by Taylor & Francis Group, LLC
CRC Press is an imprint of Taylor & Francis Group, an Informa business

Library of Congress Cataloging-in-Publication Data

Nutrition and wound healing / editor, Joseph Molnar.
p. ; cm. -- (CRC series in modern nutrition science)
Includes bibliographical references and index.
ISBN-13: 978-0-8493-1731-6 (alk. paper)
ISBN-10: 0-8493-1731-2 (alk. paper)
1. Wound healing--Nutritional aspects. 2. Nutrition. 3. Wounds and injuries--Treatment. I. Molnar, Joseph Andrew. II. Series.
[DNLM: 1. Wound Healing. 2. Nutrition. WO 185 N976 2006]

RD94.N882 2006
617.1'40654--dc22   2006018578

**Visit the Taylor & Francis Web site at
http://www.taylorandfrancis.com**

**and the CRC Press Web site at
http://www.crcpress.com**

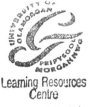

Dedication

To Nancy, Brett, and Liara for their support and understanding.

In Memoriam
for Charles R. Baxter, M.D.

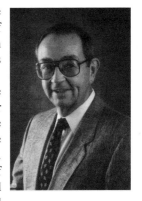

While this book has many esteemed authors, we were extremely honored to have Dr. Charles R. Baxter as one of the contributors. Unfortunately, he passed away on March 10, 2005, shortly after completing a final review of his chapter contribution.

Dr. Baxter served in the Department of Surgery at the University of Texas Southwestern Medical Center for over 40 years. During this time he served as the director of the Parkland Burn Center, the Transplant Services Center, the NIH Burn Research Center, and as the Frank H. Kidd, Jr. Professor of Surgery. He also served as the president of the American Burn Association, which he helped build, and the American Association of Surgery. Dr. Baxter published hundreds of papers and book chapters and received numerous national and international awards for the visionary work he completed in the area of burns, skin transplantation, and the care of chronic wounds. His contributions in burn care include the fluid resuscitation formula referred to as the Baxter Formula. He is also known to many throughout the world as the surgeon who cared for President John F. Kennedy one fateful day in Dallas in 1963.

While his name is on the key publications related to burn and wound care as well as nutrition, those of us who knew him as our teacher or as their physician know the real expertise of Dr. Baxter — that is, providing personal care to patients — listening, touching, and of course, joking. He is notorious for having brought a puppy into the burn unit to inspire an 8-year-old girl who had suffered a large body surface area burn. Whether you were the CEO of a large company or an indigent patient — you received the same top-notch care from Dr. Baxter. And if you didn't follow his advice, the same admonitions!

Dr. Baxter will be sorely missed by all of the people he helped train in the profession and those he touched as patients and friends. The size of Dr. Baxter's professional contributions was only surpassed by the size of his heart.

Carol Ireton-Jones, PhD, RD, LD, CNSD, FACN

George U. Liepa, PhD, FACN

Joseph A. Molnar, MD, PhD, FACS

Preface

Nutrition is of interest to everyone. For the impoverished, nutrition is an issue of obtaining enough food to survive. For some, it is a health concern in their fight against obesity and diabetes, hypertension, heart disease, and degenerative skeletal disorders that accompany this nutritional problem. For others, it is of interest so that they will not be embarrassed wearing their bathing suits. While these situations are apparent to all, we have become aware that some nutrients with less obvious outward manifestations, such as vitamins and minerals, may have consequences that are significant to our health and well-being.

Healing a wound is a high priority to the body. The complex system of wound healing presents an adaptive advantage that ensures the survival of the organism despite the decreased defense against microbial invasion. When injured, the wound is an effective parasite removing from the body what it needs. In 1794, Hunter stated that "There is a circumstance attending accidental injury which does not belong to disease — namely, that the injury done has, in all cases, a tendency to produce both the disposition and the means of cure," (Hunter, J.A., *A Treatise on the Blood, Inflammation and Gunshot Wounds*. Nicol, London, 1794, as quoted in Albina, J.E., Nutrition and wound healing, *Journal of Parenteral and Enteral Nutrition*, 18(4), 368, 1994). In this regard, the wound is not unlike the fetus during pregnancy. Indeed, pregnancy is also a condition that has a "tendency to produce both the disposition and the means of cure." Nonetheless, we have learned that pregnancy requires appropriate nutritional supplementation (i.e., folic acid) to avoid fetal distress. In a similar fashion, despite the fact that most wounds heal well without special nutritional supplementation, the clinician must be aware of those circumstances where intervention is necessary.

Malnutrition may be simply defined as a condition of too much or too little nutrition. While conditions of too little nutrition, such as starvation or total protein and calorie deprivation (marasmus), are obvious malnutrition, many often forget the opposite extreme of this — obesity is also malnutrition. Although total protein–calorie deprivation is often well tolerated, a similar condition of excessive calories with inadequate protein (kwashiorkor) is poorly tolerated and is associated with a higher mortality rate. Similarly, obesity, while not necessarily associated with any nutritional deprivation, may have serious health consequences. It is apparent that proper nutritional support of the patient with a wound requires attention to not only provide enough nutrition but also to avoid nutrient excess to avoid the "toxic" effects of the nutrient.

In the following pages, the importance of each nutrient, both macronutrients and micronutrients, to the healing wound will be systematically described. Also discussed will be the role of pharmacologic manipulation of wound healing and specific conditions associated with challenges in wound healing. The approach taken is similar with each nutrient. A discussion of the role of each nutrient in the healing process is provided, including the dangers of nutrient excess. Finally, recommendations are made for providing the nutrient in appropriate quantities for the patient with a healing wound, and directions for future research are provided. In this manner, it is hoped that this book will provide needed information for the experienced researcher, the novice, or the practicing clinician just wishing to know what to do.

Editor

Joseph A. Molnar is associate professor of plastic and reconstructive surgery at Wake Forest University School of Medicine. He earned his M.D. from Ohio State University and his Ph.D. in nutritional biochemistry and metabolism from the Massachusetts Institute of Technology while doing a research fellowship at Harvard Medical School. His clinical training in general surgery was at the University of Washington, plastic surgery education at the Medical College of Virginia, and hand fellowship and microsurgery training at the Medical College of Wisconsin. His clinical interests include the diversity of plastic surgery, wound care, reconstructive microsurgery, and hand surgery. As the associate director of the burn unit at Wake Forest, a large portion of his clinical practice deals with acute and reconstructive burn care.

Dr. Molnar's research interests relate to both nutrition and wound healing. He has studied the effect of malnutrition on collagen using stable isotopes and the clinical nutrition of burns and trauma. The author has extensive experience and publications in the use of negative pressure wound therapy and bioengineered skin substitutes both in laboratory research and in clinical application.

The author is a Fellow of the American College of Surgeons and is a member of the American Society of Parenteral and Enteral Nutrition, the American Burn Association, the International Society of Burn Injury, the Wound Healing Society, the American Association of Plastic Surgeons, and the American Society of Plastic Surgery.

Contributors

Shefali Agarwal
Strong Regional Burn Center
The University of Rochester
Rochester, New York

Vanita Ahuja
Department of Surgery
Sinai Hospital/Johns Hopkins Medical
  Institutions
Baltimore, Maryland

Adrian Barbul
Department of Surgery
Sinai Hospital/Johns Hopkins Medical
  Institutions
Baltimore, Maryland

Hemendra Basu
School of Health Sciences
Eastern Michigan University
Ypsilanti, Michigan

Thomas G. Baumgartner
Nutrition and Metabolic Support
  Service
College of Pharmacy
Gainesville, Florida

Charles R. Baxter
Department of Surgery
Burn Trauma Critical Care Division
University of Texas
Southwestern Medical Center
Dallas, Texas

C. Dustin Bechtold
Strong Regional Burn Center
The University of Rochester
Rochester, New York

Carmelle Cooper
Regional Nutrition Services
Capital Health
Edmonton, Alberta, Canada

Robert H. Demling
Trauma and Burn Center
Peter Bent Brigham Hospital
Boston, Massachusetts

Maggie L. Dylewski
Shriners Burn Hospital
Harvard Medical School
Boston, Massachusetts

Michele M. Gottschlich
Shriners Hospital
Cincinnati, Ohio

Carol Ireton-Jones
Carrollton, Texas

Tom Jaksic
Department of Surgery
Harvard Medical School
Children's Hospital Boston
Boston, Massachusetts

Patrick J. Javid
Department of Surgery
Children's Hospital Boston
Boston, Massachusetts

Christopher W. Lentz
Strong Regional Burn Center
The University of Rochester
Rochester, New York

George U. Liepa
School of Health Sciences
Eastern Michigan University
Ypsilanti, Michigan

Shayn Martin
Department of Surgery
Wake Forest University School of
  Medicine
Winston-Salem, North Carolina

Joseph A. Molnar
Department of Plastic and
  Reconstructive Surgery
Wake Forest University School of
  Medicine
Winston-Salem, North Carolina

Hannah G. Piper
Department of Surgery
Children's Hospital Boston
Boston, Massachusetts

Majida Rizk
Department of Surgery
Sinai Hospital/Johns Hopkins Medical
  Institutions
Baltimore, Maryland

Mark B. Schoemann
Strong Regional Burn Center
The University of Rochester
Rochester, New York

Perry Shen
Department of Surgery
Wake Forest University School of
  Medicine
Winston-Salem, North Carolina

Hideharu Tanaka
Burn, Trauma, and Critical Care Medicine
Kyorin University
Mitaka City, Tokyo, Japan

Edward E. Tredget
Wound Healing Research Group
Firefighter's Burn Treatment Unit
Divisions of Plastic and Reconstructive
  Surgery and Critical Care
Edmonton, Alberta, Canada

John J. Turek
Department of Basic Medical Sciences
Purdue University
West Layfayette, Indiana

Corilee A. Watters
Department of Agricultural, Food and
  Nutritional Science
University of Alberta
Edmonton, Alberta, Canada

Yong-Ming Yu
Shriners Burn Hospital
Harvard Medical School
Boston, Massachusetts

Contents

1 Overview of Nutrition and Wound Healing

Joseph A. Molnar

CONTENTS

WOUND HEALING

The process of wound healing may be best understood by dividing it into phases.[1–4] These phases are somewhat arbitrary, as they overlap in time, physiology, and cell type, with each phase not entirely completed before the next begins. Our knowledge of these phases is constantly improving, resulting in additional revision of our understanding of how these different aspects of healing interact. In addition, not all wounds heal in precisely the same manner due to differences in the etiology of the wound, presence or absence of infection, and medical or surgical interventions. Which of these components predominates depends on whether the wound is closed immediately (first intention), allowed to granulate (secondary intention), or has delayed primary closure (third intention). These processes remain more similar than different regardless of how the wound is managed. Medical and surgical interventions primarily change the time course of events. For the purposes of the present discussion, the healing process will be divided into the five components of hemostasis, inflammation, proliferation, contraction, and remodeling (Figure 1.1).

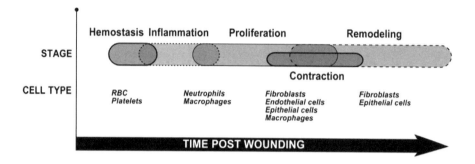

FIGURE 1.1 The process of wound healing may be considered to consist of five overlapping stages. Some authors combine one or more of these stages under a single category. The time course of these stages depends upon methods of treatment and metabolic status of the injured individual.

Hemostasis

Healing begins the instant the wound is made. When the skin is cut, the body responds with a complex mechanism that protects us from exsanguination. Vasoconstriction is almost immediate to decrease blood loss, but enough blood is released in the wound to stimulate Hageman Factor (XII) to initiate the clotting cascade.[3-5] Collagen, present in all tissues of the body and ironically the major protein of wound healing, is exposed in the wound, resulting in stimulation of the alternate complement pathway as well as platelet adherence and degranulation.[3,4,6] Along with complement and Hageman pathway stimulation, numerous additional vasoactive and chemotactic components are released. Blood fibrinogen quickly converts to fibrin, which, along with platelets, helps form what is commonly called a scab.[3,7,8] The scab ultimately provides a temporary protective barrier. The fibrin forms a pathway to aid cell migration, especially for the fibroblast, one of the major cells of the proliferative phase of wound healing.[9]

One of the most active components of the hemostatic phase of wound healing is the platelet. Platelets are present in the blood; they rapidly aggregate and degranulate in the wound. With degranulation, numerous cytokines, such as PDGF (platelet-derived growth factor) are released (Table 1.1).[3,4,6-8] PDGF is a potent cytokine with numerous functions, including being a chemoattractant for neutrophils, one of the dominant cells of the inflammatory phase (Figure 1.1).

The stage of hemostasis does more than just stop exsanguination. It also initiates the process of healing by creating a protective layer to minimize the infection risk while providing both a biochemical milieu and physical framework for the stages that follow.

Thus, the hemostatic stage prepares for and influences the onset of the next stage of healing — inflammation.

Inflammation

Overlapping with the stage of hemostasis is the stage of inflammation (Figure 1.1). While fibrin is forming and platelets are aggregating, leukocytes are coming into

TABLE 1.1
Cytokine Involvement in Wound Healing

Healing Function	Cytokine Involved
Inflammatory cell migration	PDGF
	TGF-β
	TNF-α
Fibroblast migration	PDGF
	TGF-β
	EGF
Fibroblast proliferation	PDGF
	TGF-β
	EGF
	IGF
	TNF-α
	IL-1
Angiogenesis	bFGF (FGF2)
	aFGF (FGF1)
	TGF-β
	TGF-α
	EGF
	TNF-α
	VEGF
	IL-8
	PD-ECGF
Epithelialization	EGF
	TGF-α
	KGF (FGF7)
	bFGF (FGF2)
	IGF
	HB-EGF
Collagen synthesis	PDGF
	TGF-β
	bFGF (FGF2)
	EGF

Note: PDGF = platelet-derived growth factor; TGF-β = transforming growth factor-β; TNF-α = tumor necrosis factor-α; EGF = epidermal growth factor; IGF = insulin-like growth factor; IL-1 = interleukin-1; bFGF = basic fibroblast growth factor; aFGF = acidic fibroblast growth factor; TGF-α = transforming growth factor-α; VEGF = vascular endothelial growth factor; IL-8 = interleukin-8; PD-ECGF = platelet-derived-endothelial cell growth factor; KGF = keratinocyte growth factor; and HB-EGF = heparin binding epidermal growth factor.

Source: From Lawrence, W.T., *Clin. Plast. Surg.*, 25, 321, 1998. With permission.

the wound. The initial vasoconstriction is replaced by vasodilation, but clotted vessels prevent continued blood loss. Vasodilation is the result of prostaglandin, nitric oxide, and other inflammatory mediators. The release of bradykinin, histamines, and free radicals from leukocytes leads to increased vascular permeability.

This, in turn, results in plasma fluid leak into the interstitial space as well as increased margination of white blood cells and diapedesis.[4,10–12]

This process leads to an influx into the interstitial space of macromolecules, including enzymes, antibodies to fight infection, and nutrients.[11] We have long known that glucose and oxygen are crucial to the inflammatory process. More recently, it has become apparent that even the influx of a single amino acid such as arginine to the wound site may serve as a precursor for an important mediator such as nitric oxide.[13] This is discussed in greater detail in Chapter 6. Similarly, lipids in the wound may be chemically altered by free radicals in the wound to create isoprostanes. These potent inflammatory mediators may stimulate a cascade of events in the wound.[12,14] These events are discussed in greater detail in Chapter 3.

After polymorphonuclear leukocyte influx, the monocytes are next to arrive. Monocytes become phagocytic macrophages that remove debris as well as bacteria from the wound. These macrophages secrete proteases, producing interferon and prostaglandins as well as cytokines. These cytokines, among other things, are chemoattractants for mesenchynal cells. These cells will differentiate into fibroblasts, one of the major cell types involved in the proliferative phase and in connective tissue formation.[4,11]

PROLIFERATION

In the first two stages of wound healing, the bleeding is stopped, the wound debrided, and bacteria controlled. However, none of the major components of these stages will be a significant part of the mature healed wound. The macrophages, neutrophils, lymphocytes, and platelets will become senescent, ultimately undergo apoptosis, and will themselves then be degraded to their biochemical subunits. Nonetheless, through wound preparation, the secretion of proliferative cytokines (PDGF, interleukin-1 [IL-1], fibroblast growth factor [FGF]) and chemoattractants (transforming growth factor-[TGF-β], PDGF) these cells have done their part to set the stage for the next phase of wound healing.[4,6,11,15,16] This transition to the proliferative stage is not discrete. Macrophages may remain active at altered levels throughout the healing process, secreting collagenase and elastase into the wound to aid the influx of proliferative cells and remodeling of the wound. Should the wound become infected, polymorphonuclear leukocytes will return in numbers to control the bacterial proliferation, and macrophage numbers will increase. Clearly, this will stimulate a recurrent cascade of events that maintains the wound in a more inflammatory state and interferes with progress to the next stage.

Here the clinician may alter the course of the wound healing. Removing debris surgically, either with wound care or whirlpool, lessens the job of the inflammatory stage. Maintaining bacterial control with topical or systemic antibiotics will also expedite this stage. Clearly, the ultimate intervention is closing the wound, thus making these stages as short as possible. Finally, proper systemic support (i.e., critical care) to aid tissue perfusion or metabolic support to optimize the immune response by providing substrate for energy or protein synthesis is necessary for optimal outcome in the healing wound.

In most wounds unimpeded by overwhelming necrotic tissue and infection, the proliferative phase becomes dominant several days after injury. As discussed below, this will often correspond chronologically to the "flow" or hypermetabolic phase of the metabolic response to injury. The fibrin network initiated in the hemostatic phase becomes a framework and chemoattractant for fibroblast ingrowth.[4,6,7,9] Under these circumstances, the fibroblasts actually become mobile, developing lamellipodia and advancing by "pulling" themselves forward. Once in the wound, they proliferate rapidly under the influence of facilitating cytokines such as PDGF and TGF-β (Table 1.1).[15,16]

Fibroblasts are responsible for the production of the key extracellular structural components of the healing wound. Most of the ultimate scar formed in the healing process is made of the structural protein collagen, although a variety of proteoglycans and other proteins are also present.

Collagen is one of the most complex proteins in the body, consisting of a triple alpha helix of approximately 1000 amino acids per strand depending on the collagen type (Figure 1.2).[17] Type I collagen dominates in the mature wound; it accounts for 80 to 90%, with the rest being primarily Type III.[4,18,19] Early in the healing process, the concentration of Type III may be even higher. Smaller amounts of Type IV

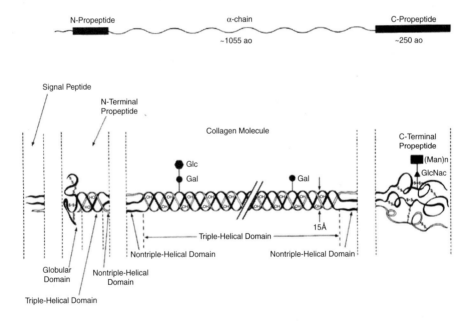

FIGURE 1.2 The collagen molecule is a complex protein that requires several nutrient cofactors for proper intracellular synthesis. It is the dominant protein of the healed wound. (From Pesciotta, D.M. and Olsen, B.R., *The Cell Biology of Collagen Secretion in Heinz Furthmayr, Immunochemistry of the Extracellular Matrix*, Vol. 2, CRC Press, Boca Raton, FL, 1982. With permission.)

(basement membrane), Type V (blood vessels), and Type VII (epidermal basement membrane anchoring fibers) may be present as well.[18]

The amino acid structure of collagen is unusual, consisting of the repeating triplet structure of glycine –X–Y. Approximately 20 to 25% of the "Y" position is either proline or hydroxyproline. Hydroxyproline is found almost exclusively in collagen and is made from the posttranslational hydroxylation of proline. This requires the mixed function oxygenase prolyl hydroxylase as well as the cofactors of ferrous iron, α-ketoglutarate, free molecular oxygen, and vitamin C.[17] A similar process also creates the amino acid hydroxylsine from lysine, an amino acid crucial to proper collagen cross-linking. This cross-linking is essential to impart the tensile strength and decreased turnover as seen in the mature collagen molecule.

It is clear that these amino acid substrates must be present in adequate amounts for normal wound healing. Without adequate available amino acids and cofactors such as vitamin C, there would be inadequate collagen. Without adequate quantities of collagen, the wounds will be weak, leading to dehiscence. This phenomenon will be discussed in more detail in Chapter 8.

The proliferative phase also involves the influx of endothelial cells and neovascularization. In some wounds left to granulate and heal by secondary intention, this process will dominate, leading to beefy-red vascular tissue. This process, like the fibroblast migration and proliferation, requires large amounts of energy compared to the quiescent wound that is mature. This process of angiogenesis is under the strict control of cytokines being stimulated by FGF-2 and vascular endothelial growth factor (VEGF), among others.[19–21] Proliferating endothelial cells must be properly aligned on the fibrin–fibrinogen matrix to form vascular sprouts and channels to create the new vessels.

While epithelialization is another component of the proliferative phase, it may dominate in certain wounds, such as superficial burns. Basal epithelial cells present in the wound edge or in the epidermal appendages such as hair follicles begin to migrate across the wound edge in the early days of wound healing. Again, this is under cytokine control, such as by TGF-β, EGF (epidermal growth factor), KGF (keratinocyte growth factor), and FGF-7 (Table 1.1).[4,19,22] As the cells proceed across a newly produced collagen matrix, they produce a new basement membrane essential to normal epithelial cell activity.

CONTRACTION

Contraction is a process of wound healing whereby the wound essentially shrinks by recruiting adjacent tissue and pulling it into the wound. This process is intimate with the phases of proliferation and remodeling, because the key effector cell is the fibroblast (Figure 1.1). More specifically, the cell involved is the myofibroblast as first described by Gabbiani et al.[19,23] While motor function is present in all fibroblasts as well as in other cells such as leukocytes, these cells are modified in a way that moves the edges of the wound toward the center of the wound, rather than just being motile and moving themselves. This process is independent of collagen synthesis, but collagen in the extracellular matrix aids in locking the cells in place, thus augmenting the contraction process.[4] Stimulation of this process is under control of TGF-β as well as of other cytokines.

Depending on the location and origin of the wound, contraction may be a major process in wound closure. In animals, such as the rat, with a *panniculus carnosus*, contraction may dominate the process of wound healing such that it may interfere with use of this animal as an experimental model of human wound healing. The back of the human hand has loose mobile tissue, similar to the skin of a rat, which readily allows the process of contraction to be a major contributor to the healing process. The result will potentially interfere with use of the hand should the contraction process render the skin too tight. The same forces may be less effective on the palm of the hand or the sole of the foot, where the skin connections render the skin more stable.

REMODELING

Thus far in the process of healing, the wound is characterized by a high level of metabolic activity. This allows for the extensive proliferation of inflammatory cells, epithelial cells, endothelial cells for angiogenesis, and fibroblasts actively laying down the collagen matrix of the healed wound. During the remodeling phase, the nutritional requirements of wound healing will be diminishing. Initially the wound is a soft, cellular structure lacking strength. Subsequently, through the process of remodeling, the scar is transformed to the final mature healed wound with tensile approaching that of the uninjured tissue.

The phase of remodeling represents an entirely different aspect of the healing process. While hemostasis may take minutes, inflammation days, and proliferation weeks, the remodeling phase may continue for months or years. Instead of progressively increased collagen synthesis, in a net sense, collagen accretion decreases to a balance between synthesis and degradation, except in abnormal states such as keloid or hypertrophic scars. The initial mixture of Type I and Type III collagen is slowly changed into a wound with primarily Type I collagen. The amount of ground substance decreases, and collagen cross-linking increases.[4,19]

These processes appear to be under the control of interferon, matrix metalloproteinases, TGF-β, PDGF, and IL-1, among others.[4,19,20] Although such enzymes may control the collagen type and the synthesis and degradation rates, they likely have less to do with the degree of collagen cross-linking. Collagen cross-linking starts with the hydroxylation of lysine to make hydroxylysine. Once the initial cross-links are formed, the maturation of the cross-link to the more mature cross-link appears not to be under enzymatic control.[24] This suggests that certain aspects of the maturation process occur as a direct result of the chemical structure of the collagen molecule rather than of enzymatic control. This may provide a certain metabolic efficiency for changes in an extracellular molecule less directly accessible to intracellular enzymes.

While not as rapidly changing as the phases preceding it, the remodeling phase is equally important. As we will see, under certain disease states, such as scurvy, the balance of synthesis and degradation is crucial to maintain a healed wound even years after the original injury. This is discussed in Chapter 8 in greater detail.

NUTRITION AND THE METABOLIC RESPONSE
TO INJURY

Cuthbertson described the metabolic response to injury as consisting of an "ebb" phase and a "flow" phase.[25,26] The "ebb" phase is the period of traumatic shock or hypometabolism during the first few hours or days after injury. This phase is soon replaced by the "flow" phase that is a period of hypermetabolism that may last for weeks or months depending on the nature of the injury and obstacles to recovery. In the case of minor injury, such as elective surgery, both of these phases may be relatively brief and of minor magnitude. In the case of multiple trauma or large percent body surface area burns, both ebb and flow may be of maximum magnitude and duration. In this latter group of patients, nutritional support becomes critical, because the potential to deplete the body's nutrient reserves is high. On the contrary, in a patient of good preoperative nutritional status undergoing routine elective surgery, it is unlikely that perioperative nutritional support will have a measurable effect on outcome of the healing wound.[26–28]

The wound is an effective parasite on the substrate available in the rest of the body. Much like the human fetus, the wound demands high priority of circulating nutrients. In a teleological sense, this would be expected, because healing of the wound is crucial to the survival of the organism. During periods of metabolic stress, the body is able to effectively catabolize the carcass (muscle, skin, bone) to support visceral protein synthesis of acute phase proteins, immunoglobulins, inflammatory cells, and collagen, needed to fight infection and heal the wound.[25,26,29–31] In the case of proteins, intricate shuttling mechanisms have developed to allow redistribution of the substrate from the periphery to the viscera (Figure 1.3 and Figure 1.4). Although this has been well studied in the case of protein, it is likely that similar mechanisms apply to other nutrients.[26,29,32] As seen in Figure 1.4, glucose and protein metabolism are intricately linked in the glucose–alanine cycle so that energy needs and amino acid needs are met simultaneously. This could also apply to micronutrients. Because a large percentage of body zinc stores are found in the skin, it would not be surprising that if the skin proteins are catabolized, this might also allow mobilization of skin zinc to provide cofactors for enzymatic activity in other parts of the body.

Clearly, though, in patients with chronic malnutrition the situation is entirely different. These individuals may have inadequate reserves with which to respond appropriately to the metabolic demands of even a minor trauma. This is similar to the described conversion of individuals with marasmus (protein–calorie malnutrition) to kwashiorkor (a more severe form of protein–calorie malnutrition characterized by protein deficiency greater than the caloric deficiency) with the onset of infection.[33] These marginally compensated individuals lack the reserve to respond to infection and may ultimately succumb to the infection that might otherwise not be life threatening. Deficiency of even a single micronutrient such as vitamin C may lead to disastrous results in the healing process. This is discussed in Chapter 8 in greater detail.

Nutrients may be arbitrarily divided into "macronutrients" and "micronutrients." However, the difference between these categories is not well defined. Macronutrients

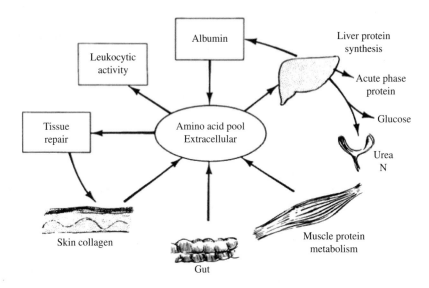

FIGURE 1.3 The metabolic process of injury results in a peripheral to visceral redistribution of nutrients. The carcass is effectively catabolized to contribute to a systemic amino acid pool to support wound healing and the manufacture of acute phase reactants. (From Molnar, J.A., Wolfe, R.R., and Burke, J.F., in *Nutritional Support of Medical Practice*, 2nd ed., Harper & Row, Philadelphia, 1983, adapted from Benotti et al., *Crit. Care Med.*, 7, 520, 1979. With permission.)

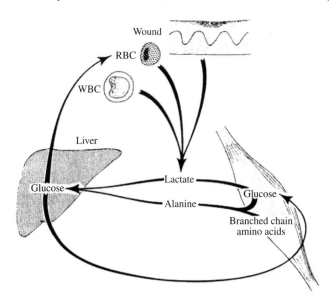

FIGURE 1.4 The glucose–alanine cycle effectively supports the metabolic needs of the healing wound by shuttling amino acids from the carcass to the liver to support gluconeogenesis. This mechanism is an example of the complex interrelationships between nutrients. (From Molnar, J.A., Wolfe, R.R., and Burke, J.F., in *Nutritional Support of Medical Practice*, 2nd ed., Harper & Row, Philadelphia, 1983. With permission.)

include carbohydrates, protein, and fat. Micronutrients include all the vitamins and trace elements and have also been described as those nutrients consumed in quantities less than some arbitrary level per day.[34] As will be discussed below, when some micronutrients are consumed in what might be considered pharmacologic quantities, these quantitative distinctions become blurred. For the purposes of this text, micronutrients will be defined as all nutrients other than carbohydrates, fats, and proteins.

MACRONUTRIENTS

Macronutrients provide the energy for all body functions as well as the major building blocks for all tissues and reparative processes (Table 1.2). As will be discussed in Chapter 2 and Chapter 3, carbohydrate and fat may both be used to support the energy needs of the organism, although certain cells may be obligate carbohydrate consumers. This is especially true in the healing wound, with a density of inflammatory cells and fibroblasts that use carbohydrate as an energy source.[35,36] Studies suggest that, even when carbohydrates are readily available, a substantial percentage of the total energy needs are met by fat.[37] These findings are discussed in greater detail in Chapter 3 and Chapter 11. In addition, fats provide the building blocks for the cell membrane and certain inflammatory mediators. Carbohydrates may minimize the burden for fat intake by providing substrate for fatty acid synthesis, except for essential fatty acids that must be obtained from dietary sources.

Protein is the third component of macronutrients. Amino acids provide the major structural building blocks of all proteins in the body, including collagen, the major protein of the healing wound. Amino acids are necessary for the cell membrane and enzymes and cytokine production in the healing wound. In the inflammatory and proliferative phases, amino acid requirements in the wound will be maximal due to the high level of enzymatic activity and the high rate of cell turnover.

Protein metabolism is closely interrelated to carbohydrate and fat metabolism. Glucose and fatty acid metabolites may be used as substrate for endogenous amino acid synthesis (Figure 1.4). Conversely, metabolites of amino acid breakdown may be deaminated to provide gluconeogenic precursors and substrate for fatty acid production. However, much like the fatty acids that cannot be synthesized by the human body, certain amino acids are essential or conditionally essential and must, therefore, be obtained through the diet. This concept is discussed in greater detail in Chapter 4.

MICRONUTRIENTS

Micronutrients function primarily as cofactors in biochemical reactions and, as such, are critical to all of the activities of macronutrients. Protein synthesis cannot continue without adequate quantities of vitamin B_6, zinc, and copper.[26,37,38] Collagen synthesis will be impaired without vitamin C, iron, and copper. Carbohydrate utilization is impaired without chromium and manganese. Vitamin B_{12}, folate, and zinc are essential for nucleic acid metabolism and, thus, are essential in the healing wound with rapid cellular proliferation.

TABLE 1.2
Function of Some Key Nutrients Involved in Wound Healing

Nutrient	Specific Compound	Contribution of Wound Healing
Proteins	Amino acids	Needed for platelet function, neovascularization, lymphocyte formation, fibroblast proliferation, collagen synthesis, and wound remodeling
		Required for certain cell-mediated responses, including phagocytosis and intracellular killing of bacteria
		Gluconeogenic precursors
Carbohydrates	Glucose	Energy substrate of leukocytes and fibroblasts
Fats	Fatty acids	Serve as building blocks for prostaglandins, isoprostanes
	Cholesterol	that are inflammatory mediators; energy source for some cell types
		Are constituents of triglycerides and fatty acids contained in cellular and subcellular membranes
Vitamins	Vitamin C	Hydroxylates proline and lysine in collagen synthesis
		Free radical scavenger
		Is a necessary component of complement that functions in immune reactions and increases defenses to infection
	Vitamin B complex	Serves as cofactor of enzyme systems
		Required for antibody formation and white blood cell function, essential for nucleic acid metabolism
	Vitamin A	Enhances epithelialization of cell membranes
		Enhances rate of collagen systhesis and cross-linking of newly formed collagen
		Antagonizes the inhibitory effects of glucocorticoids on cell membranes
	Vitamin D	Necessary for absorption, transport, and metabolism of calcium
		Indirectly affects phosphorus metabolism
	Vitamin E	Free radical scavenger
	Vitamin K	Needed for synthesis of prothrombin and clotting factors VII, IX, and X
		Required for synthesis of calcium-binding protein
Minerals	Zinc	Stabilizes cell membranes; enzyme cofactor
		Needed for cell mitosis and cell proliferation in wound repair
	Iron	Needed for hydroxylation of proline and lysine in collagen synthesis
		Enhances bactericidal activity of leukocytes
		Hemoglobin oxygen transport to wound
	Copper	Integral part of the enzyme lysyloxidase, which catalyzes formation of stable collagen cross-links

Source: Modified from Schumann, D., *Nurs. Clin. North Am.*, 14, 683, 1979. With permission.

Micronutrients are ubiquitous in a normal diet, and therefore, severe deficiencies are uncommon without pathologic stress. In many cases, they are only cofactors in chemical reactions, not altered or consumed, so they may ultimately be reutilized. However, with certain micronutrients, we have come to recognize the value of intake orders of magnitude greater than needed for cofactors of biochemical reactions. Vitamin C, for instance, in large quantities may be a useful free-radical scavenger, as discussed in greater detail in Chapter 8.[39,40] Vitamin A in large quantities may be useful to offset the adverse effects of corticosteroids on wound healing.[38,41,42] In Chapter 9, this is discussed in greater detail.

NUTRIENT TOXICITY

Malnutrition may be defined as a state of nutrient deficiency or excess. This fact is often overlooked when providing nutrition, despite the fact that some of the adverse effects of nutrient excess are evident to everyone. Carbohydrate excess, for example, clearly may lead to a state of obesity, with the well-recognized risks of cardiovascular disease, diabetes, and shorter life expectancy. What is less obvious is that carbohydrate excess in the critically ill patient may also result in liver damage and the inability to wean from ventilators.[26] In Chapter 2 and Chapter 11, this will be discussed in greater detail. Other nutrients, such as vitamin A, have the potential for toxicity that is even less obvious but equally dangerous.[38,42] This is discussed in greater detail in Chapter 9. It is apparent that in providing nutrition to stimulate healing, the caregiver cannot assume that "more is better."

In the chapters that follow, not only will the need for nutritional supplementation to optimize healing be evaluated, but also how to optimize that supplementation to avoid the consequences of nutrient excess will be addressed.

REFERENCES

1. Lawrence, W.T., Physiology of the acute wounds, *Clin. Plast. Surg.*, 25, 321, 1998.
2. Phillips, S.J., Physiology of wound healing and surgical wound care, *ASAIO J.*, S2, 2000.
3. Orgill, D. and Demling, R.H., Current concepts and approaches to wound healing, *Crit. Care Med.*, 16, 899, 1988.
4. Monaco, J.L. and Lawrence, W.T., Acute wound healing: An overview, *Clin. Plast. Surg.*, 30, 2003.
5. Ryan, G.B. and Manjo, G., Acute inflammation — a review, *Am. J. Pathol.*, 86, 183, 1987.
6. Wakefield, T.W., Hemostasis, in *Surgery: Scientific Principals and Practice*, 3rd ed., Greenfield, L.J., Mulholland, M.W., Oldham, K.T., Zelenock, G.B., and Lillemoe, K.D., Eds., Lippincott Williams & Wilkins, Philadelphia, 2001, chap. 4, p. 86.
7. Clark, R.A. et al., Fibronectin and fibrin provide a provisional matrix for epidermal all migration during wound re-epithelization, *J. Invest. Derm.*, 79, 264, 1982.
8. Herndon, D.N., Nguten, T.T., and Gilphin, D.A., Growth factors; local and systemic, *Arch. Surg.*, 128, 1227, 1993.
9. Postlethwaite, A.E. et al., Induction of fibroblast chemotaxis by fibronectin, *J. Exp. Med.*, 153, 494, 1981.

10. Martin, P.M., Wooley, J.H., and McCluskey, J., Growth factors and cutaneous wound repair, *Prog. Growth Factor Res.*, 4, 25, 1992.

11. Barbul, A., Role of the immune system, in *Wound Healing: Biochemical and Clinical Aspects*, Cohen, I.K., Diegelmann, R.F., and Lindblad, W.B., Eds., W.B. Saunders, Philadelphia, 1992, chap. 17, p. 282.

12. Robson, M.C. and Heggers, J.P., Eicosanoids, cytokines and free radicals, in *Wound Healing: Biochemical and Clinical Aspects*, Cohen, I.K., Diegelmann, R.F., and Lindblad, W.B., Eds., W.B. Saunders, Philadelphia, 1992, chap. 18, p. 292.

13. Williams, J.Z. and Barbul, A., Nutrition and wound healing, *Surg. Clin. N. Am.*, 83, 571, 2003.

14. Morrow, J.D. et al., The isoprostanes: unique prostaglandin-like products of free-radical initiated lipid peroxidation, *Drug Metab. Rev.*, 31, 117, 1999.

15. Seppä, H. et al., Platelet derived growth factor chemotactic for fibroblasts, *J. Cell. Biol.*, 92, 584, 1982.

16. Postlethwaite, A.E. et al., Stimulation of the chemotactic migration of human fibroblasts by transforming growth factor-, *J. Exp. Med.*, 165, 251, 1987.

17. Pesciotta, D.M. and Olsen, B.R., The cell biology of collagen secretion, in *Immunochemistry of the Extracellular Matrix*, Furthmayer, H., Ed., CRC Press, Boca Raton, FL, 1992, chap. 2, p. 1.

18. Miller, E.J., Collagen types: structure, distribution and functions, in *Collagen Volume II: Biochemistry and Biomechanics*, Nimni, Marcel E., Ed., CRC Press, Boca Raton, FL, 1988, p. 139.

19. Diegelmann, R.F., Lindblad, W.J., and Cohen, I.K., Fibrogenic processes during tissue repair, in *Collagen Volume II: Biochemistry and Biomechanics*, Nimni, Marcel E., Ed., CRC Press, Boca Raton, FL, 1998, p. 113.

20. Gospodarowicz, D., Newfield, G., Schweigerer, L., Fibroblast growth factor: structural and biologic properties, *J. Cell. Physiol.*, 5, 15, 1987.

21. Gospodarowicz, D., Abraham, J., and Schilling, J., Isolation and characterization of a vascular endothelial cell mitogen produced by pituitary derived follicular stellate cells, *Proc. Natl. Acad. Sci. USA*, 86, 7311, 1989.

22. Werner, S. et al., Large induction of keratinocyte growth factor expression in the dermis during wound healing, *Proc. Natl. Acad. Sci. USA*, 89, 6896, 1992.

23. Gabbianni, G., Ryan, G.B., and Majno, G., Presence of modified fibroblasts in granulation tissue and their possible role in wound contraction, *Experientia*, 27, 549, 1971.

24. Molnar, J.A., Skin collagen turnover in healthy and protein calorie malnourished rats. Doctorate thesis, Massachusetts Institute of Technology, 1985.

25. Cuthbertson, D.P., Observations on the disturbance of metabolism produced by injury to the limbs, *Quart. J. Med.*, 1, 233, 1932.

26. Molnar, J.A. and Burke, J.F., Nutritional aspects of surgical physiology, in *Surgical Physiology*, Burke, J.F., Ed., W.B. Saunders, Philadelphia, 1983.

27. Albrina, J.E., Nutrition and wound healing, *J. Parenteral and Enteral Nutr.*, 336, 1994.

28. Clark, M., Plank, L.D., and Hill, G.L., Wound healing associated with severe surgical illness, *World J. Surg.*, 24, 648, 2000.

29. Cuthbertson, D.P., The disturbance of metabolism produced by bony and non-bony injury with notes on certain abnormal conditions of bone, *Biochem. J.*, 24, 1244, 1930.

30. Cuthbertson, D.P. and Tilstone, W.J., Nutrition of the injured, *Am. J. Clin. Nutr.*, 24, 911, 1968.

31. Molnar, J.A., Wolfe, R.R., and Burke, J.F., Burns: metabolism and nutritional therapy in thermal injury, in *Nutritional Support of Medical Practice*, 2nd ed., Schneider, H.A., Anderson, C.E., and Coursin, D.B., Eds., Harper & Row, Philadelphia, 1983

32. Cuthbertson, D.P. et al., Effects of severity, nutrition, and environmental temperature on protein, potassium, zinc and creatinine, *Brit. J. Surg.*, 59, 68, 1972.

33. Bhattacharyya, A.K., Protein-energy malnutrition (kwashiorkor-marasmus syndrome): terminology, classification and evolution, *Wld. Rev. Nutr. Diet*, 47, 80, 1986.

34. Ettinger, S., Macronutrients: carbohydrates, proteins and lipids, in *Krause's Food Nutrition and Diet Therapy*, 10th ed., Mahan, L., and Escott-Stump, S., Eds., W.B. Saunders, Philadelphia, 2000.

35. Hunt, T.K., The physiology of wound healing, *Ann. Emerg. Med.*, 17, 1265, 1988.

36. Whitney, J.D. and Heitkemper, M.M., Modifying perfusion, nutrition, and stress to promote wound healing in patients with acute wounds, *Heart and Lung*, 28, 123, 1999.

37. Smith, J.S., Austen, W.G., and Souba, W.W., Nutrition and metabolism, in *Surgery: Scientific Principles and Practice*, 3rd ed., Greenfield, L.J., Mullholland, M.J., and Oldham, K.T., Eds., Lippincott Williams & Wilkins, Philadelphia, 2001.

38. Demling, R.A. and DeBiasse, M.A., Micronutrients in critical illness, *Crit. Care Clin.*, 11, 651, 1995.

39. Matsuda, T. et al., Effects of high dose vitamin C administration on postburn microvascular fluid and protein flux, *J. Burn Care Rehabil.*, 14, 624, 1993.

40. Tanaka, H. et al., Vitamin C administration reduces resuscitation fluid volume in severely burned patients. A randomized prospective study, *Arch. of Surg.*, submitted for publication.

41. Thompson, C.W., Nutrition and adult wound healing, *Nutrition Week*, January 18, 2003.

42. Petry, J.J., Surgically significant nutritional supplements, *Plast. Reconstr. Surg.*, 97, 233, 1996.

2 Carbohydrates and Wound Healing

Carol Ireton-Jones and George U. Liepa

CONTENTS

The role of carbohydrates in wound healing predominately relates to the provision of energy substrates to fuel the body to allow re-epithelialization and recovery. In this chapter, the basic structure and function of carbohydrates, the essential role of carbohydrates, and energy needs and energy metabolism in wound healing will be reviewed.

STRUCTURE AND FUNCTION

Carbohydrates are defined as compounds that are composed of simple sugars (monosaccharides). They were initially named this because they contain both carbon (carbo) and H_2O (water), as shown in Figure 2.1.

Until recently, most medical textbooks focused primarily on the nutrient/energy roles played by three simple sugars (glucose, fructose, and galactose), three disaccharides (sucrose, lactose, and maltose), as well as the fiber/energy roles of complex carbohydrates (cellulose, glycogen, and starch). Over 200 simple carbohydrates are now known to be produced by plants. Eight of these carbohydrates (galactose, glucose, mannose, *N*-acetylneuraminic acid, fructose 6, *N*-acetylglucosamine, *N*-acetylglucosamine, and xylose) are now recognized as being essential for health, and new roles for carbohydrates are constantly being discovered (1).

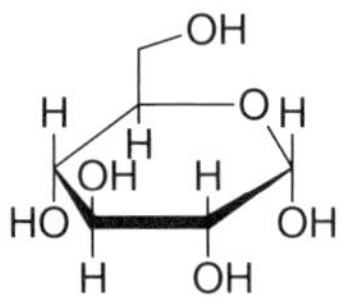

FIGURE 2.1 Glucose.

CARBOHYDRATES, ENERGY METABOLISM, AND WOUND HEALING

In general, calories are needed to supply the energy that is necessary for wound healing. Nutritional support generally includes some form of carbohydrates (parenteral dextrose, and enteral lactose, oligosaccharides, etc.). Glucose is a critical nutrient, especially in patients who have experienced significant trauma, such as a burn, as it is required for cellular growth, fibroblastic mobility, and leukocyte activity. As the metabolic rate increases, there is a concomitant increase in the conversion of amino acids to glucose and an increased rate of hepatic gluconeogenesis if adequate carbohydrate substrates are not provided.

Carbohydrates have been shown to impact wound healing in a variety of ways. Historically, carbohydrates have been viewed as an energy source for patients who are recovering from wounds. Differences have been noted in regards to carbohydrate requirements of patients who suffer from acute traumatic wounds (i.e., burns), acute iatrogenic wounds (i.e., incisions), and chronic wounds (i.e., diabetic wounds) (2). Under normal circumstances, the body increases glucose production via the liver and kidneys. This increase in gluconeogenesis is stimulated by a variety of hormones, including glucagons, epinephrine, and norepinephrine. Skin cells are glucose dependent for energy in cutaneous wound healing (3). Although adequate glucose levels are vital for wound healing, excessively high levels (hyperglycemia) have a negative impact on this process.

CARBOHYDRATE REQUIREMENTS/ENERGY METABOLISM

In healthy adults, carbohydrate intake should account for 45 to 60% of total consumed calories. Carbohydrate requirements for patients with burn injuries greater than 25% of the body surface area have been recommended at levels up to 60 to 65% of total energy requirement (4,5). Carbohydrate is the key nonprotein energy source for the patient with burns, in particular. In a study by Hart and colleagues of 14 pediatric burn patients, it was shown that the administration of a high-carbohydrate diet (rather then fat) was associated with an improved net balance of skeletal muscle protein across the leg via an apparent protein sparing effect of the high-carbohydrate diet and a concomitant decrease in protein breakdown (6). Protein is needed in adequate amounts approaching 20 to 25% of the total caloric needs, leaving exogenous fat as the balance of caloric need at 20% or less of total calories due to potential immunosuppressive effects.

Hyperglycemia is a complication of excessive carbohydrate (glucose) provision and must be addressed in reference to the higher percentages of carbohydrate need suggested. Clearly, there is a hyperglycemic effect in the flow phase of burn injury as well as in critically ill patients who may also have a wound. Although short-term hyperglycemia accompanies the stress response to injury, persistent hyperglycemia is a problem that has commonly been associated with poor wound healing and immunity (7). Pediatric burn patients with poor glucose control experienced reduced skin graft take and subsequent mortality. Total caloric intake should be evaluated, as hypercaloric feeding may be associated with hyperglycemia. Further, because carbohydrate is a key substrate in burn wound healing, internal insulin production may be enhanced. Insulin, an anabolic hormone, has positive effects on nitrogen utilization. The use of exogenous insulin has been shown to lead to a decrease in peripheral muscle wasting and an increase in lean body mass and bone mass. Exogenous insulin may be used to control hyperglycemia, but care must be taken to assure that the dextrose or total calorie provision is not excessive.

Van den Berghe studied two different levels of insulin therapy in critically ill adult intensive care unit patients (ICUs) (8). One group received intensive insulin therapy to control blood glucose levels in the range of 80 to 110 mg/dL, and the other group received insulin only when blood glucose levels exceeded 200 mg/dL. A significant difference in intensive care mortality risk (43% reduction), infection (46% reduction in risk of severe infection), and a 35% reduction in prolonged antibiotic therapy requirement were seen in the intensive insulin therapy group. The author concluded that maintaining normoglycemia (blood glucose levels of less than 110 mg/dL) in adult surgical intensive-care patients is associated with positive outcomes. Krinsley utilized an insulin protocol involving intensive monitoring and treatment to maintain blood glucose levels of less than 140 mg/dL in a study of 800 critically ill adult patients and saw improved glycemic control, which was associated with decreased mortality, organ dysfunction, and length of ICU stay (9). Thomas and colleagues demonstrated the benefit of euglycemic hyperinsulinemia with exogenous insulin maintained throughout the hospital course in decreasing muscle catabolism and preserving lean body mass in pediatric patients with major burns (10). These studies demonstrate the importance of careful attention to glycemic control in the ICU population and can be extrapolated to the acute and chronic care setting.

Excessive glucose administration can be as deleterious as inadequate nutrition support for reasons other than exacerbation of hyperglycemia. Burn patients have accelerated gluconeogenesis, glucose oxidation, and plasma clearance of glucose (11).

Excessive glucose intake in the face of a traumatic injury or sepsis is associated with increased carbon dioxide production and hepatic steatosis (12,13). Burke and Wolfe evaluated whole-body protein synthesis and rate of glucose oxidation in 18 patients who were severely burned and determined the optimal glucose infusion rate to be 5 mg/kg/min (13). They concluded that exceeding the maximal infusion rate for glucose does not enhance protein synthesis but is associated with increased deposition of fat in the liver, as noted on autopsy, as well as the above-mentioned increased rates of carbon dioxide production that are associated with ventilatory challenges, including prolonged ventilator dependence. Interestingly, these authors also found that an enteral diet high in carbohydrate and low in fat compared to a diet high in fat and low in carbohydrate resulted in decreased protein degradation, although protein synthesis was unaltered (14).

Respiratory quotient (RQ) can be utilized as an indicator of energy fuel utilization. The RQ is the ratio of oxygen consumed to carbohydrate produced in the Kreb's cycle. In clinical practice, RQs are most often determined during the measurement of energy expenditure using indirect calorimetry (15). The amount of oxygen consumed and the amount of carbon dioxide produced for each major nutrient type occurs at a fixed RQ, ranging from 0.7 for fat oxidation to 0.8 for protein oxidation to 1.0 for glucose oxidation. A diet of mixed nutrient intake — protein, carbohydrate, and fat — will produce an RQ of ~0.85. Net fat synthesis is indicated by an RQ greater than 1.0 (16). RQs greater than 1.0 can occur when carbohydrate (glucose) intake or total caloric intake is excessive. The effect is probably a function of excessive glucose intake. Ireton-Jones and Turner examined the RQs of patients receiving intensive nutrition support to assess the frequency with which net fat synthesis occurred, as determined by RQs greater than 1.0 (15). They found RQs to be significantly lower in patients fed enterally or parenterally with a mixed substrate formulation including glucose (carbohydrate), protein, and fat as compared to glucose and protein alone. This indicated that the route of administration, enteral or parenteral, did not influence energy nutrient utilization determined using RQ. It is important to carefully manage carbohydrate intake, whether given enterally or parenterally, to avoid the deleterious effects of overfeeding, which include hepatic steatosis and increased carbon dioxide production, leading to ventilatory compromise, especially in the critically ill patient.

Many patients who experience wounds are diabetic and are, therefore, predisposed to carbohydrate metabolism abnormalities. As such, their blood glucose concentrations may be significantly above what is recommended as an acceptable range. While these patients are not critically ill, when they experience a wound, and have higher blood glucose levels, their risk for increased infections and delayed wound healing is increased. Animal studies have shown impaired wound healing due to fibroblast dysfunction, which can be assumed to occur in the diabetic human patient. Careful attention to the dietary carbohydrate intake and maintenance of euglycemia through oral and intravenous hypoglycemic agents may be underrated and extremely important in enhancing the healing process. Anabolic agents have been used to attempt to improve wound healing (17). Insulin therapy to maintain euglycemia may also exert an anabolic effect in the nonacute setting.

ENERGY METABOLISM/CALORIC NEEDS

It is generally recognized that energy needs rise with the increased demands for wound healing (18). Although energy needs increase, this increase may not be at a level as significant as initially thought. Studies have shown that energy needs are variable and are not necessarily related to burn wound size, although nitrogen balance is related to the size of the open burn wound (19,20). Hart demonstrated that body surface area (BSA) burned increased catabolism until 40% BSA was reached and then did not increase significantly after that (21). Hart also demonstrated that ventilatory status is associated with energy expenditure in patients with burns, as has been shown previously; however, this data also showed a correlation between energy expenditure and burn size (22). In the critical care literature, various equations are used to predict energy expenditure. For burnpatients alone, there are more than seven equations that can be used (5,20,23).

In the critically ill or injured patient, energy expenditure can be measured using indirect calorimetry (24). Indirect calorimetry is the measurement of oxygen consumption and carbon dioxide production during respiratory gas exchange to determine energy expenditure (15). It is based on the principle that the energy released by oxidative processes and by anaerobic glycolysis is ultimately transformed into heat or external work. Indirect calorimetric measurements are usually done using portable machines called metabolic measurement carts that allow portability of the measurement equipment inside the hospital. Energy expenditures of ventilator-dependent and spontaneously breathing patients can be measured by indirect calorimetry. Smaller, handheld versions of the indirect calorimeter are available; however, these are only useful in measuring the energy expenditures of spontaneously breathing patients (25). Measuring a patient's energy expenditure allows the clinician to tailor the nutrition support regimen to the individual patient's needs. In addition, because critically ill patients have many variables that affect their energy expenditure during recovery, measurement of energy expenditure during recovery is preferable to the use of a static energy expenditure equation.

However, when indirect calorimetry is not available, an equation must be used to estimate energy expenditure. It is important to avoid both underfeeding and overfeeding in the critically injured patient. Hart recommended an energy intake of 1.2 times measured resting metabolic rate (22). The resting metabolic rate in critically ill patients is higher than that of a healthy individual, even one with a wound. Therefore, energy needs of the critically ill should be separated from those of the healthy individual. Examples of equations that can be used to predict the energy expenditures of critically ill patients are found in Table 2.1 (26–28).

Patients who are not critically ill make up a large number of patients who will have wounds. It is important to be as accurate as possible in estimating the energy needs of these individuals as well. These patients may have comorbidities, such as diabetes, renal disease, or obesity, that further complicate the wound healing process as well as the decision of the calorie provision. Energy expenditure studies have not focused on the ambulatory care patient with a wound. In a study conducted in a tertiary care setting of acute and intensive care patients of various diagnoses, the presence of a burn did not make a difference in the energy expenditures of patients who were spontaneously breathing; however, in those who were ventilator dependent, it did (26). While the need for adequate and effective nutrient and energy intake is extremely important in the patient with a wound, there may only be a small effect on overall energy expenditure. For the non-ICU and ambulatory care patient, there are two equations that are

TABLE 2.1
Energy Expenditure Equations for Critically Ill or Injured Individuals

Ireton-Jones Equations[a]

Ventilator Dependent:
$$IJEE(v) = 1784 - 11(A) + 5(W) + 244(G) + 239(T) + 804(B)$$

Spontaneously Breathing:
$$IJEE(s) = 629 - 11(A) + 25(W) - 609(O)$$

where

IJEE = kcal/day

A = age (years)

W = actual weight (kg)

G = gender (male = 1, female = 0)

T = trauma

B = burn

O = obesity (if present = 1, absent = 0)

No additional factor is added for activity or injury.

Kcal/Kg[b]

25 kcal/kg using usual or current body weight

Mifflin[c]

M:
$$RMR \ (kcal/day) = 10(W) + 6.25(H) - 5(A) + 5$$

F:
$$RMR \ (kcal/day) = 10(W) + 6.25(H) - 5(A) - 161$$

where

H = height (cm)

W = actual weight (kg)

A = age (years)

Use with stress factors:

Mild: RMR × 1

Moderate: RMR × 1.2 – 1.3

Moderate: RMR × 1.2 – 1.3

Severe: RMR × 1.4 – 1.5

[a]From Ireton-Jones C, Jones J. Improved equations for estimating energy expenditure in patients: the Ireton-Jones equations. *Nutr. in Clin. Prac.*, 17 (4), 236–239, 2002. With permission.
[b]From McCowen KC, Friel C, Sternberg J, Chan S, Forse RA, Burke PA, Bistrian BR. Hypocaloric total parenteral nutrition: effectiveness in prevention of hyperglycemia and infectious complications — a randomized clinical trial. *Crit. Care Med.*, 28 (11), 3606–3611, 2000. With permission.
[c]From Mifflin MD, St. Jeor ST, Hill LA, et al. A new predictive equation for resting energy expenditure in healthy individuals. *Am. J. Clin. Nutr.*, 51, 241–247, 1990. With permission.

recommended for consideration, and these are listed in Table 2.2. It is important to note that for obese patients, the actual body weight is used in these energy equations. For morbidly obese patients, there are many challenges to the care of the patient, including mobility. Maximization of nutrients with a concomitant decrease in energy (calories) may be useful to meet health goals. A qualified dietitian should always be involved in the management of a patient with wounds, especially those who are obese.

CARBOHYDRATES, WOUND HEALING, AND IMMUNE FUNCTION

An early phase of wound healing involves an inflammatory response in which inflammatory cells migrate into wound sites. Neutrophils first move into the wound to defend against invading bacteria. After neutrophils kill invading organisms via free radical

---

TABLE 2.2
Energy Expenditure Equations for Healthy Individuals

Mifflin

M:

$$RMR \ (kcal/day) = 10(W) + 6.25(H) - 5(A) + 5$$

F:

$$RMR \ (kcal/day) = 10(W) + 6.25(H) - 5(A) - 161$$

where

H = height (cm)
W = actual weight (kg)
A = age (years)

Use with activity factors:
Mild: RMR × 1.1
Moderate: RMR × 1.2 – 1.3
Intense: RMR × 1.4 – 1.5

Ireton-Jones Equations

Spontaneously Breathing:
$$IJEE(s) = 629 - 11(A) + 25(W) - 609(O)$$

where

IJEE = kcal/day
A = age (years)
W = actual weight (kg)
O = obesity (if present = 1, absent = 0)

No additional factor is added for activity or injury.

---

release and the secretion of proinflammatory cytokines, macrophages move into the wound (29). These cells also secrete cytokines, chemokines, and growth factors and control leukocyte recruitment. During all of this cell adhesion, migration and proliferation is regulated by cell-surface carbohydrates. Specifically, β-4-galactosylated carbohydrate chains synthesized by β-4Gal-I play a critical role in the wound healing process (30).

Carbohydrates provide energy to wound cells, which helps in cell proliferation and phagocytic activity; however, more recently, carbohydrates have also been shown to play a variety of non-energy-related roles via their functions as communication or recognition markers when they are formed into glycoproteins or glycolipids. These roles become extremely important after a trauma, when the body must mobilize an immune response.

Carbohydrates have been found to play a significant role as components of glycoproteins in cell communication and have also been shown to have a wide variety of other critical roles (structural, lubricant, transport, immunologic, hormonal, and enzymatic). Over the past 20 years, glycoproteins have been shown to be altered by dietary intake of carbohydrates. Mannose and galactose have been shown to be directly used in the synthesis of glycoproteins by the liver and small intestine. Recent reviews indicate that when humans are fed only glucose, liver dysfunction is more common, and that the feeding of a variety of carbohydrates seems to alleviate some of these problems (31,32).

Recent work by Mori et al. showed that skin wound healing was impaired in mice that were β-1,4-galactosyltansferase deficient (28). Mice that were deficient in this key glycoprotein showed significantly delayed wound healing as well as reduced re-epithelialization, collagen synthesis, and angiogenesis. The authors speculate that the immune system is impacted, because both neutrophils and macrophages migrate into the wound site during wound healing, and this process is closely related to cell adhesion through interactions with selectins and their ligands. Chemokines were also shown to be reduced, and they have critical roles as chemoattractants for neutrophils and oncocytes/macrophages.

More detailed work regarding the role played by carbohydrates in wound healing has been done by studying rats that were either immunocompromised or aged. In this study, cutaneous cells were shown to depend on carbohydrates metabolism for wound healing. The key intermediate steps in energy metabolism that were altered included a decrease in the activity of the regulatory enzymes hexokinase and citrate synthase. These enzymes were altered, and this, in turn, impacted upon energy availability for cellular activity in the repair process (33). In this particular model, it appears that insulin and glucose uptake is less of an issue, and the problem lies more in a disturbed enzymatic role in the cutaneous cells.

CARBOHYDRATES IN WOUND CARE

Carbohydrates have been discussed predominately in relation to energy sources and fuel for metabolic processes. Sucrose, table sugar, has been used as an adjunct to antibiotics in treating deep wound infections. Filling infected wounds with sugar has been practiced for centuries in some countries (34). In a study by DeFeo in Italy, nine patients who had undergone heart surgery and developed sternal infections were treated with redebridement, and the wound was filled with granulated sugar four times a day. Fever ceased within 4.3 ± 1.3 days, and complete wound healing occurred in 58.8 ± 32.9 days (35). Sugar treatment was concluded to be reasonable and effective in patients with mediastinitis refractory to closed irrigation treatment. In another study using a carbohydrate derivative, 43 pediatric patients with partial thickness burns that had been treated with β-glucan collagen (BGC) matrix as the primary wound dressing were evaluated retrospectively (36). The BGC wound dressing combined the carbohydrate β-glucan with collagen. When BGC was applied to debrided burn wounds in this pediatric population (average age 5.5 yr), almost 80% of the subjects had the BGC remain intact while the wound healed underneath, with excellent cosmetic results, minimal analgesic requirements, and no need for repetitive dressing changes. It was concluded that BGC markedly simplifies wound care for the family and patient and seems to significantly decrease postinjury pain.

RECOMMENDATIONS FOR CARBOHYDRATE INTAKE

Carbohydrates are important as the key energy nutrient for the patient with wounds. In patients who are critically ill or injured, a rate of no more than 5 mg/kg/min of carbohydrate (and especially dextrose) is recommended. For patients who are receiving an oral or enteral diet, carbohydrate appears to be well tolerated when adequate protein is also provided. Whether patients are receiving their nutrients enterally (oral or tube feeding) or parenterally, care should be taken to assure that excessive total calories are avoided. Measurement of energy needs using indirect calorimetry is preferable for determining energy needs. However, if this is not available, energy expenditure can be determined using a predictive equation. Special attention must be paid to monitoring to assure that the provision of carbohydrates is contributing to the attainment of positive outcomes.

Appropriate nutritional assessment and advice should, therefore, be an integral part of all wound management (37).

PROBLEMS RELATED TO EXCESS CARBOHYDRATE INTAKE

Carbohydrates are necessary in the diet for the maintenance of good health. As with other nutrient groups, excessive intake of certain carbohydrates (i.e., refined carbohydrates; high in starch/glucose and low in fiber) can have deleterious effects on health in general as well as on wound healing. Recently, the relationship between dietary fat and obesity has been questioned. Mean fat intake has decreased in the United States for the past three decades, while obesity has continued to rise (38). During this same time period, an increased intake of refined carbohydrates has been documented (39). It has been suggested that a high intake of refined carbohydrates may be a contributor to the national trend toward obesity. Ludwig et al. have suggested that high glycemic index (GI) foods that rapidly increase the body's sugar level (i.e., white bread and waffles) induce hormonal and metabolic changes that lead to overeating (40). Obesity, in turn, has been associated with increases in coronary heart disease, adult onset diabetes, and hypertension, as well as poor wound healing. In general, obese patients have an increased frequency of wound infections and impaired healing. This is thought to be due to the fact that adipose tissue is poorly vascularized, resulting in a decrease in blood flow to the wound and impairment in the delivery of nutrients. Obese patients have also been shown to have a higher incidence of surgical wound dehiscence, possibly because their operations can be more technically difficult, and they are prone to hematoma formation (41). Clearly, prevention of obesity is key; however, practitioners should be aware of the effects of obesity on wound healing.

Excessive quantities of carbohydrates can also have a negative impact in the hospital setting. Even moderate degrees of hyperglycemia may result in an increased incidence of infection and adverse outcomes (42). Persistent hyperglycemia has been associated with poor wound healing and immunity (7). Excessive amounts of glucose have been positively correlated with increased carbon dioxide production and hepatic steatosis in traumatized and septic patients (12,13). Diabetic subjects who suffer from wounds need to be especially careful in regard to the regulation of glucose intake and the maintenance of euglycemia (17).

RECOMMENDATIONS FOR FUTURE RESEARCH

Further research is needed to determine if differing types of carbohydrates can be used as energy fuel substrates for wound healing. Varying the absolute level of carbohydrate intake has been studied, with levels as much as 82% of total calories being acceptable. In addition, determining the timing of nutrition intervention and the route of administration continue to be challenges in patients needing critical care and in those requiring chronic wound care. Further research into alternate nutritive sources may also be useful.

REFERENCES

1. Murray, R.K., Glycoproteins, in *Harper's Biochemistry*, 25th ed., Murray, R.K., Granner, D.K., Mayes, K.K., Mayes, P.A., and Rodwell, W.V., Eds., Stamford, CT.
2. Wilson, J.A. and Clark, J.J., Advances in skin and wound care, *J. Prev. and Wound Healing*, 17 (8), 426–435, 2004.
3. Gupta, A. and Raghubir, R., Energy metabolism in the granulation tissue of diabetic rats during cutaneous wound healing, *Mol. Cell. Biochem.* 270 (1–2), 71, 2005.
4. Gottschlich, M.M., Nutrition in the burned pediatric patient, in *Handbook of Pediatric Nutrition*, Queen, P.M. and Lang, C.E., Eds., Aspen, Gaithersburg, MD, 1993, pp. 536–559.
5. Mayes, T. and Gottschlich, M.M., Burns and wound healing, in *The Science and Practice of Nutrition Support*, Gottschlich, M.M., Fuhrman, M.P., Hammond, K.A., Holcombe, B.J., and Seidner, D., Eds., Kendall/Hunt, Dubuque, IA, 2001, pp. 391–420.

6. Hart, D., Wolf, S.E., Zhang, X.J., Chinkes, D.L., Buffalo, M.C., Matin, S.I., DebRoy, A., Wolfe, R.R., and Herndon, D.N., Efficacy of a high-energy carbohydrate diet in catabolic illness, *Crit. Care Med.*, 29 (7), 1318–1324, 2001.

7. Gore, D.C., Chinkes, D., Heggers, J., Herndon, D.N., Wolf, S.E., and Desai, M., Association of hyperglycemia with increased mortality after severe burn injury, *Trauma*, 51 (3), 540–544, 2001.

8. Van den Berghe, G.H., Role of intravenous insulin therapy in critically ill patients, *Endocr. Pract.*, 10 (Suppl. 2), 17–20, 2004.

9. Krinsley, J.S., Effect of an intensive glucose management protocol on the mortality of critically ill adult patients, *Mayo Clin. Proc.*, 79 (8), 992–1000, 2004.

10. Thomas, S.J., Morimoto, K., Herndon, D.N., Ferrando, A.A., Wolfe, R.R., Klein, G.L., and Wolf, S.E., The effect of prolonged euglycemic hyperinsulinemia on lean body mass after severe burn, *Surgery*, 132 (2), 341–347, 2002.

11. Tredget, E.E. and Yu, Y.M., The metabolic effects of thermal injury, *World J. Surg.*, 16 (1), 68–79, 1992.

12. Ireton-Jones, C. and Turner, W.W., The use of respiratory quotient to determine the efficacy of nutrition support regimens, *J. Am. Diet. Assoc.*, 87 (2), 180–183, 1987.

13. Burke, J.F., Wolfe, R.R., Mullany, C.J., Matthews, D.E., and Bier, D.M., Glucose requirements following burn injury, *Ann. Surg.*, 190 (3), 274–285, 1979.

14. Hart, D.W., Wolf, S.E., Zhang, X.J., Chinkes, D.L., Buffalo, M.C., Matin, S.I., DebRoy, M.A., Wolfe, R.R., and Herndon, D.N., Efficacy of a high carbohydrate diet in critical illness, *Crit. Care Med.*, 29 (7), 1318–1324, 2001.

15. Ireton-Jones, C., Estimating energy requirements, in *Nutritional Considerations in the Intensive Care Unit. Science, Rationale, Practice*, Shikora, S., Martindale, R., and Schwaitzberg, S., Eds., Kendall/Hunt, Dubuque, IA, 2003, pp. 31–39.

16. Elia, M. and Livesey, G., Theory and validity of indirect calorimetry during net lipid synthesis, *Am. J. Clin. Nutr.*, 47 (4), 591–607, 1988.

17. Demling, R.H. and DeSanti, L., Oxandrolone induced lean mass gain during recovery from severe burns is maintained after discontinuation of the anabolic steroid, *Burns*, 29 (8), 793–797, 2003.

18. Burdge, J.J., Conkright, J.M., and Ruberg, R.L., Nutritional and metabolic consequences of thermal injury, *Clin. Plast. Surg.*, 13 (1), 49–55, 1986.

19. Ireton, C.S., Turner, W.W. Jr., Cheney, J.C., Hunt, J.L., and Baxter, C.R., Do changes in burn size affect measured energy expenditures? *J. Burn Care Rehabil.*, 6 (5), 419–421, 1985.

20. Ireton-Jones, C.S., Turner, W.W., Liepa, G.U., et al., Equations for the estimation of energy expenditures in patients with burns with special reference to ventilatory status, *J. Burn Care Rehabil.*, 13 (3), 330–333, 1992.

21. Hart, D.W., Wolf, S.E., Chinkes, D.L., Gore, D.C., Mlcak, R.P., Beauford, R.B., Obeng, M.K., Lal, S., Gold, W.F., Wolfe, R.R., and Herndon, D.N., Determinants of skeletal muscle catabolism after severe burn, *Ann. Surg.*, 232 (4), 455–465, 2000.

22. Hart, D.W., Wolf, S.E., Chinkes, D.L., Gore, D.C., and Micak, R.P., Energy expenditure and caloric balance after burn: increased feeding leads to fat rather than lean mass accretion, *Ann. Surg.*, 235 (1), 152–161, 2002.

23. Dickerson, R.N., Gervasio, J.M., Riley, M.L., Murrell, J.E., Hickerson, W.L., Kudsk, K.A., and Brown, R.O., Accuracy of predictive methods to estimate resting energy expenditure of thermally-injured patients, *J. Parenteral Enteral Nutr.*, 26 (1), 17–29, 2002.

24. McClave, S., Snider, H., and Ireton-Jones, C., Can we justify continued interest in indirect calorimetry? *Nutr. in Clin. Pract.*, 17 (3), 133–136, 2002.

25. Compher, C., Hise, M., Sternberg, A., and Kinosian, B.P., Comparison between the MedGem and Delatrac resting metabolic rate measurements, *Eur. J. Clin. Nutr.*, 59 (10), 1136–1141, 2005.

26. Ireton-Jones, C. and Jones, J., Improved equations for estimating energy expenditure in patients: the Ireton-Jones equations, *Nutr. in Clin. Prac.*, 17 (4), 236–239, 2002.

27. McCowen, K.C., Friel, C., Sternberg, J., Chan, S., Forse, R.A., Burke, P.A., and Bistrian, B.R., Hypocaloric total parenteral nutrition: effectiveness in prevention of hyperglycemia and infectious complications — a randomized clinical trial, *Crit. Care Med.*, 28 (11), 3606–3611, 2000.

28. Mifflin, M.D., St. Jeor, S.T., Hill, L.A., et al., A new predictive equation for resting energy expenditure in healthy individuals, *Am. J. Clin. Nutr.*, 51 (2), 241–247, 1990.

29. Stadelmann, W.K., Digenis, A.G., and Tobin, G.R., Impediments to wound healing, *Am. J. Surg.*, 176 (2A Suppl.), 39S–47S, 1998.

30. Mori, R., Kondo, T., Nishie, T., Ohshima, T., and Asano, M., Impairment of skin wound healing in β-1,4-galactosyltransferase-deficient mice with reduced leukocyte recruitment, *Am. J. Pathol.*, 164 (4), 1303–1314, 2004.

31. Martin, A., Rambal, C., Berger, V., Perier, S., and Louisot, R., Availability of specific sugars for glycoconjugate biosynthesis: a need for further investigation in man, *Biochemie*, 80 (1), 75–86, 1998.

32. Berger, V., Perier, S., Pachiaudi, C., Normand, S., Louisot, P., and Martin, A., Dietary specific sugars for serum protein enzymatic glycosylation in man, *Metabolism*, 47 (12), 1499–1503, 1998.

33. Gupta, A., Manhas, N., and Raghubir, R., Energy metabolism during cutaneous wound healing in immunocompromised and aged rats, *Mol. Cell Biochem.*, 259 (1–2), 9–14, 2004.

34. Beadling, L., A bag of sugar. Surgeons find that ordinary table sugar is a sweet adjunct to conventional treatment of deep wound healing, *Today's Surg. Nurse*, 19 (3), 28–30, 1997.

35. DeFeo, M., Gregorio, R., Renzulli, A., et al. Treatment of recurrent postoperative mediastinitis with granulated sugar, *J. Cardiovasc. Surg.* (Torino), 41 (5), 715–719, 2000.

36. Delatte, S.J., Evans, J., Hebra, A., et al., Effectiveness of -glucan collagen for treatment of partial thickness burns in children, *J. Pediatr. Surg.*, 36 (1), 113–118, 2001.

37. Patel, G.K., The role of nutrition in the management of lower extremity wounds, *Int. J. Low Extrem. Wounds*, 4 (1), 12–22, 2005.

38. Baschetti, R., Low-fat diets and HDL cholesterol, *Am. J. Clin. Nutr.*, 68 (5), 1143, 1998.

39. Stephen, A.M., Sieber, G.M., Gerster, Y.A., and Morgan, D.R., Intake of carbohydrate and its components — international comparisons, trends overtime, and effects of changing to low-fat diets, *Am. J. Clin. Nutr.*, 62, 851S–867S, 1995.

40. Ludwig, D.S., Majzoub, J.A., Al-Zaharani, A., Dallal, G.E., Blanco, I., and Roberts, S.B., High glycemic index foods, overeating and obesity, *Pediatrics*, 103 (3), 26–40, 1999.

41. Armstrong, M., Obesity as an intrinsic factor effecting wound healing, *J. Wound Care*, 7 (5), 220–221, 1998.

42. Pomposelli, J.J. and Bistrian, B.R., Is total parenteral nutrition immunosuppressive? *New Horiz.*, 2 (2), 224–229, 1994

3 Fat and Wound Healing

John J. Turek

CONTENTS

INTRODUCTION

Fats are unique among the macronutrients in that they function as both energy stores and signaling molecules. They are also unique in that the cell membranes in tissues and organs largely reflect the fatty acid composition of the diet.[1] Polyunsaturated fatty acids (PuFA) can alter the formation of eicosanoids,[2–4] cytokines,[5,6] and enzymes of cell activation, such as protein kinase C[7]; change membrane receptor expression;[8,9] and also influence the expression of numerous genes.[10–12] Therefore, no other nutrient class has the capability of causing such a profound functional change in cells throughout the body. Because there is a significant storage capacity for this macronutrient, a consideration of the role of fat in the healing process needs to take into account both dietary and stored fat. The fatty acids (Figure 3.1) incorporated into cellular phospholipids and adipose tissue could be considered to be a type of dietary memory. Physiological and healing processes may be influenced when fatty acids are released from membranes via phospholipase or if they are mobilized from adipocytes for energy. In addition to the storage function, white adipose tissue (WAT) is a source of proinflammatory cytokines, such as tumor necrosis factor-α (TNF-α) and interleukin-6 (IL-6)[13] and other bioactive molecules, such as leptin and adiponectin, currently referred to as adipokines.[14–16] Taken collectively, the products of fat metabolism and homeostasis may be viewed as being one of the key regulators of inflammation and the healing process. This property takes on further significance if one considers that individuals suffering from poor wound healing often have additional complicating factors characterized by dysfunctions in lipid metabolism (e.g., diabetes in combination with obesity).

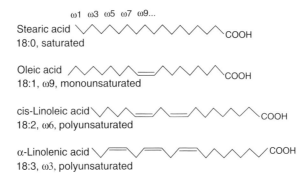

FIGURE 3.1 Examples of the structure for saturated, monounsaturated, and polyunsaturated fatty acids. No double bonds are present in saturated fatty acids. Monounsaturated fatty acids have a single double bond, and polyunsaturated fatty acids have two or more double bonds. Humans can insert a double bond at carbon atoms 4, 5, 6, and 9 numbered from the carboxyl terminal. The ω numbers of the carbon atoms in the fatty acid side chain are numbered from the methyl end of the molecule (ω-1, ω-2, ω-3, etc.).

FAT METABOLISM AND ENERGY METABOLISM IN THE WHOLE BODY

Fat in the diet is almost completely absorbed in the intestine. The process of digestion begins with the introduction of salivary and then gastric lipases.[17,18] The majority of lipolysis then occurs in the small intestine with the addition of pancreatic lipase in combination with a colipase.[19] Bile salts and phospholipids secreted by the liver then emulsify the hydrolyzed fat for absorption by the enterocytes. Approximately 90 to 95% of dietary fats are in the form of triacylglycerols (TAGs) (Figure 3.2). TAGs are composed of three fatty acid side chains attached to a glycerol skeleton, and they are the primary concentrated store of metabolic energy found in adipose cells and tissues. The fatty acids on the glycerol backbone are usually different and often consist of two saturated fatty acids and one unsaturated fatty acid side chain. Pancreatic lipase cleaves fatty acids from the TAGs at the *sn*-1 and *sn*-3 positions, with the result being free fatty acids and 2-monoacylglycerol. These components are then absorbed by the enterocyte. The TAGs are then reassembled and packaged into chylomicrons along with cholesterol, phospholipids, and apoproteins. Shorter-chain fatty acids (< 12 carbon) may be bound to albumin and directly transported to the liver as nonesterifed fatty acids (NEFAs).[20,21]

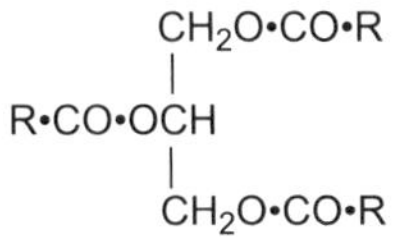

$$CH_2O\cdot CO\cdot R$$
$$|$$
$$R\cdot CO\cdot OCH$$
$$|$$
$$CH_2O\cdot CO\cdot R$$

FIGURE 3.2 Triacylglycerols consist of a glycerol backbone with three fatty acid side chains (R). Removal of the fatty acid from the middle carbon would yield 1,3-diacylglycerol. Removal of the fatty acids from the two end carbons would yield 2-monoacylglycerol.

In addition to TAGs, the other dietary fat components consist largely of glycerophospholipids and cholesterol esters. The glycerophospholipids (Figure 3.3) are primarily in the form of phosphatidylcholine (~70%) and phosphatidylethanolamine.[22] Pancreatic phospholipase A_2 hydrolyzes the ester-bond-linking fatty acids to the *sn-2* position of phospholipids.[23] The resulting lysophospholipids are absorbed and may be reesterified and packaged into intestinal lipoproteins in combination with cholesterol and TAGs. The cholesterol esters are hydrolyzed by cholesterol ester hydrolase to yield free fatty acids and cholesterol.[24] The free fatty acids are readily absorbed, but the cholesterol needs to be incorporated into micelles with fatty acids, monoacylglycerols, lysophospholipids, and conjugated bile acids for it to be absorbed.

After absorption and repackaging, fat is distributed to the body by chylomicrons, which first enter the lymphatic circulation before making their way to the blood. In the capillary beds of muscle and adipose tissue, the chylomicrons come in contact with the enzyme lipoprotein lipase, which hydrolyzes fatty acids from the TAGs. The fatty acids may be oxidized by the tissues for energy, taken up by adipose tissue and reesterified into TAGs, or circulated back to the liver bound to albumin. The chylomicron remnant consists primarily of cholesterol esters and contains apolipoprotein E (apo E) on its surface. The remnant is cleared by the liver, which has receptors for apo E.

There is also an endogenous pathway in the body for the synthesis and distribution of lipids needed in energy metabolism. Saturated fatty acids may be synthesized in the liver from acetyl-CoA derived from glucose metabolism. These fatty acids may be stored as TAGs or packaged in very low-density lipoproteins (VLDLs) in combination with cholesterol, phospholipids, and lipoproteins. The TAG-enriched VLDL particles are released into the blood circulation, and the TAGs are utilized in the same manner as those from chylomicrons. As TAGs are removed, the VLDL particles transition first to an intermediate-density lipoprotein, and then to low-density lipoprotein (LDL) particles. The LDL particles contain apolipoprotein B-100 (apo B-100) on the surface, and this is also cleared via the liver, which has receptors for this ligand.

Fatty acids of all classes can ultimately be oxidized to carbon dioxide and water. However, each of the different dietary lipid classes has preferential routes of utilization and localization in different tissue compartments. The long-chain saturated fatty acids (LC-SFA > 16 carbon) may by oxidized in muscle mitochondria to supply

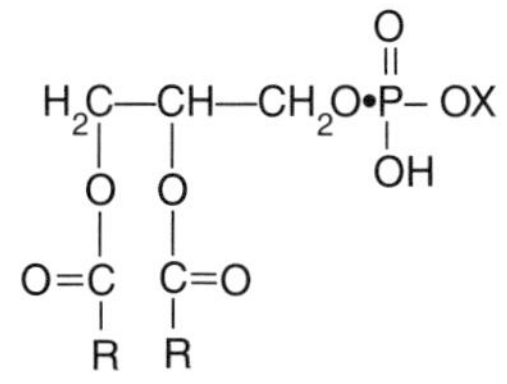

$$H_2C-CH-CH_2O \bullet \overset{\overset{\displaystyle O}{\|}}{P}-OX$$

FIGURE 3.3 Phospholipids are amphipathic molecules with two fatty acid side chains (R) and a phosphorylated alcohol head group. Linked to the phosphate group is an additional polar group (X) that may consist of choline, ethanolamine, serine, or inositol.

ATP, but they are also readily stored in adipocyte TAGs. One reason for this is that LC-SFAs require carnitine acyltransferase for transport into the mitochondria for oxidation,[25] so they are, therefore, more readily incorporated into TAGs. Some saturated fatty acids, like stearic acid (18:0), will be stored in TAGs or will be desaturated and converted to monounsaturated fatty acids (MuFAs), such as oleic acid (18:1; ω-9), before storage or β-oxidation.[26] Medium-chain fatty acids (8 to 14 carbon) are preferentially β-oxidized in liver mitochondria, because they do not require enzyme transport into the mitochondria. The MuFA are readily utilized for energy by β-oxidation in mitochondria but may also be stored in adipocyte TAGs.[27] The long-chain ω-3 and ω-6 PuFAs (> 18 carbon) (Figure 3.4) are a significant component of cellular phospholipids but may also occur, to some degree, in TAGs. This lipid class is considered essential, because mammals do not have the enzymatic ability to insert a *cis* double bond at the ω-3 or ω-6 position of a fatty acid chain, and therefore, these must be acquired from the diet. The types, amounts, and ratios of these nutrients in the diet have been the subject of extensive research due to the fact that they are the source of eicosanoids, which participate in control of the inflammatory response. The parent compounds for each of these fatty acid classes (linoleic acid, 18:2, ω-6 and α-linolenic acid, 18:3, ω-3) compete for δ-6-desaturase and elongase enzymes, and the 20-carbon ω-3 and ω-6 PuFA, eicosapentaenoic acid (EPA, 20:5; ω-3) and arachidonic acid (AA, 20:4; ω-6) compete for cyclooxygenase/lipoxygenase enzymes, which influences the amounts and types of eicosanoids formed from these nutrients. Arachidonic acid is a major component of mammalian membranes. Arachidonic acid is readily formed via elongation and desaturation of linoleic acid or by retroconversion of adrenic acid by removal of a two-carbon unit.

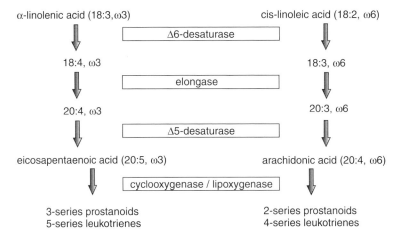

FIGURE 3.4 The parent compounds for the essential ω-3 and ω-6 fatty acids are18 carbon fatty acids that may be desaturated and elongated to form the longer-chain polyunsaturated fatty acids. Arachidonic acid (20:4, ω-6) and eicosapentaenoic acid (20:5, ω-3) are substrates for cyclooxygenase and lipoxygenase enzymes that result in the formation of eicosanoids from these fatty acids.

Likewise, EPA is readily formed from α-linolenic acid, but retroconversion from the highly unsaturated docosahexaenoic acid (DHA, 22:6; ω-3) requires removal of both a double bond and a two-carbon unit. The β-oxidation pathway in the peroxisomes is utilized for catalyzing the oxidation of very-long-chain fatty acids, and the highly unsaturated ω-3 fatty acids stimulate peroxisomal β-oxidation.[28,29] In the liver, the acetyl-CoA generated by β-oxidation is used to produce acetoacetate and β-hydroxybutyrate (ketone bodies), which the brain may use as an alternative energy source. There have been conflicting reports about the ability to store these fatty acids in adipocyte TAGs, especially the longer-chain ω-3 PuFA. One study found differences in postprandial storage of fatty acids in adipose tissue, with the amount of MuFA being > ω-6 PuFA > saturated > ω-3 PuFA.[30] Some reports indicate minimal storage ability for EPA,[31,32] whereas others provide evidence for long-chain ω-3 PuFA (EPA and DHA) in adipose tissue.[33,34] The possibility of ω-3 and ω-6 PuFA being released from adipocyte TAGs during wound healing could be significant if the nutritional status was such that there was mobilization of TAG fatty acid stores for energy metabolism (e.g., hypermetabolic state).

In nature, trans-fatty acids occur in small amounts in dairy products and in some plant oils. Currently, there are attempts to reduce the amount of these fats in prepared foods, but they are still a significant energy source in the Western diet due to the consumption of hydrogenated vegetable oils,[35] and therefore should be mentioned in this section. Trans fatty acids behave very much like saturated fats, and they are transported in a manner similar to other fatty acids and can be found within the cholesterol ester, triacylglycerol, and phospholipid fractions of lipoproteins.[36] There is evidence that the content of adipose tissue trans fatty acid is a reflection of diet content.[37,38] These fats are associated with a greater risk of ischemic heart disease than even saturated fat.[39,40] The effects on wound healing by this class of fatty acids are currently unknown.

Glucose and fatty acids are the main oxidative fuels in the body and account for a majority of oxidative metabolism. There are still many questions that need to be answered about the interaction of glucose and fatty acid metabolism, especially the differences that may exist between the resting and exercise states. However, an understanding of energy metabolism in the body requires an examination of how these two pathways interact. Lipolysis and lipogenesis in adipose tissue and fatty acid oxidation in liver and skeletal muscle may be influenced by the type of fat, as indicated above, but they are also under the control of several hormones and transcription factors that regulate fatty acid metabolism Adipose tissue contains a hormone-sensitive lipase that is suppressed by insulin. An elevation in blood glucose stimulates insulin secretion, which suppresses the release of NEFA from adipose tissue TAGs. However, when insulin levels fall, the hormone-sensitive lipase activates so that NEFA may be released. Beyond this simple explanation of what has come to be known as the glucose–fatty acid cycle,[41–43] it is evident from many studies that the interaction between glucose and fatty acid metabolism involves additional levels of regulatory control and cross talk that influence utilization of these energy sources. If carbohydrate/glucose is the primary energy source, then glucose oxidation is promoted along with storage of energy as glycogen and TAGs, and fatty acid oxidation is inhibited. However, in the presence of adequate insulin, free fatty acids compete with glucose for uptake by peripheral tissues, so that the presence of free fatty acids promotes fatty acid oxidation and inhibition of glucose oxidation. Low insulin levels elevate lipolysis rates, and the free fatty acids actually enhance endogenous glucose output.[42] This effect of fatty acids on glucose metabolism is likely due to a direct action of fatty acids upon the pancreatic β-cell, by influencing glucose-stimulated insulin secretion. Initially, fatty acids may potentiate the effects of glucose on the β-cell, but prolonged exposure (> 12 h) to high fatty acid concentrations can then result in inhibition.[26]

In addition to insulin, the adipocyte-derived hormones leptin and adiponectin are involved in fatty acid metabolism, as well as the recently identified acylation-stimulating protein (ASP). Leptin directly inhibits fatty acid synthesis[44,45] and increases the release and oxidation of fatty acids by activating hormone-sensitive lipase.[46] Leptin also has multiple additional metabolic and endocrine functions. Leptin functions in immunoregulation, inflammation, and hematopoiesis,[47] and regulates food intake by communicating with the hypothalamus about the degree of fat stores and changing eating behavior accordingly to maintain a level of homeostasis.[48] It may also regulate TAG homeostasis by restricting TAG storage primarily to adipocytes and sparing nonadipocytes.[49] Leptin deficiency may lead to hyperglycemia, hyperinsulinemia, and insulin resistance.[50] A review of the role of leptin in lipid metabolism provides more information on this topic.[51] A possible role for leptin in wound healing will be discussed in the section on fat metabolism in the healing wound. Adiponectin stimulates fatty acid oxidation and affects glucose metabolism by increasing insulin sensitivity. This hormone also may suppress inflammation.[14,52] Additional research is needed to understand the role of ASP in fat metabolism, but the data indicate it may augment fat storage by increasing TAG synthesis and by decreasing intracellular lipolysis.[13]

In addition to hormonal effects on glucose and fatty acid metabolism, there are several transcription factors that regulate metabolism. Polyunsaturated ω-3 and ω-6 fatty acids are known to inhibit hepatic lipogenesis by inhibiting transcription of a number of genes necessary for lipid synthesis (fatty acid synthase, acetyl-CoA carboxylase, and stearoyl-CoA desaturase).[53] This effect is currently known to be mediated, in part, by a family of membrane-bound transcription factors called sterol regulatory element-binding proteins (SREBPs) that occur as three iso-forms.[54–57] Fatty acid homeostasis in cellular phospholipids is mediated by SREBPs. The cholesterol content of cell membranes serves as a feedback mechanism on the activity of SREBPs. When cholesterol content is adequate, the SREBPs are inactive and remain bound to endoplasmic reticulum (ER) membranes. Sterol depletion in the membrane is a signal for SREBPs to move to the Golgi in ER transport vesicles, and this process is initiated by an SREBP cleavage activating protein that functions both as a sterol sensor and an escort protein. In the Golgi, the release of the active amino-terminal portion of the SREBPs from the membrane is mediated initially by a serine protease and then a zinc metalloprotease before translocation to the nucleus. In addition to regulating sterol content of membrane phospholipids, SREBPs modulate the action of insulin on adipocyte gene expression by activating genes for cholesterol, fatty acid, and TAG synthesis[58] and suppressing genes for fatty acid oxidation.[59] Peroxisome proliferator-activated receptors (PPARs) are members of the superfamily of ligand-activated nuclear transcription factors. This family of receptors was first recognized as regulators for the synthesis, adipocyte storage, and oxidation of fatty acids. A secondary effect of their action on lipid metabolism is modulation of glucose homeostasis. A detailed analysis of PPARs activity may be found in several reviews on the subject.[60,61] The three PPAR subtypes are: PPARα, PPARβ/δ, and PPARγ.[62,63] PPARα is expressed primarily in liver and skeletal muscle; PPARγ is found in adipose tissues[64]; and PPARβ/δ is ubiquitous in most cell types.[65] PPARs are activated by many LC-SFA, PuFA, and eicosanoids.[11] When activated, PPARs affect gene transcription by binding to response elements of target genes. Many of the response elements are associated with genes encoding proteins of fatty acid metabolism, such as fatty acid synthase, acyl-CoA oxidase, lipoprotein lipase, and phosphoenolpyruvate carboxykinase.[66,67] Activation of PPARγ helps regulate glucose homeostasis by directing fatty acids derived from TAGs toward adipose tissue rather than muscle, which has the result of increasing muscle glucose metabolism. Activation of PPARδ in adipose tissue induces genes needed for fatty acid oxidation.[68,69] Beyond these effects of energy metabolism, this class of receptors is now recognized to have an additional role in inflammation and immune regulation.[70,71]

FAT METABOLISM IN THE HEALING WOUND

The need for proper nutrition to facilitate wound healing is a well-established paradigm in medicine.[72–79] However, an understanding of the molecular, biochemical, and cellular processes that occur during wound healing is complicated by the fact that there are multiple types of both acute and chronic wounds. Acute wounds (e.g., surgical, trauma, or burns) require a different treatment regimen than chronic wounds (e.g., venous, pressure, or diabetic ulcers). Moreover, individuals with chronic wounds often have underlying disease or complicating factors that present additional challenges to healing (e.g., diabetes, obesity, frail geriatric patients). Although we have a good level of understanding about the effects of wounds on whole body energy metabolism, this data cannot be directly extrapolated to metabolism in the wound. The reason for this is that the wound functions within its own metabolic microenvironment. Tissue blood flow (perfusion) and oxygen tension may be lower than non-wound tissue, and the recruitment of inflammatory cells into the wound can influence local metabolism.[80] Application of some newer technologies (e.g., *in vivo* nuclear magnetic resonance spectroscopy[81] and genomic/proteomic profiling of wound fluids) should provide insights into localized, *in vivo* metabolism, in the future. In the meantime, an analysis and synthesis of the literature on this topic is probably best approached by considering the general nutritional requirements for wound healing and the potential role of fats to modulate the healing response.

The healing process for most wounds requires an increase in caloric intake over basal levels. This is especially true in severely injured, burned, or critical patients in whom the stress response has placed them in a hypermetabolic state.[82,83] Induction of the stress response via the hypothalamus is initiated by proinflammatory cytokines and results in increased levels of the stress hormones (e.g., glucagon, cortisol, and catecholamines). These hormones then result in a protein-catabolic state as well as increased lipolysis. To meet the increased caloric demand, the accepted approach is to provide a diet high in protein and fat, as these are also needed for the synthesis of new tissues. Research has shown that injured or stressed patients utilize protein for only about 20% of the energy requirement, with glucose and fatty acids being the major energy suppliers.[84,85] Therefore, both dietary fat and fatty acids released from adipose tissue are readily utilized during wound healing and are potential modulators of the healing response.

Wound healing may be divided into an inflammatory phase, a proliferative (fibroblastic) phase, and a remodeling (maturation) phase.[86,87] In acute wounds, the inflammatory phase begins with vasoconstriction followed by vasodilation.[88] This response is mediated, in part, by lipid-derived mediators, such as thromboxane A_2 (vasoconstrictor) and prostacylin (vasodilator), which are products of cyclooxygenase enzyme metabolism of arachidonic acid. The vasoconstriction stems blood loss and allows clotting to occur, and the vasodilation begins the process of fluid and cellular infiltration necessary to initiate the healing process. Inflammation can be a two-edged sword, and the healing process can be delayed by either excessive inflammation, such as might occur in a septic wound, or the inability to mount an adequate inflammatory response (e.g., immunosuppressed patients). Depending upon the nature of the wound, the inflammatory phase during normal healing lasts from several days to weeks. Inflammation persisting beyond this initial period is considered to be chronic[89] and may be due to foreign material in the wound or sepsis. In the next stage of healing (proliferative or fibroblastic phase), there is reepithelialization (for cutaneous wounds), neovascularization, and production of connective tissue fibers by fibroblasts. This stage may last up to 1 month, but again, this may be shorter or longer depending upon the nature of the wound. During the remodeling phase, which can last up to 1 year, there is progressive deposition of and remodeling of extracellular matrix material. This includes the turnover of collagen types, with type III reticular fiber collagen predominating early in the healing process, which is then replaced by type I collagen.

During all phases of wound healing, lipids, or mediators derived or regulated by lipids, are likely to influence metabolism in the wound. During the inflammatory phase, eicosanoids derived from ω-3 and ω-6 fatty acids via cyclooxygenase and lipoxygenase enzymes systems as well as cytokines play a central role as mediators of inflammation (see section on essential fatty acids). The eicosanoids derived from ω-6 PuFA are the more potent mediators of pain and inflammation, and those from ω-3 PuFA are less proinflammatory. The two-series prostanoids and four-series leukotrienes are derived from arachidonic acid. The three-series prostanoids and five-series leukotrienes are derived from eicosapentaenoic acid. In humans, ω-3 fatty acids also lead to decreased production of proinflammatory cytokines by peripheral blood monocytes.[6] Oxidative stress likely influences the wound healing and local metabolism throughout the healing process. The vasoconstriction/vasodilation that occurs at the time of wound creation can produce ischemia-reperfusion injury in the tissues due to the generation of reactive oxygen species (ROS) (e.g., superoxide, hydrogen peroxide, hydroxyl and peroxyl radicals). Likewise, neutrophils that infiltrate the wound during the early stages of inflammation and monocyte/macrophages that appear later in the healing process are an abundant source of ROS. So how do

ROS relate to fat metabolism in the wound? The longer-chain PuFAs are known to be more susceptible to oxidation than LC-SFA or MuFA. This susceptibility to oxidation has often led investigators to hypothesize that these fats, although essential and beneficial for many disease states, could lead to increased lipid peroxidation in tissues. An examination of the literature will find that some *in vivo* studies do associate dietary PuFA with increased oxidative stress.[90] However, there are also many studies that indicate that dietary PuFA, especially the ω-3 fatty acids, actually decrease oxidative stress.[91–94] Additional research is necessary to determine if PuFA content of cellular phospholipids and WAT at the time of wounding, or whether PuFAs supplied in the diet (oral, parenteral, enteral) are a significant factor, beneficial or otherwise, in wound oxidative stress. Because oxidative stress is known to be one of the factors capable of inducing apoptosis in cells,[95–97] it could influence the course of wound healing. This fact becomes especially pertinent when one considers the nonenzymatically derived products of PuFA. The effects of cyclooxygenase and lipoxygenase metabolites have been well characterized, but in recent years a new class of prostanoids derived from long-chain PuFA, called isoprostanes, was iden-tified.[98–100] The isoprostanes are nonenzymatically derived from PuFA and are pro-duced via lipid peroxidation in much greater quantities *in vivo* than prostaglandins generated by cyclooxygenase. The isoprostanes are associated with oxidative damage to tissues, and an additional product of the isoprostane pathway is the formation of isoketals. Isoketals may be formed from fatty acids esterified to phospholipids in the cell membrane. After formation, the isoketals rapidly adduct to membrane pro-teins, and they can alter membrane function.[101,102] Oxidative stress could therefore influence wound metabolism by fostering the production of lipid-derived mediators, which could in turn lead to apoptosis of cells in the wound. One *in vitro* study found that proliferating fibroblasts at a wound margin were more susceptible to oxidative stress and induction of apoptosis. The authors suggested that their findings could be applicable to wounds that fail to heal.[103] Chronic wounds are often characterized by hypoxia, and evidence for oxidative stress has been found in chronic venous ulcers. Elevated levels of allantoin:uric acid percentage ratio, a marker of oxidative stress, were found in the wound fluid from chronic leg ulcers compared to both plasma and acute surgical wound fluid. The elevated percentage ratio was correlated with wound fluid neutrophil elastase.[104]

The previously mentioned endocrine function of WAT may also play a role in wound metabolism during the early stages of wound healing. Leptin production increases during inflammation.[47] Interestingly, leptin activity has been detected in the fluids of experimental wounds in pigs during the first few days following injury,[105] and it was suggested by the authors that this hormone may function in an autocrine and paracrine manner during wound healing. The significance and role of leptin derived from fat stores located in the vicinity of acute and chronic wounds will require more research. However, leptin has been shown to have antiapoptotic activ-ities for a number of cell types, to inhibit the hypothalamic–pituitary axis stress response,[106] and to promote the secretion of proinflammatory cytokines.[107] All of these leptin functions have a role in modulating the healing process.

Another previously mentioned regulator of lipid metabolism, PPARs, may also function in wound healing. PPARα and PPARβ are both activated in cutaneous wounding.[108–110] PPARα is activated in the early inflammation phase of the healing,[108] and PPARβ functions to protect keratinocytes from apoptosis and also may regulate keratinocyte migration via potentiation of transcription factor NF-κB activity and matrix-metalloprotease-9 (MMP-9) production.[111]

ESSENTIAL FATTY ACIDS AND OTHER SPECIFIC FATTY ACIDS

In the context of wound healing, the obvious role for essential fatty acids is on modulation of inflammation and the immune response.[112–114] An examination of the literature in this area will uncover some conflicting data as to the benefits of essential ω-3 and ω-6 fatty acids in wound healing. One study in essential fatty acid deficient (EFAD) rats found that the healing rate of partial-thickness cutaneous burns was significantly decreased compared to controls.[115] However, this study also found that healed single dorsal skin incisions were stronger in control animals, but there was no difference between the groups when ventral skin incisions with underlying fascial incisions were measured. These results would suggest that the type of wound or wound location and regional environment (adipose tissue?) may influence healing. Another study on cutaneous wound healing in EFAD rats concluded that essential fatty acids were not necessary for cutaneous wound repair.[116] In this study, there was no difference in maximal breaking strength or cellular inflammatory infiltration when compared to controls. An additional cutaneous wound healing study found that rats fed a diet enriched in ω-3 fatty acids produced wounds that were weaker in tensile strength compared to those from rats fed a diet containing ω-6 fatty acids.[117] Fish oil was found to inhibit connective tissue proliferation in a rat model of liver wound healing,[118] but the effect could be blocked by treatment with the antioxidant α-lipoic acid. This latter result again raises the question of the role of oxidative stress in the wound and the susceptibility of essential fatty acids to lipid peroxidation. It is clear from many studies that there is a close relationship between antioxidants and lipid peroxidation *in vivo*. Antioxidants that have been shown to reduce lipid peroxidation and modify the effects of fatty acids include vitamins C[119] and E,[120] selenium compounds,[121,122] and the previously mentioned α-lipoic acid.[118] Therefore, to properly understand and interpret the data on the effects of essential fatty acids, the antioxidant status of the patient or the model system needs to be considered. To make conclusions about the effects of essential fatty acids, the stage of wound healing and the type of wound need to be considered. The data suggest that in the early stages of wound healing, the anti-inflammatory effects of ω-3 fatty acids or other lipid mixtures[123] may delay wound healing. However, burn patients have lower levels of arachidonic acid and ω-3 fatty acids in their plasma following burn injury,[124] and supplementation with ω-3 fatty acids seems to be beneficial for these patients,[125] or for those in a hypermetabolic state.[126]

The cardiovascular risk factors associated with saturated fatty acids are well documented. This lipid class is not metabolized to any bioactive molecules and is, therefore, considered to be more or less neutral to the inflammation process. Studies have shown that diets containing stearic acid had no effect on *in vivo* thromboxane

A$_2$ or prostacyclin biosynthesis.[127] When comparing the effects of diets enriched in lauric plus myristic acid or palamitic acid to stearic acid in healthy young men, it was found that palmitic acid increased factor VII coagulant activity compared to those enriched with stearic acid. However, stearic acid increased fibrinogen concentration compared to the lauric plus myristic acid diet.[128] It is unknown if these modest affects on clotting factors could be a factor in the early stages of wound healing.

The monounsaturated fatty acids are an excellent source of energy and appear to provide modest benefits in improving plasma lipoprotein profiles in high risk groups. In one study in healthy young men, diets high in MuFA (33% of total fatty acids in the diet) resulted in reduced platelet aggregatory response compared to a moderate MuFA diet (16% of total fatty acids in the diet).[129] MuFA may also be able to modify the lipolysis rates in adipocytes. Some research indicates that dietary MuFA may lower the antilipolytic activity of insulin better than PuFA. A study in rats demonstrated an increased baseline and adrenaline-stimulated lipolytic activity and a decreased antilipolytic capacity of insulin in animals with an increase in MuFAs in their tissues.[130] Rats fed MuFAs have also been shown to have increased glycemic tolerance compared to those fed a diet containing saturated fatty acids. Rats fed MuFA had increased secretion of the antidiabetic hormone, glucagon-like peptide-1 (GLP-1), as determined by immunoreactive methods.[131] These results suggest that MuFA may be beneficial as part of the nutrient regimen for diabetic patients.

CONSEQUENCES OF INADEQUATE FAT INTAKE ON THE HEALING WOUND

Healthy humans have the capacity to thrive on very diverse combinations and ratios of protein, carbohydrate, and fat. The same is basically true for the patient with a healing wound so long as energy requirements are adequately met. As discussed above, wound healing will occur for some wounds even in the presence of essential fatty acid deficiency. Wounds due to surgery without underlying trauma, or lacerations to cutaneous tissue appear to heal well independent of nutrition, although inadequate nutrition prior to surgery is a risk factor for a poor surgical outcome.[132] On the other hand, the healing of pressure sores/ulcers and burns appears to be more sensitive to nutritional status.[133] Clearly, there are different mechanisms at play for these different types of wounds. The first question, though, is under what scenario would there be inadequate fat intake? One likely cause is fat malabsorption. Fat malabsorption can be idiopathic, due to a number of diseases,[134–136] or can be a consequence of intestinal surgery, such as a bowel resection.[137] In these instances, it is possible for a patient to be in negative energy balance if sufficient calories are not supplied via protein and carbohydrate sources. A negative energy balance would impair wound healing and immune function and quickly lead to malnutrition in hypermetabolic patients. Another condition in which inadequate fat intake can occur is in patients receiving fat-free parenteral nutrition.[138,139] In these instances, the glucose supplied by parenteral nutrition inhibits the release of fatty acids from adipose tissue, and patients can become essentially fatty acid deficient and manifest the scaly skin associated with EFAD. Elderly patients are also potentially at greater risk, because they appear to have a decreased ability to adjust their metabolism (e.g., resting energy expenditure) in response to lower caloric intake.[140] There may be benefits to an "inadequate" fat intake for burn injuries. Immunosuppression is a common outcome of burn-injured patients. A study in rats found that a low-fat diet (1% fat) compared to a high-fat diet (25% fat) prevented immunosuppression as measured by *in vitro* splenocyte proliferation.[141] A followup study from the same laboratory group found that the type of fatty acid in the diet did not influence the degree of immunosuppression, and that nitric oxide release by macrophages was the cause of reduced T-cell activity.[142]

CONSEQUENCES OF FAT EXCESS ON THE HEALING WOUND

Overfeeding carbohydrate or fat can result in fatty infiltration of the liver, and a high-fat/low-carbohydrate diet moves the metabolic state toward a ketogenic condition that could be problematic for patients with kidney or liver problems. As with underfeeding, the human body has the ability to adapt to an excess of calories from multiple macronutrient sources. In two groups of normal men fed an excess (5 MJ/d for 21 d) of carbohydrate or fat, both groups had the same level of fat storage.[143] A small study performed in lean and obese women tested overfeeding with fat, glucose, fructose, or sucrose, and no significant difference in fat balance was observed.[144] Elevated leptin levels were observed in short-term studies of overfeeding[145] and also of overfeeding of carbohydrates but not fat.[146] If there is a fat excess, then it is important to consider the type of fat and the possible consequences. For the healing wound, there is no data to suggest that an excess of saturated or monounsaturated fatty acids is either harmful or beneficial. However, an excess or imbalance in PuFA could impact the immune system. The anti-inflammatory effects of ω-3 PuFA in humans are well documented.[6,147] However, mice fed high levels of ω-3 PuFA (~38% of calories) had decreased production of interleukin-12 and gamma interferon by splenocytes.[148] Therefore, if there is an excess of ω-3 PuFA in the diet, the anti-inflammatory benefits of these fats may turn into immunosuppression. This result could be a complicating factor for patients who have healing wounds and are fighting local or systemic infection. Also, a high fat diet is often not advisable for burn patients because the fat may exacerbate the immunosuppression often experienced by these patients.[149] Likewise, an excess of ω-6 PuFA may exacerbate inflammation that needs to be brought under control.

RECOMMENDATIONS TO OPTIMIZE FAT INTAKE

Dietary reference intakes for macronutrients have recently been published.[150] Significantly, for the first time these recommendations include amounts of ω-3 PuFA for infants as well as adults. For ω-6 PuFA, it is recommended that men between the ages of 19 and 50 years receive 17 g/d of linoleic acid and that women in the same age group receive 12 g/d. The requirements drop to 14 g/d for men older than

50 years of age and to 11 g/d for women over 50 years of age. For ω-3 PuFA, it is recommended that men older than 19 years of age receive 1.6 g/d of α-linolenic acid, and women older than 19 years of age receive 1.1 g/d. Based upon these amounts, the recommended ω-6:ω-3 ratio for men up to 50 years of age is approximately 10.6:1, and changes to 8.75:1 for men over age 50. For adult women up to 50 years of age, the ratio is 10.9:1, and it then changes to 10:1 for women over 50 years of age. Research on ω-6 and ω-3 PuFA has found that it is the ratio of these two essential fatty acid classes in the diet that determines the systemic and metabolic effects.[1] In the past century, there was a large increase in the amount of ω-6 fatty acids found in the Western diet due to the increasing use of plant seed oils. The increased intake of these oils led to ω-6:ω-3 ratios in the Western diet in excess of 15:1.[1] The new recommended levels for these PuFAs recognize the excess of ω-6 and the need for ω-3 PuFA, but the ratios may not be low enough to realize some of the therapeutic effects of ω-3 PuFA. For cardiovascular- and inflammatory-related diseases such as asthma and rheumatoid arthritis, ω-6:ω-3 PuFA ratios less than 5:1 have been shown to be beneficial. The optimal ω-6:ω-3 PuFA ratio for wound healing is unknown. However, these fatty acids could be used as adjuvants to the healing process by modulating inflammation if needed. The use of these nutrients will largely depend upon the nature of the wound, the stage in the healing process, and the existence of any underlying disease states. It is clear that in the early stages of wound healing, an adequate inflammatory response is needed to initiate the healing process, and ratios of ω-6:ω-3 less than 10:1 may not be advisable. During the proliferative and remodeling stages of wound healing, there may be benefits to varying the ω-6:ω-3 ratios or the type of PuFA, but research is still needed before any recommendations can be made. With respect to the other fatty acid classes, there are no recommended amounts in the new dietary reference intakes, as these are not considered essential nutrients. However, there are some general principles that can be followed. The first is that trans-fatty acids in the diet should be minimized, as there are no requirements or benefits, and likely only harmful effects.[39] Saturated fatty acids are an excellent energy source, but there is no dietary requirement, because they can be synthesized endogenously from carbohydrate energy sources. Monounsaturated fatty acids may be a better alternative as a fat energy source, because they are readily utilized and do not have the negative cardiovascular affects associated with saturated fatty acids. Therefore, the current data suggest that the need for dietary lipids to supply the components for tissue growth and remodeling as well as energy is best met primarily by monounsaturated fatty acids with varying amounts of ω-6 and ω-3 PuFA. The best ratio of ω-6:ω-3 PuFA to use as an adjuvant to the healing process remains to be determined. The amount of fat to include in treating wound patients needs to be determined in the context of energy expenditure and the nature of the wound.[151]

FUTURE DIRECTIONS

Fats/lipids are an extremely diverse class of molecules that includes the fatty acids and all their metabolic derivatives, glycerophospholipids, glycolipids, neutral lipids, sphingolipids, and sterols. The recognition that this class of molecules functions not only as nutrients but also as signaling molecules has given rise to the new field of lipidomics, which seeks to profile this vast group. Many of the lipid derivatives are now known to be involved in regulating various stages of cell growth, and the implications extend far beyond wound healing and will likely have significant impact in cancer biology and autoimmune disease. There are several fields that will likely spur advances in wound healing in the next decade. An understanding of the healing process (inflammation, proliferation, and remodeling) in acute and chronic wounds will benefit from genomic, proteomic, and lipidomic profiling of wound tissue and wound fluids. This will undoubtedly lead to the identification of target molecules and pathways for pharmacological intervention to enhance healing, especially in chronic wounds. This profiling will also lead to a better understanding of how nutrients may be used as adjuvants to the healing process. In our laboratory, we have used gene expression profiling of fibroblasts grown in media containing varying ratios of ω-6 and ω-3 fatty acids, and we have found that PuFA are capable of altering gene expression for a number of growth factors, integrins, matrix metallo-proteases, and transcription factors (manuscript submitted and currently under review). Moreover, many of the genes affected by PuFA are responsive to different ω-6:ω-3 ratios. An example of one gene that displays an interesting expression pattern in response to different fatty acid ratios is Adamts1 (A disintegrin and metalloproteinase with thrombospondin motifs 1). Adamts1 is a matrix metallopro-tease that has antiangiogenic properties (e.g., blocks neovascular response induced by growth factors) and also has been shown to inhibit endothelial cell proliferation *in vitro*.[152] In 3T3-Swiss fibroblasts incubated with an ω-3 as the primary fatty acid in the medium, the cells have a level of expression for this protein that is 60% of the level for the β-actin housekeeping gene. The level drops to 30% of β-actin expression at an ω-6:ω-3 ratio of 1:25, it increases back to 60% at an ω-6:ω-3 ratio of 1:10, and then drops back to 30% if the fatty acid source is primarily an ω-6 fatty acid. The process of collagen production and turnover is a necessary component of the healing process, and PuFA are capable of affecting *in vitro* collagen pro-duction by fibroblasts.[153] There are situations when increasing the production of healthy collagen is desirable (e.g., healing torn ligaments or tendons) and other instances where collagen production needs to be minimized or controlled to prevent organ fibrosis.[154,155] The fact that PuFA can alter the *in vitro* expression of pro-duction of extracellular matrix molecules offers the prospect that ω-6:ω-3 ratios could be used to enhance or suppress various biological processes necessary for healing, but more research is clearly necessary to determine if this is a viable approach.

REFERENCES

1. Simopoulos, A.P., The importance of the ratio of omega-6/omega-3 essential fatty acids, *Biomed. Pharmacother.*, 56, 365, 2002.
2. Abeywardena, M.Y., McLennan, P.L., and Charnock, J.S., Differences between *in vivo* and *in vitro* production of eicosanoids following long-term dietary fish oil supplementation in the rat, *Prost. Leuk. Essent. Fatty Acids*, 42, 159, 1991.

3. Hardard'ottir, I., Whelan, J., and Kinsella, J.E., Kinetics of tumour necrosis factor and prostaglandin production by murine resident peritoneal macrophages as affected by dietary n-3 polyunsaturated fatty acids, *Immunology*, 76, 572, 1992.

4. Mathias, M.M. and Dupont, J., Quantitative relationships between dietary linoleate and prostaglandin (eicosanoid) biosynthesis, *Lipids*, 11, 791, 1985.

5. Turek, J.J., Schoenlein, I.A., and Bottoms, G.D., The effect of dietary n-3 and n-6 fatty acids on tumor necrosis factor-α production and leucine aminopeptidase levels in rat peritoneal macrophages, *Prost. Leuk. Essent. Fatty Acids*, 43, 141, 1991.

6. Meydani, S.N. et al., Oral (n-3) fatty acid supplementation suppresses cytokine production and lymphocyte proliferation: comparison between young and older women, *J. Nutr.*, 121, 547, 1991.

7. May, C.L., Southworth, A.J., and Calder, P.C., Inhibition of lymphocyte protein kinase C by unsaturated fatty acids, *Biochem. Biophys. Res. Comm.*, 195, 823, 1993.

8. Opmeer, F.A., Adolfs, M.J.P., and Bonta, I.L., Regulation of prostaglandin E_2 receptors *in vivo* by dietary fatty acids in peritoneal macrophages from rats, *J. Lip. Res.*, 25, 262, 1984.

9. Awazu, M. et al., Dietary fatty acid modulates glomerular atrial natriuretic peptide receptor, *Kidney Int.*, 42, 265, 1992.

10. Clarke, S.D. et al., Fatty acid regulation of gene expression. Its role in fuel partitioning and insulin resistance, *Ann. N.Y. Acad. Sci.*, 827, 178, 1997.

11. Kliewer, S.A. et al., Fatty acids and eicosanoids regulate gene expression through direct interactions with peroxisome proliferator-activated receptors alpha and gamma, *Proc. Natl. Acad. Sci. U.S.A.*, 94, 4318, 1997.

12. Reseland, J.E. et al., Reduction of leptin gene expression by dietary polyunsaturated fatty acids, *J. Lipid Res.*, 42, 743, 2001.

13. Fruhbeck, G. et al., The adipocyte: a model for integration of endocrine and metabolic signaling in energy metabolism regulation, *Am. J. Physiol. Endocrinol. Metab.*, 280, E827, 2001.

14. Milan, G. et al., Resistin and adiponectin expression in visceral fat of obese rats: effect of weight loss, *Obes. Res.*, 10, 1095, 2002.

15. Mora, S. and Pessin, J.E., An adipocentric view of signaling and intracellular trafficking, *Diabetes Metab. Res. Rev.*, 18, 345, 2002.

16. Fliers, E. et al., White adipose tissue: getting nervous, *J. Neuroendocrinol.*, 15, 1005, 2003.

17. Hamosh, M., Lingual and gastric lipases, *Nutrition*, 6, 421, 1990.

18. Carriere, F. et al., Secretion and contribution to lipolysis of gastric and pancreatic lipases during a test meal in humans, *Gastroenterology*, 105, 876, 1993.

19. Brockman, H., Pancreatic lipase: physiological studies, in *Intestinal Lipid Metabolism*, Mansbach, III, C.M., Tso, P., and Kuksis, A., Eds., Kluwer Academic/Plenum, New York, 2001, p. 61.

20. Tso, P., Gastrointestinal digestion and absorption of lipid, *Adv. Lipid Res.*, 21, 143, 1985.

21. Tso, P. and Fujimoto, K., The absorption and transport of lipids by the small intestine, *Brain Res. Bull.*, 27, 477, 1991.

22. Akesson, B., Content of phospholipids in human diets studied by the duplicate-portion technique, *Br. J. Nutr.*, 47, 223, 1982.

23. Sternby, B. et al., Pancreatic lipolytic enzymes in human duodenal contents. Radioimmunoassay compared with enzyme activity, *Scand. J. Gastroenterol.*, 26, 859, 1991.

24. Howles, P.N., Hui, D.Y., Cholesterol esterase, in *Intestinal Lipid Metabolism*, Mansbach, III, C.M., Tso, P., and Kuksis, A., Eds., Kluwer Academic/Plenum, New York, 2001, p. 119.

25. McGarry, J.D. and Brown, N.F., The mitochondrial carnitine palmitoyltransferase system. From concept to molecular analysis, *Eur. J. Biochem.*, 244, 1, 1997.

26. Grill, V. and Qvigstad, E., Fatty acids and insulin secretion, *Br. J. Nutr.*, 83 (Suppl 1), S79, 2000.

27. Summers, L.K. et al., Uptake of individual fatty acids into adipose tissue in relation to their presence in the diet, *Am. J. Clin. Nutr.*, 71, 1470, 2000.

28. Wanders, R.J. et al., Peroxisomal fatty acid alpha- and beta-oxidation in humans: enzymology, peroxisomal metabolite transporters and peroxisomal diseases, *Biochem. Soc. Trans.*, 29, 250, 2001.

29. Wanders, R.J. and Tager, J.M., Lipid metabolism in peroxisomes in relation to human disease, *Mol. Aspects Med.*, 19, 69, 1998.

30. Nirgiotis, J.G. et al., Low-fat, high-carbohydrate diets improve wound healing and increase protein levels in surgically stressed rats, *J. Pediatr. Surg.*, 26, 925, 1991.

31. Sinclair, H. and Gale, M., Eicosapentaenoic acid in fat, *Lancet*, 1, 1202, 1987.

32. Wood, D.A. et al., Linoleic and eicosapentaenoic acids in adipose tissue and platelets and risk of coronary heart disease, *Lancet*, 1, 177, 1987.

33. Leaf, D.A. et al., Incorporation of dietary *n*-3 fatty acids into the fatty acids of human adipose tissue and plasma lipid classes, *Am. J. Clin. Nutr.*, 62, 68, 1995.

34. Marckmann, P. et al., Biomarkers of habitual fish intake in adipose tissue, *Am. J. Clin. Nutr.*, 62, 956, 1995.

35. Dupont, J., White, P.J., and Feldman, E.B., Saturated and hydrogenated fats in food in relation to health, *J. Am. Coll. Nutr.*, 10, 577, 1991.

36. Vidgren, H.M. et al., Divergent incorporation of dietary trans fatty acids in different serum lipid fractions, *Lipids*, 33, 955, 1998.

37. Chen, Z.Y. et al., Similar distribution of trans fatty acid isomers in partially hydrogenated vegetable oils and adipose tissue of Canadians, *Can. J. Physiol. Pharmacol.*, 73, 718, 1995.

38. Garland, M. et al., The relation between dietary intake and adipose tissue composition of selected fatty acids in US women, *Am. J. Clin. Nutr.*, 67, 25, 1998.

39. Stender, S. and Dyerberg, J., Influence of trans fatty acids on health, *Ann. Nutr. Metab.*, 48, 61, 2004.

40. Valenzuela, A. and Morgado, N., Trans fatty acid isomers in human health and in the food industry, *Biol. Res.*, 32, 273, 1999.

41. Randle, P.J., Regulatory interactions between lipids and carbohydrates: the glucose fatty acid cycle after 35 years, *Diabetes Metab. Rev.*, 14, 263, 1998.

42. Ferrannini, E. et al., Effect of fatty acids on glucose production and utilization in man, *J. Clin. Invest.*, 72, 1737, 1983.

43. Kelley, D.E. et al., Interaction between glucose and free fatty acid metabolism in human skeletal muscle, *J. Clin. Invest.*, 92, 91, 1993.

44. William, W.N., Jr., Ceddia, R.B., and Curi, R., Leptin controls the fate of fatty acids in isolated rat white adipocytes, *J. Endocrinol.*, 175, 735, 2002.

45. Wang, M.Y., Lee, Y., and Unger, R.H., Novel form of lipolysis induced by leptin, *J. Biol. Chem.*, 274, 17541, 1999.

46. Steinberg, G.R., Bonen, A., and Dyck, D.J., Fatty acid oxidation and triacylglycerol hydrolysis are enhanced after chronic leptin treatment in rats, *Am. J. Physiol. Endocrinol. Metab.*, 282, E593, 2002.

47. Fantuzzi, G. and Faggioni, R., Leptin in the regulation of immunity, inflammation, and hematopoiesis, *J. Leukoc. Biol.*, 68, 437, 2000.

48. Salvador, J., Gomez-Ambrosi, J., and Fruhbeck, G., Perspectives in the therapeutic use of leptin, *Expert Opin. Pharmacother.*, 2, 1615, 2001.

49. Unger, R.H., Zhou, Y.T., and Orci, L., Regulation of fatty acid homeostasis in cells: novel role of leptin, *Proc. Natl. Acad. Sci. U.S.A.*, 96, 2327, 1999.

50. Shimomura, I. et al., Decreased IRS-2 and increased SREBP-1c lead to mixed insulin resistance and sensitivity in livers of lipodystrophic and ob/ob mice, *Mol. Cell*, 6, 77, 2000.

51. Reidy, S.P. and Weber, J., Leptin: an essential regulator of lipid metabolism, *Comp. Biochem. Physiol. A Mol. Integr. Physiol.*, 125, 285, 2000.

52. Havel, P.J., Control of energy homeostasis and insulin action by adipocyte hormones: leptin, acylation stimulating protein, and adiponectin, *Curr. Opin. Lipidol.*, 13, 51, 2002.

53. Jump, D.B. and Clarke, S.D., Regulation of gene expression by dietary fat, *Annu. Rev. Nutr.*, 19, 63, 1999.

54. Brown, M.S. and Goldstein, J.L., The SREBP pathway: regulation of cholesterol metabolism by proteolysis of a membrane-bound transcription factor, *Cell*, 89, 331, 1997.

55. Brown, M.S. and Goldstein, J.L., Sterol regulatory element binding proteins (SREBPs): controllers of lipid synthesis and cellular uptake, *Nutr. Rev.*, 56, S1, 1998.

56. Brown, M.S. and Goldstein, J.L., A proteolytic pathway that controls the cholesterol content of membranes, cells, and blood, *Proc. Natl. Acad. Sci. U.S.A.*, 96, 11041, 1999.

57. Goldstein, J.L., Rawson, R.B., and Brown, M.S., Mutant mammalian cells as tools to delineate the sterol regulatory element-binding protein pathway for feedback regulation of lipid synthesis, *Arch. Biochem. Biophys.*, 397, 139, 2002.

58. Horton, J.D., Goldstein, J.L., and Brown, M.S., SREBPs: activators of the complete program of cholesterol and fatty acid synthesis in the liver, *J. Clin. Invest.*, 109, 1125, 2002.

59. Foretz, M. et al., Sterol regulatory element binding protein-1c is a major mediator of insulin action on the hepatic expression of glucokinase and lipogenesis-related genes, *Proc. Natl. Acad. Sci. U.S.A.*, 96, 12737, 1999.

60. Rosen, E.D. et al., Transcriptional regulation of adipogenesis, *Genes Dev.*, 14, 1293, 2000.

61. Morrison, R.F. and Farmer, S.R., Hormonal signaling and transcriptional control of adipocyte differentiation, *J. Nutr.*, 130, 3116S, 2000.

62. Issemann, I. and Green, S., Activation of a member of the steroid hormone receptor superfamily by peroxisome proliferators, *Nature*, 347, 645, 1990.

63. Kliewer, S.A. et al., Differential expression and activation of a family of murine peroxisome proliferator-activated receptors, *Proc. Natl. Acad. Sci. U.S.A.*, 91, 7355, 1994.

64. Barak, Y. et al., PPAR gamma is required for placental, cardiac, and adipose tissue development, *Mol. Cell*, 4, 585, 1999.

65. Braissant, O. et al., Differential expression of peroxisome proliferator-activated receptors (PPARs): tissue distribution of PPAR-alpha, -beta, and -gamma in the adult rat, *Endocrinology*, 137, 354, 1996.

66. Frohnert, B.I., Hui, T.Y., and Bernlohr, D.A., Identification of a functional peroxisome proliferator-responsive element in the murine fatty acid transport protein gene, *J. Biol. Chem.*, 274, 3970, 1999.

67. Frohnert, B.I. and Bernlohr, D.A., Regulation of fatty acid transporters in mammalian cells, *Prog. Lipid Res.*, 39, 83, 2000.
68. Wang, Y.X. et al., Peroxisome-proliferator-activated receptor delta activates fat metabolism to prevent obesity, *Cell*, 113, 159, 2003.
69. Tanaka, T. et al., Activation of peroxisome proliferator-activated receptor delta induces fatty acid beta-oxidation in skeletal muscle and attenuates metabolic syndrome, *Proc. Natl. Acad. Sci. U.S.A.*, 100, 15924, 2003.
70. Zhang, X. and Young, H.A., PPAR and immune system — what do we know?, *Int. Immunopharmacol.*, 2, 1029, 2002.
71. Trifilieff, A. et al., PPAR-α and γ- but not -δ agonists inhibit airway inflammation in a murine model of asthma: *in vitro* evidence for an NF-κB-independent effect, *Br. J. Pharmacol.*, 139, 163, 2003.
72. Pollack, S.V., Wound healing: a review. III. Nutritional factors affecting wound healing, *J. Dermatol. Surg. Oncol.*, 5, 615, 1979.
73. Scholl, D. and Langkamp-Henken, B., Nutrient recommendations for wound healing, *J. Intraven. Nurs.*, 24, 124, 2001.
74. Brylinsky, C.M., Nutrition and wound healing: an overview, *Ostomy Wound Manage.*, 41, 14, 1995.
75. Trujillo, E.B., Effects of nutritional status on wound healing, *J. Vasc. Nurs.*, 11, 12, 1993.
76. Thomas, D.R., Specific nutritional factors in wound healing, *Adv. Wound Care*, 10, 40, 1997.
77. Stotts, N.A. and Wipke-Tevis, D., Nutrition, perfusion, and wound healing: an inseparable triad, *Nutrition*, 12, 733, 1996.
78. Thomas, D.R., Nutritional factors affecting wound healing, *Ostomy Wound Manage.*, 42, 40, 1996.
79. Mazzotta, M.Y., Nutrition and wound healing, *J. Am. Podiatr. Med. Assoc.*, 84, 456, 1994.
80. Falcone, P.A. and Caldwell, M.D., Wound metabolism, *Clin. Plast. Surg.*, 17, 443, 1990.
81. Ennis, W.J. and Meneses, P., 31P NMR spectroscopic analysis of wound healing: the effect of hydrocolloid therapy, *Adv. Wound Care*, 9, 21, 1996.
82. Barton, R.G., Nutrition support in critical illness, *Nutr. Clin. Pract.*, 9, 127, 1994.
83. Wilmore, D.W., Metabolic response to severe surgical illness: overview, *World J. Surg.*, 24, 705, 2000.
84. Duke, J.H., Jr. et al., Contribution of protein to caloric expenditure following injury, *Surgery*, 68, 168, 1970.
85. Long, C.L. et al., A physiologic basis for the provision of fuel mixtures in normal and stressed patients, *J. Trauma*, 30, 1077, 1990.
86. Gilmore, M.A., Phases of wound healing, *Dimens. Oncol. Nurs.*, 5, 32, 1991.
87. Kirsner, R.S. and Eaglstein, W.H., The wound healing process, *Dermatol. Clin.*, 11, 629, 1993.
88. Lawrence, W.T., Physiology of the acute wound, *Clin. Plast. Surg.*, 25, 321, 1998.
89. Lazarus, G.S. et al., Definitions and guidelines for assessment of wounds and evaluation of healing, *Arch. Dermatol.*, 130, 489, 1994.
90. Jenkinson, A. et al., Dietary intakes of polyunsaturated fatty acids and indices of oxidative stress in human volunteers, *Eur. J. Clin. Nutr.*, 53, 523, 1999.
91. Barbosa, D.S. et al., Decreased oxidative stress in patients with ulcerative colitis supplemented with fish oil omega-3 fatty acids, *Nutrition*, 19, 837, 2003.

92. Kikugawa, K. et al., Protective effect of supplementation of fish oil with high *n*-3 polyunsaturated fatty acids against oxidative stress-induced DNA damage of rat liver *in vivo*, *J. Agric. Food Chem.*, 51, 6073, 2003.

93. Mabile, L. et al., Moderate intake of *n*-3 fatty acids is associated with stable erythrocyte resistance to oxidative stress in hypertriglyceridemic subjects, *Am. J. Clin. Nutr.*, 74, 449, 2001.

94. Mori, T.A. et al., Effect of omega 3 fatty acids on oxidative stress in humans: GC-MS measurement of urinary F2-isoprostane excretion, *Redox. Rep.*, 5, 45, 2000.

95. Kannan, K. and Jain, S.K., Oxidative stress and apoptosis, *Pathophysiology*, 7, 153, 2000.

96. Curtin, J.F., Donovan, M., and Cotter, T.G., Regulation and measurement of oxidative stress in apoptosis, *J. Immunol. Methods*, 265, 49, 2002.

97. Lee, Y.J. et al., Oxidative stress-induced apoptosis is mediated by ERK1/2 phosphorylation, *Exp. Cell Res.*, 291, 251, 2003.

98. Morrow, J.D. et al., The isoprostanes: unique prostaglandin-like products of free-radical-initiated lipid peroxidation, *Drug Metab. Rev.*, 31, 117, 1999.

99. Nourooz-Zadeh, J. et al., F4-isoprostanes: a novel class of prostanoids formed during peroxidation of docosahexaenoic acid (DHA), *Biochem. Biophys. Res. Comm.*, 242, 338, 1998.

100. Awad, J.A. et al., Isoprostanes — prostaglandin-like compounds formed *in vivo* independently of cyclooxygenase: use as clinical indicators of oxidant damage, *Gastroenterol. Clin. North Am.*, 25, 409, 1996.

101. Morrow, J.D. et al., A series of prostaglandin F2-like compounds are produced *in vivo* in humans by a non-cyclooxygenase, free radical-catalyzed mechanism, *Proc. Natl. Acad. Sci. U.S.A.*, 87, 9383, 1990.

102. Brame, C.J. et al., Modification of proteins by isoketal-containing oxidized phospholipids, *J. Biol. Chem.*, 14, 13447, 2004.

103. Takahashi, A., Aoshiba, K., and Nagai, A., Apoptosis of wound fibroblasts induced by oxidative stress, *Exp. Lung Res.*, 28, 275, 2002.

104. James, T.J. et al., Evidence of oxidative stress in chronic venous ulcers, *Wound Repair Regen.*, 11, 172, 2003.

105. Marikovsky, M. et al., Appearance of leptin in wound fluid as a response to injury, *Wound Repair Regen.*, 10, 302, 2002.

106. Heiman, M.L. et al., Leptin inhibition of the hypothalamic-pituitary-adrenal axis in response to stress, *Endocrinology*, 138, 3859, 1997.

107. Loffreda, S. et al., Leptin regulates proinflammatory immune responses, *FASEB J.*, 12, 57, 1998.

108. Michalik, L. et al., Impaired skin wound healing in peroxisome proliferator-activated receptor (PPAR) and PPAR mutant mice, *J. Cell Biol.*, 154, 799, 2001.

109. Tan, N.S. et al., Peroxisome proliferator-activated receptor (PPAR)-β as a target for wound healing drugs: what is possible?, *Am. J. Clin. Dermatol.*, 4, 523, 2003.

110. Kuenzli, S. and Saurat, J.H., Peroxisome proliferator-activated receptors in cutaneous biology, *Br. J. Dermatol.*, 149, 229, 2003.

111. Di Poi, N. et al., Antiapoptotic role of PPAR in keratinocytes via transcriptional control of the Akt1 signaling pathway, *Mol. Cell*, 10, 721, 2002.

112. Yaqoob, P., Fatty acids as gatekeepers of immune cell regulation, *Trends Immunol.*, 24, 639, 2003.

113. Calder, P.C., Dietary fatty acids and the immune system, *Nutr. Rev.*, 56, S70, 1998.

114. Calder, P.C., Dietary fatty acids and the immune system, *Lipids*, 34 (Suppl), S137, 1999.

115. Hulsey, T.K. et al., Experimental wound healing in essential fatty acid deficiency, *J. Pediatr. Surg.*, 15, 505, 1980.

116. Porras-Reyes, B.H. et al., Essential fatty acids are not required for wound healing, *Prost. Leuk. Essent. Fatty Acids*, 45, 293, 1992.

117. Albina, J.E., Gladden, P., and Walsh, W.R., Detrimental effects of an omega-3 fatty acid-enriched diet on wound healing, *J. Parenter. Enteral Nutr.*, 17, 519, 1993.

118. Arend, A. et al., Lipoic acid prevents suppression of connective tissue proliferation in the rat liver induced by *n*-3 PUFAs. A pilot study, *Ann. Nutr. Metab.*, 44, 217, 2000.

119. Kelley, D.S. and Daudu, P.A., Fat intake and immune response, *Prog. Food Nutr. Sci.*, 17, 41, 1993.

120. Allard, J.P. et al., Lipid peroxidation during *n*-3 fatty acid and vitamin E supplementation in humans, *Lipids*, 32, 535, 1997.

121. Meltzer, H.M. et al., Supplementary selenium influences the response to fatty acid-induced oxidative stress in humans, *Biol. Trace Elem. Res.*, 60, 51, 1997.

122. Beharka, A.A. et al., Mechanism of vitamin E inhibition of cyclooxygenase activity in macrophages from old mice: role of peroxynitrite, *Free Radic. Biol. Med.*, 32, 503, 2002.

123. Politis, M.J. and Dmytrowich, A., Promotion of second intention wound healing by emu oil lotion: comparative results with furasin, polysporin, and cortisone, *Plast. Reconstr. Surg.*, 102, 2404, 1998.

124. Pratt, V.C. et al., Fatty acid content of plasma lipids and erythrocyte phospholipids are altered following burn injury, *Lipids*, 36, 675, 2001.

125. De Souza, D.A. and Greene, L.J., Pharmacological nutrition after burn injury, *J. Nutr.*, 128, 797, 1998.

126. Jeschke, M.G. et al., Nutritional intervention high in vitamins, protein, amino acids, and omega3 fatty acids improves protein metabolism during the hypermetabolic state after thermal injury, *Arch. Surg.*, 136, 1301, 2001.

127. Blair, I.A., Dougherty, R.M., and Iacono, J.M., Dietary stearic acid and thromboxane-prostacyclin biosynthesis in normal human subjects, *Am. J. Clin. Nutr.*, 60, 1054S, 1994.

128. Tholstrup, T. et al., Fat high in stearic acid favorably affects blood lipids and factor VII coagulant activity in comparison with fats high in palmitic acid or high in myristic and lauric acids, *Am. J. Clin. Nutr.*, 59, 371, 1994.

129. Smith, R.D. et al., Long-term monounsaturated fatty acid diets reduce platelet aggregation in healthy young subjects, *Br. J. Nutr.*, 90, 597, 2003.

130. Soriguer, F. et al., Monounsaturated *n*-9 fatty acids and adipocyte lipolysis in rats, *Br. J. Nutr.*, 90, 1015, 2003.

131. Rocca, A.S. et al., Monounsaturated fatty acid diets improve glycemic tolerance through increased secretion of glucagon-like peptide-1, *Endocrinology*, 142, 1148, 2001.

132. Daley, J. et al., Risk adjustment of the postoperative morbidity rate for the comparative assessment of the quality of surgical care: results of the National Veterans Affairs Surgical Risk Study, *J. Am. Coll. Surg.*, 185, 328, 1997.

133. Pinchcofsky-Devin, G.D. and Kaminski, M.V., Jr., Correlation of pressure sores and nutritional status, *J. Am. Geriatr. Soc.*, 34, 435, 1986.

134. Desai, H.G., Merchant, P.C., and Antia, F.P., Malabsorption in cirrhosis of liver. Relationship of fecal fat and vitamin B_{12} excretion, *Indian J. Med. Sci.*, 27, 673, 1973.

135. Murphy, J., Laiho, K., and Wootton, S., Fat malabsorption in cystic fibrosis patients, *Am. J. Clin. Nutr.*, 70, 943, 1999.

136. Poles, M.A. et al., HIV-related diarrhea is multifactorial and fat malabsorption is commonly present, independent of HAART, *Am. J. Gastroenterol.*, 96, 1831, 2001.

137. Leth, R.D. et al., Malabsorption of fat after partial gastric resection. A study of pathophysiologic mechanisms, *Eur. J. Surg.*, 157, 205, 1991.

138. Jeppesen, P.B. et al., Essential fatty acid deficiency in patients with severe fat malabsorption, *Am. J. Clin. Nutr.*, 65, 837, 1997.

139. Jeppesen, P.B., Hoy, C.E., and Mortensen, P.B., Differences in essential fatty acid requirements by enteral and parenteral routes of administration in patients with fat malabsorption, *Am. J. Clin. Nutr.*, 70, 78, 1999.

140. Das, S.K. et al., An underfeeding study in healthy men and women provides further evidence of impaired regulation of energy expenditure in old age, *J. Nutr.*, 131, 1833, 2001.

141. Jobin, N. et al., Improved immune functions with administration of a low-fat diet in a burn animal model, *Cell Immunol.*, 206, 71, 2000.

142. Borde, V.D., Bernier, J., and Garrel, D.R., Effects of dietary fatty acids on burn-induced immunosuppression, *Cell Immunol.*, 220, 116, 2002.

143. Lammert, O. et al., Effects of isoenergetic overfeeding of either carbohydrate or fat in young men, *Br. J. Nutr.*, 84, 233, 2000.

144. McDevitt, R.M. et al., Macronutrient disposal during controlled overfeeding with glucose, fructose, sucrose, or fat in lean and obese women, *Am. J. Clin. Nutr.*, 72, 369, 2000.

145. Kolaczynski, J.W. et al., Response of leptin to short-term and prolonged overfeeding in humans, *J. Clin. Endocrinol. Metab.*, 81, 4162, 1996.

146. Dirlewanger, M. et al., Effects of short-term carbohydrate or fat overfeeding on energy expenditure and plasma leptin concentrations in healthy female subjects, *Int. J. Obes. Relat. Metab. Disord.*, 24, 1413, 2000.

147. Kremer, J.M., *n*-3 fatty acid supplements in rheumatoid arthritis, *Am. J. Clin. Nutr.*, 71, 349S, 2000.

148. Fritsche, K.L., Anderson, M., and Feng, C., Consumption of eicosapentaenoic acid and docosahexaenoic acid impair murine interleukin-12 and interferon- production *in vivo*, *J. Infect. Dis.*, 182 (Suppl 1), S54, 2000.

149. Mayes, T., Enteral nutrition for the burn patient, *Nutr. Clin. Pract.*, 12, S43, 1997.

150. Trumbo, P. et al., Dietary reference intakes for energy, carbohydrate, fiber, fat, fatty acids, cholesterol, protein and amino acids, *J. Am. Diet. Assoc.*, 102, 1621, 2002.

151. Collins, N., Estimating caloric needs to promote wound healing, *Adv. Skin Wound Care*, 15, 140, 2002.

152. Iruela-Arispe, M.L., Carpizo, D., and Luque, A., ADAMTS1: a matrix metalloprotease with angioinhibitory properties, *Ann. N.Y. Acad. Sci.*, 995, 183, 2003.

153. Hankenson, K.D. et al., Omega-3 fatty acids enhance ligament fibroblast collagen formation in association with changes in interleukin-6 production, *Exp. Biol. Med.*, 223, 88, 2000.

154. Tomashefski, J.F., Jr., Pulmonary pathology of acute respiratory distress syndrome, *Clin. Chest. Med.*, 21, 435, 2000.

155. Ghosh, A.K., Factors involved in the regulation of type I collagen gene expression: implication in fibrosis, *Exp. Biol. Med.*, 227, 301, 2002.

4 Protein and Wound Healing

Maggie L. Dylewski and Yong-Ming Yu

CONTENTS

Wound healing is a dynamic, interactive process involving soluble mediators, blood cells, extracellular matrix, and parenchymal cells. The healing process of the wound can be divided into three phases — inflammation, tissue formation, and tissue remodeling — that overlap in time. Many aspects of the detailed mechanisms of this pathophysiological processes, and hence, the approaches to modulate the healing process, are still under extensive investigation. However, this complicated healing process, including the various morphological changes, can also be viewed as a complicated metabolic process (i.e., the utilization of various substrates by the cells in the area of injury for the recovery of their normal lives and functions, including the protein synthesis and degradation in the repairing of the wound and the renewal of tissues). All these regional metabolic processes are also associated with the whole body metabolic status of the host under the conditions of health and severe trauma, such as thermal injury.

Because the process of healing in different tissues is more similar than different, in this chapter the focus will be on the metabolic changes of the skin with wound healing. The mechanisms described for skin would be similar in other tissues, such as muscle, because the major protein of the healing wound is collagen (see Chapter 1). By discussing skin, one may also explore the unique aspect of skin wound healing — epithelialization.

In every living subject, the cellular and protein components of skin undergo a constant degradation and regeneration process. This self-renewal process of the skin involves two components: cell proliferation, mostly among the fibroblasts and keratinocytes; and protein synthesis and degradation within the cells. From the metabolic point of view, the former component is related to the metabolic turnover of DNA and the latter is associated with the turnover of skin proteins. After injury, both metabolic processes are accelerated for repairing the wounded skin and restoring its normal function. In severely injured patients, the metabolic process of wound healing proceeds under a state of the severely altered whole body energy and protein metabolism — hypermetabolic response and severe protein catabolism. Therefore, understanding the relationship between the metabolism in the regional wound and the whole body is an important aspect in managing wound healing. Such a relationship will be discussed based on clinical observations and the recent laboratory *in vivo* experimental data on the simultaneous measurements on both whole body and skin protein metabolism under different physiological and pathophysiological conditions.

EXPERIMENTAL MODELS EXPLORING METABOLIC PROCESSES IN SKIN AND WHOLE BODY *IN VIVO*

The knowledge of energy and substrate metabolism in skin *in vivo* and its relationship to altered whole body metabolic status in health and disease has not been fully elucidated due to the lack of an appropriate experimental approach in obtaining simultaneous measurements of metabolic processes in both sites in a living animal. The development of *in vivo* experimental models using a stable isotope technique has significantly expanded our knowledge of the functional metabolism of proteins and DNA in the skin and its relationship with the whole body status of protein metabolism. Therefore, it is worthwhile to briefly review some of the major *in vivo* metabolism models used for this purpose.

IN VIVO QUANTITATIVE ESTIMATE OF COLLAGEN TURNOVER AS AN INDICATOR OF THE DYNAMIC METABOLIC PROCESS OF WOUND HEALING

The first series of investigations was focused on quantitative evaluation of the collagen turnover rate *in vivo*. Early investigations defining the model concentrated on the evaluation of skin, because 70 to 90% of the protein of skin is collagen, it is readily available for sampling with minimal harm to the animal, and skin is the largest organ of the body and represents approximately 10 to 12% of the body weight of the animal.[1-3] Finally, collagen is the major protein of the healing wound and alteration of collagen synthesis rate reflects the process of wound healing. In order to measure how fast the collagen was formed and degraded, the collagen would first be labeled with stable isotopes, and then observed to see how fast the labeled collagen is replaced by the newly synthesized collagen in subsequent hours or days (decay kinetic model). In a series studies by Molnar et al.,[26-28] rats were exposed to pure $^{18}O_2$ in a chamber for 36 h. The major peptide structure of a collagen molecule is mostly the repeated units of glycine-X-Y; where X may be any amino acid, and Y is approximately 25% proline or hydroxyproline[4] (see Chapter 1). As there is no transfer RNA for hydroxyproline, the only source of this amino acid is from the posttranslational hydroxylation of the peptide-bound proline. After the animals constantly inhale $^{18}O_2$-containing air, the proline residue of the newly synthesized collagen would become ^{18}O labeled hydroxyproline from the incorporation of free molecular oxygen into the hydroxyl group. After 36 h, about 7 to 10% of the protein-bound proline became ^{18}OH-hydroxyproline. By sequential biopsy of the skin at different time points, the turnover rate of collagen protein can be accurately measured based on the fractional change in the abundance of the protein-bound ^{18}O-hydroxyproline. The results revealed that in a healthy rat, soluble collagen synthesis is about 95 mg/d, about 55% of the newly synthesized soluble collagen per day is subsequently matured into insoluble collagen, and 45% of the soluble collagen is degraded into amino acids, which is equivalent to less than 30 mg/d. Using this method, further studies revealed that in protein malnourished rats (where the animals received only 1/6 of the adequate amount of total protein intake for 180 d), the rates of collagen synthesis, degradation, and maturation were reduced to only 11, 16, and 16%, respectively, of those seen in well-nourished healthy controls.[3]

These studies provided strong evidence that whole body nutritional status has significant impact on skin collagen metabolism and, hence, the healing process of the wound. They support the clinical observations that improving whole body protein nutritional status accelerates the wound healing process in severely burned patients and other surgical patients. It should be noted that, because ^{18}OH-hydroxyproline does not reincorporate into collagen after this amino acid is released from collagen degradation, scientifically, the ^{18}O inhalation method has provided the most accurate estimate of collagen metabolism. Other approaches to label collagen using either [^2H]-or [^{13}C]proline as probes always underestimated the rate of collagen metabolism due to the fact that proline can be released and reincorporated into collagen proteins. In Molnar's study, the simultaneous use of $^{18}O_2$ and [$^2H_2$]proline tracers revealed that the underestimate could be 44%.[1] So far, the $^{18}O_2$ method is the most accurate and least harmful approach with which to determine collagen metabolic rate. It could potentially be applied to investigations in human subjects and burn patients.

EXPERIMENTAL MODELS FOR ASSESSING THE DYNAMICS OF SKIN DNA AND PROTEIN METABOLISM

Zhang et al.,[5-9] from the Metabolic Unit of Shriners Hospital in Galveston, Texas, established a unique animal model with which to estimate the *in vivo* pathways of skin DNA metabolism and protein metabolism by using stable isotope labeled glucose, glycine, and phenylalanine tracers. Their work provided the opportunity to quantify whole body protein metabolism, skin protein metabolism, and skin DNA metabolism simultaneously in a living animal. This has been a major contribution to the knowledge of the *in vivo* aspects of skin protein and cellular turnover, their impact on the wound healing process, and their relationship to whole body nutritional status.

DNA METABOLISM

The formation of new skin cells is accompanied by the synthesis of DNA; hence, these are the dynamics of quantifying the rate of DNA turnover. DNA (e.g., adenosine) can be synthesized from the *de novo* synthesis starting from the formation of the nucleotide base; the *de novo* synthesis of deoxyribose and its reaction with intact base; and the reuse of intact deoxyribonucleotides, the so-called deoxyribonucleoside salvage pathway. These pathways are graphically shown in Figure 4.1. Traditionally, DNA synthesis had been measured *in vitro* using either ^{3}H-thymidine or bormode-oxyuridine as the tracer. These tracers are toxic and are not suitable for application to the measurement of the *in vivo* DNA synthesis rate. More importantly, these tracers determine only the deoxyribonucleoside salvage pathway, which does not include the rate of the *de novo* synthesis of DNA starting from the formation of nucleotides, described as above. Studies have demonstrated that the deoxyribose (dR) of deoxyadenosine (dA) and deoxyguanine (dG) is derived almost entirely from extracellular glucose, the reuse of free dR from degradated DNA does not occur, and that of the dA and dG is minor:[10–12] therefore, the *de novo* nucleotide synthesis pathway predominates in the synthesis of deoxyadenosine (dA) and deoxyguanosine (dG).[13–15]

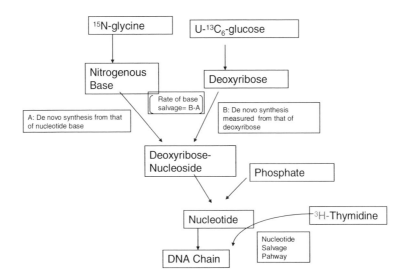

FIGURE 4.1 Pathways of nucleotide synthesis and the model of quantifying the DNA synthesis rate *in vivo*.

Based on the above considerations, Zhang et al.[16] used [^{15}N]-glycine as a precursor to estimate the *de novo* synthesis rate of the nucleotide base and, simultaneously, [U-^{13}C$_6$]glucose for the *de novo* synthesis rate of purine nucleotide. [^{15}N]-glycine incorporated into the newly synthesized nucleotide base,[15] and the [U-^{13}C$_6$]glucose yielded 13C-labeled ribose,[17] which subsequently formed the ^{13}C-ribose-labeled nucleotide. ^{13}C-ribose-labeled nucleotide is regarded as an approximation of total DNA synthesis.[16,17] The difference between the synthesis rates of ^{13}C-ribose-labeled deoxynucleotide and the [^{15}N]-labeled deoxynucleotide represents the nucleotide base salvage pathway.[16] Thus, the investigators successfully measured the fractional rate of total DNA *de novo* synthesis of rabbit skin at approximately 3% per day, and they found that the rate of DNA synthesis starting from the *de novo* nucleotide base was 2.5% per day. Hence, about 0.5% (= 3% – 2.5%) DNA synthesis occurs *via* the base salvage pathway. The established animal and isotope model is a novel approach with which to quantify the metabolic marker of cell proliferation in the skin, simultaneously with the rate of protein synthesis, and the influence of whole body nutritional status under various physiological and pathophysiological conditions.

DETERMINATION OF PROTEIN SYNTHESIS AND DEGRADATION RATES IN THE EPIDERMIS AND DERMIS

Intact skin is composed of dermis and epidermis, which have different structure, function, and turnover/growth rates.[12] The dermis serves as a base physically and nutritionally supporting the epidermis, whereas the epidermis exerts the barrier function of the skin. Hence, it is important to develop experimental methods not only to quantify protein synthesis in the whole skin, but also to differentiate the metabolic regulation of these two components of the skin, under various physiological and pathophysiological conditions. Using rabbit ear as a skin model, Zhang et al.[5] found that the dermal protein contains 75.7% of the total cutaneous phenylalanine and 97.9% of the total cutaneous proline; the remaining 24.3% of phenylalanine and 2.1% of proline reside in the epidermal protein. Taking advantage of the different distribution of amino acids in these two proteins, the investigators were able to use stable isotope L-[ring-^{13}C$_6$]phenylalanine and [^{15}N]proline tracers to estimate the *in vivo* rates of protein synthesis and breakdown distinctively in the dermis and epidermis layers of the skin tissue. Their results indicate that for rabbit skin, the synthesis rate of dermal skin was about 9 mg per 100 g wet weight per day with the same rate of protein breakdown, indicating that skin protein maintains its homeostasis in normal physiological conditions, including short periods of fasting. In addition, the synthesis and breakdown rate of epidermal protein was approximately ten times that found in the dermal protein. It is likely that such a quick turnover rate is of pivotal importance in the wound healing process after injury. Their studies also demonstrated a significant transport of amino acids from dermis to epidermis, supporting the notion that an intact dermis is essential in the overall process of wound repair.

Physiological Regulation of Wound Metabolism and Wound Healing Process in Relation to Whole Body Metabolic State

With the established metabolism models described above, it was then possible to assess the effect of whole body protein nutritional status and its relationship with the regional wound healing process.

Using this model, Zhang et al.[16] reported that the synthesis of DNA and proteins in skin proceeded independently, because the fractional synthesis of whole skin DNA from the *de novo* nucleotide synthesis pathway was about $3.26 \pm 0.593\%$ per day, with DNA synthesis in dermis $3.08 \pm 1.86\%$ per day ($P = 0.38$); however, the fractional synthesis rates of whole skin protein were distinctively $5.35 \pm 4.42\%$ per day, which was greater ($P < 0.05$) than that of the dermal proteins at $2.91 \pm 2.52\%$ per day. The results indicate that cell division and protein synthesis are likely regulated by different mechanisms.

This animal model also allows for a simultaneous quantitative evaluation of protein metabolism in the skin and muscle tissues and their possible relationship in health and disease. It was found that in healthy animals, 64 h of fasting resulted in negative muscle protein balance. Nutritional support with an amino acid mixture and lipid significantly improved muscle protein balance, although it remained in a negative state. Amino acid and lipid feeding plus the use of insulin resulted in a positive protein balance in muscle. Despite the positive and negative responses seen in muscle, protein kinetics in skin protein maintained a balanced state under all these circumstances in healthy animals.[6] The data further indicate that the stability of skin protein metabolism was maintained through a mechanism in the efficient reutilization, or recycling, of the amino acids released from protein breakdown for protein synthesis in the skin.[6] Therefore, under healthy conditions, skin maintains the homeostasis of its protein mass in response to short-term changes in nutritional status and hormonal environment, in contrast to the responses seen in muscle protein metabolism. These findings are also supported by those of Cherel et al.,[18] who reported that skin protein mass of healthy rats remained unchanged even after 5 d of fasting. Therefore, skeletal muscle is a mobilizable source of amino availability in the body, but skin is not. This *in vivo* skin metabolism model can further be applied to investigate the difference in the regulation of skin and muscle protein metabolism under various physiological and pathological conditions, including thermal injury and other critical illness.

After inducing a scar burn to the ear skin, the rates of both protein synthesis and breakdown in the wounded skin were increased, with the increment in proteolysis significantly exceeding protein synthesis, resulting in negative protein balance. Providing insulin combined with glucose and amino acids infusion to maintain a euglycemia and eu-amino acidemia,[7,8] the investigators found that when the insulin was given at a dose similar to that used in the above-mentioned healthy animals,[6] protein metabolism in the burned skin tissue changed from negative to positive balance, mainly due to the inhibition of proteolysis. The observed change in skin was in parallel to the improvement of skeletal muscle protein balance. It appears that after thermal injury, combined use of the anabolic agent insulin and a nutrient supply improved both skin and muscle protein metabolism; hence, improvement of whole body nutritional status is accompanied by positive skin protein balance. However, the investigators reported that short-term infusion of growth hormone did not result in improvement of protein metabolism in the skin or in the muscle.[7] It is interesting to note that the anabolic effect of insulin on thermal-injured skin required a simultaneous supplementation of amino acids, providing either amino acids alone or insulin alone, but this did not have a positive effect on skin protein metabolism.[8] These observations on the regulation of skin protein metabolism after burn injury seem to be similar to those seen in muscle tissues of healthy subjects. It was reported that the anabolic effects of insulin on whole body protein metabolism also required a simultaneous exogenous amino acid supplementation.[19,20]

The effect of a specific nutrient on skin and whole body protein metabolism was also investigated on the same animal model. It was found that leucine-enriched amino acid feeding simultaneously improved protein metabolism in both muscle and skin.[9]

The application of the stable isotope tracer method and animal models allows for the *in vivo* investigation of the quantitative and dynamic changes in skin, muscle, and whole body protein metabolism. The above studies revealed the following:

1. In healthy conditions, the biochemistry of cell proliferation (DNA synthesis) and protein synthesis in the skin are differently regulated.
2. Protein synthesis rates in the epidermis are about ten times those in the dermis, indicating that a very active metabolic process for wound repair occurs in the epidermis component of the skin, and also stressing the importance of an intact dermis in transporting nutrients and in supporting epidermis protein synthesis.
3. In healthy animals, skin protein metabolism is maintained in a dynamically stable condition in response to short-term changes in nutritional status (starvation, amino acid and insulin) as compared to the immediate responses seen in muscle protein. However, prolonged malnutrition results in a reduced rate of collagen protein synthesis accompanied by poor protein nutrition states.
4. After thermal injury, the injured skin is in negative protein balance, in parallel with the net loss of protein from whole body and muscle tissues, and hence, a negative nitrogen balance is also found in skin tissue. Insulin combined with glucose and exogenous amino acid supply and leucine-enriched amino acid feeding improves both skin and muscle protein metabolism.

These findings provide direct evidence that in an injured condition, improvement of whole body protein nutritional status parallels protein anabolism in the wound protein. Hence, nutritional support is important in the wound healing process, and the modulation of anabolic factors and nutrients in the feeding formula would help promote not only whole body but also skin protein metabolism. A positive protein balance in the skin would accelerate the wound healing process.

The findings from animal models further support the following clinical practice and observations.

EFFECT OF LOW-PROTEIN DIET ON THE WOUND

Proper wound healing requires sufficient dietary protein intake. Protein inadequacy impedes wound healing by prolonging the inflammatory phase; impairing fibroplasias, collagen, and proteoglycan syntheses; and impairing wound remodeling.[21,22] Animals consuming diets deficient in protein demonstrated decreased wound integrity and strength compared to animals receiving adequate dietary protein.[23] Additionally, protein-deficient animals experienced impaired collagen deposition, decreased skin and fascial wound breaking strength, and increased wound infection rates.[23]

A clinical trial assessing wound healing among subjects of varying nutritional states showed that subjects with low serum protein (< 6.5 g/dl) or serum albumin (< 3.5 g/dl) levels had decreased wound strength compared to those with higher serum protein and (> 6.5 g/dl) serum albumin (> 3.5 g/dl) levels.[24] Surgical patients with mild protein-energy malnutrition (defined as 90 to 95% usual body weight) or severe protein-energy malnutrition (defined as < 90% usual body weight) had lower healing rates compared to well-nourished patients. Specifically, patients with protein-energy malnutrition produced less hydroxyproline compared to well-nourished patients.[25]

EFFECT OF HIGH-PROTEIN DIET ON THE WOUND

High-protein diets are associated with increased healing of pressure ulcers. Malnourished elderly male patients who received a high protein diet (2.1 ± 0.9 g/kg) for 8 weeks had a significant decline in total truncal pressure ulcer surface area (-4.2 ± 7.1 cm^2) compared to those who received a low-protein diet (1.4 ± 0.5 g/kg) (-2.1 ± 11.5 cm^2)[6]. Additionally, among subjects with Stage IV ulcers, total truncal pressure ulcer surface area decreased by -7.6 ± 5.8 cm^2 in the high-protein group compared to a decline of -3.2 ± 16.4 cm^2 in the low-protein group. Dietary protein intake was significantly correlated with the change in ulcer area.[26]

IMPORTANCE OF SPECIFIC AMINO ACIDS

The role of single amino acids in promoting wound healing has gained interest over the past several decades. Arginine and glutamine have been the focus of most current research. Details on these two amino acids are discussed elsewhere (Chapter 5 and Chapter 6). Several other amino acids may influence wound healing. Methionine functions in fibroblast proliferation and collagen synthesis. Cysteine participates in collagen synthesis as a cofactor.[27] Historical trials showed a positive effect of sulfur amino acids, such as methionine and cysteine, on wound healing in protein-deficient rats.[29,38] However, clinical data have not been obtained in human subjects so far to support these findings.

Nutritional support enriched with valine, leucine, and isoleucine, the branched-chain amino acids, has been used to treat liver disease, and also to protect liver function during sepsis, trauma, and burns. Branched-chain amino acids are the major nitrogen source for glutamine and alanine synthesis in muscle. Following injury, branched-chain amino acids support protein synthesis and decrease protein catabolism. Although branched-chain amino acids have been shown to retain nitrogen during sepsis, trauma, and burns,[30–32] there appears to be no benefit for wound healing.[33]

RECOMMENDATIONS FOR PROTEIN INTAKE TO OPTIMIZE WOUND REPAIR

Conventional guidelines for protein intake to promote wound healing aim at promoting positive nitrogen balance or, at the very least, maintaining nitrogen balance. Protein kinetic studies provide greater insight into protein dynamics with respect to protein synthesis and protein breakdown. More specifically, protein breakdown is less amenable to exogenous protein during inflammation. Therefore, some lean body mass loss can be expected despite adequate protein intake. However, dietary protein can improve protein economy by increasing the rate of protein synthesis. This, in turn, can enhance increased structural and functional protein synthesis.

Recommended protein intakes for healthy adults and children as well as those with specific clinical conditions are presented in Table 4.1. Major surgery can increase protein requirements by 10%, and pressure ulcers can increase protein requirements by 56 to 88%.[34] Specifically, the National Pressure Ulcer Advisory Panel recommends 1.25 to 1.5 g/kg/d for patients with severe pressure ulcers.[35]

Severe injuries, such as multiple traumas or burns, are characterized by an increased amino acid efflux from the skeletal muscle[36] to accommodate amino acid needs for tissue repair, acute-phase protein production, cellular immunity, and gluconeogenesis. Inadequate protein intake compromises wound healing, muscle

---

TABLE 4.1
Recommended Protein Intakes for Specific Clinical Conditions

Clinical Condition	Protein Recommendation (g/kg/day)
Healthy adult[a]	0.8–1
Healthy children[a]	–
7–12 months	1.20
1–3 years	1.05
4–8 years	0.95
9–13 years	0.95
14–18 years	0.85
Severe pressure ulcers[b]	1.25–1.5
Burns (adult)[c]	1.2–1.5
Burns (children)	2.5–3.0

[a] See also Cohen, A. et al., *J. Biol. Chem.,* 258, 12334, 1983.
[b] See also Chen, P. and Abramson, F.P., *Anal. Chem.,* 70, 1664, 1998.
[c] See also Zhang, X.J. et al., *J. Nutr.,* 134, 2401, 2004.

---

function, and the immune system.[37] Severe protein malnutrition, when body cell mass losses exceed 40%, may result in death.[38]

Therefore, the objective of protein therapy during burn injuries is to minimize net protein catabolism, promote wound healing, and preserve lean body mass. Although protein requirements are significantly elevated in adult burn patients, it should be noted that protein intake greater than 1.5 g of protein per kilogram per day has not been shown to provide any advantage and can result in increased concentrations of urea and ammonia (see Chapter 5). In addition, excess protein intake may compromise bone health by promoting hypercalciuria. Specifically, excess dietary protein intake induces low-grade metabolic acidosis and subsequently decreases renal tubular reabsorption of calcium,[39] increases cell-mediated bone resorption,[40] and increases direct physiochemical dissolution of bone.[41]

For children with severe burn injuries, protein intake at 2.5 to 3 g of protein per kilogram is sufficient to promote wound healing.[42] However, protein intake equal to 4 to 5 g of protein per kilogram may also help maintain lean body mass. This may be particularly important in larger burns characterized by elevated protein losses via the wound. Protein intake over 5 g/kg may be harmful. This is of utmost concern in very young children if intake exceeds the renal solute load (see Chapter 13).

FUTURE DIRECTIONS IN CLINICAL NUTRITIONAL SUPPORT IN RELATION TO WOUND HEALING

Current clinical research has focused on the role of ornithine and ornithine α-ketoglutarate on wound healing. Dietary ornithine supplementation increased wound breaking strength and collagen deposition in mice.[43] Results from two randomized control trials demonstrated that ornithine α-ketoglutarate, a salt formed of two molecules of ornithine and one molecule of α-ketoglutarate, increased wound healing in burn patients.[44,45] Further research is needed to reinforce these findings.

With regard to the specific nutrient requirement in burn injury, one amino acid of special interest is proline. Posttranslational modification of proline on collagen molecule is important to collagen formation and wound healing. The interstitial proline content has been found to be related to wound healing.[46] Metabolically, proline is a nutritionally dispensable amino acid. Its formation and disposal are closely related to the metabolism of ornithine and glutamate (Figure 4.2). Ornithine is one of the components of the urea cycle, and glutamate availability is closely related to the metabolism of α-glutarate, an intermediate of the tricarboxylic acid (TCA) cycle (Figure 4.3). In patients with thermal injuries, hypermetabolism and increased nitrogen loss indicate an accelerated TCA cycle and accelerated urea cycle activities, which "drains" both ornithine and glutamate. Because proline occupies one corner of the metabolic "triangle" interrelating these three amino acids, the *de novo* synthesis of tissue proline is likely to be compromised in the burn condition. This notion is supported by three facts:

1. Stable isotope tracer studies by Jaksic et al. revealed a negative proline balance in patients with burns, suggesting a status of proline depletion.[47]

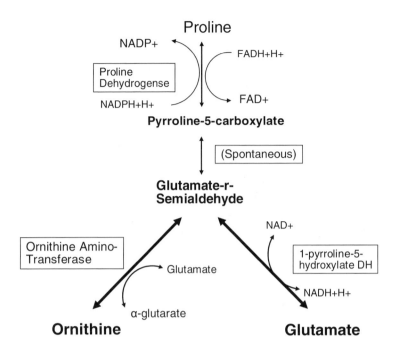

FIGURE 4.2 The "triangle" relationship among proline, ornithine, and glutamate.

2. Tracer studies by Yu et al. revealed an accelerated ornithine disposal via TCA cycle combined with limited arginine formation in severely burned patients.[48]
3. Studies also revealed a reduced tissue glutamine availability after thermal injury.[49] Therefore, the availability of proline is likely to be limited for protein synthesis including collagen. Further studies are warranted on exploring the provision of proline or its precursors ornithine and or glutamate/glutamine on whole body proline metabolism and its relation to protein metabolism in the wound healing process.

TOXICITY OF PROTEIN EXCESS

Protein nutrition is important in wound healing, but providing an excess of protein does not necessarily further help the wound healing process. Instead, this may cause serious metabolic complications. It is worth mentioning that the amount of protein intake for severely burned patients is at the level of 1.5g/kg/day. This level of protein intake has been suggested from clinical observations.[50,51] Stable isotope studies using multiple labeled amino acids have indicated that in severely burned patients, the oxidation rates of individual essential amino acids are around 150% of their corresponding levels observed in healthy subjects.[52] Increasing the feeding from 1.5g/kg/day to 2.5g/kg/day does not provide further benefit to whole body nitrogen economy.[53] This finding is in agreement with the clinical observations that

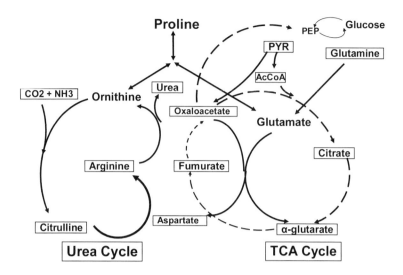

FIGURE 4.3 Relationship among flutamate, proline, and ornithine, with the coupling of urea and the tricarboxylic acid (TCA) cycle.

improved nitrogen sparing does not occur when protein intake exceeded this level.[54] Thus, the tracer kinetic findings have provided further quantitative evidence to support the notion that an adequate amount of protein intake for these patients should be about 1.5g/kg/day.

Protein overfeeding is not only unnecessary, but may lead to potential complications. In critically ill patients, the major complication of protein overfeeding is acidosis and azotemia.[55] In surplus protein feeding, the nitrogen of the amino acids is deaminated and produces ammonia and then urea. Increased renal urea excretion requires obligatory water excretion. Overfeeding protein with inadequate water can produce a state of hypertonic dehydration or "tube feeding syndrome."

Increased gluconeogenesis from amino acids in patients who are severely burned also contributes to the overload of urea nitrogen. Ureagenesis in the liver consumes up to 1000 mmol of HCO_3/day in humans as a result of $2NH_4^+ + 2HCO_3 =>$ urea + $CO_2 + 3H_2O$. In a recent study, Hosch et al.[56] revealed that in experimental human subjects, the rate of ureagenesis was correlated negatively with plasma HCO_3^- concentration over a wide range. Therefore, ureagenesis is an acidifying process. Overproduction of ureagenesis in critically ill patients may contribute adversely to the homeostasis of the acid–base balance of the patients.

Therefore, along the course of providing nutritional support to patients, a comprehensive evaluation of the clinical parameters to assess tolerance, weaning and ventilator parameters, organ function, visceral proteins, volume status, glucose tolerance, and other biochemical markers such as blood urea nitrogen (BUN), ammonia and urinary urea nitrogen, or even indirect calorimetry measurements are necessary to adjust feeding regimens to adequate levels. For patients with a tendency toward or early signs of impaired renal function, the responses to protein intake should be more closely monitored.

In summary, improving whole body protein nutritional status is an important factor in supporting the wound healing process. While this has been observed clinically, recent *in vivo* studies confirmed the metabolic relationship between whole body nutritional status and wound protein synthesis. Providing adequate nutrition plus using certain anabolic factors are an important aspect in taking care of the wounds of surgical patients.

REFERENCES

1. Molnar, J.A. et al., Synthesis and degradation rates of collagens *in vivo* in whole skin of rats, studied with $^{18}O_2$ labeling, *Biochem. J.,* 240, 431, 1986.
2. Molnar, J.A. et al., Relative and absolute changes in soluble and insoluble collagen pool size in skin during normal growth and with dietary protein restriction in rats, *Growth,* 51, 132, 1987.
3. Molnar, J.A. et al., Synthesis and degradation of collagens in skin of healthy and protein-malnourished rats *in vivo*, studied by $^{18}O_2$ labeling, *Biochem. J.,* 250, 71, 1988.
4. Lehninger, A.L., *Biochemistry,* 2nd ed., Worth, New York, 1975.
5. Zhang, X.J. et al., Measurement of protein metabolism in epidermis and dermis, *Am. J. Physiol. Endocrinol. Metab.,* 284, E1191, 2003.
6. Zhang, X.J. et al., Metabolism of skin and muscle protein is regulated differently in response to nutrition, *Am. J. Physiol.,* 274, E484, 1998.
7. Zhang, X.J. et al., Insulin but not growth hormone stimulates protein anabolism in skin wound and muscle, *Am. J. Physiol.,* 276, E712, 1999.
8. Zhang, X.J. et al., Anabolic action of insulin on skin wound protein is augmented by exogenous amino acids, *Am. J. Physiol. Endocrinol. Metab.,* 282, E1308, 2002.
9. Zhang, X.J., Chinkes, D.L., and Wolfe, R.R. Leucine supplementation has an anabolic effect on proteins in rabbit skin wound and muscle, *J. Nutr.,* 134, 3313, 2004.
10. Neese, R.A. et al., Measurement *in vivo* of proliferation rates of slow turnover cells by $2H_2O$ labeling of the deoxyribose moiety of DNA, *Proc. Natl. Acad. Sci. U.S.A.,* 99, 15345, 2002.
11. Joseph, J. and Towsnsend, F.J., The healing of defects in immobile skin in rabbits, *Br. J. Surg.,* 48, 557, 1961.
12. Orland, G.F., Structure of the skin, in *Physiology, Biochemistry and Molecular Biology of the Skin*, 2nd ed., Vol. 1, Goldsmith, L.A., Ed., Oxford University Press, New York, 1991.
13. Reichard, P., Interactions between deoxyribonucleotide and DNA synthesis, *Annu. Rev. Biochem.,* 57, 349, 1988.
14. Cohen, A. et al., Purine and pyrimidine metabolism in human T lymphocytes. Regulation of deoxyribonucleotide metabolism, *J. Biol. Chem.,* 258, 12334, 1983.
15. Chen, P. and Abramson, F.P., Measuring DNA synthesis rates with [1-13C]glycine, *Anal. Chem.,* 70, 1664, 1998.
16. Zhang, X.J. et al., Fractional synthesis rates of DNA and protein in rabbit skin are not correlated, *J. Nutr.,* 134, 2401, 2004.
17. Macallan, D.C. et al., Measurement of cell proliferation by labeling of DNA with stable isotope-labeled glucose: studies *in vitro*, in animals, and in humans, *Proc. Natl. Acad. Sci. U.S.A.,* 95, 708, 1998.
18. Cherel, Y. et al., Whole-body and tissue protein synthesis during brief and prolonged fasting in the rat, *Clin. Sci. (London),* 81, 611, 1991.

19. Flakoll, P.J. et al., Use of amino acid clamps to investigate the role of insulin in regulating protein breakdown *in vivo, J. Parenter. Enteral Nutr.*, 15, 81S, 1991.

20. Valarini, R. et al., Anabolic effects of insulin and amino acids in promoting nitrogen accretion in postoperative patients, *J. Parenter. Enteral Nutr.*, 18, 214, 1994.

21. Ruberg, R.L., Role of nutrition in wound healing, *Surg. Clin. N. Am.*, 64, 705, 1984.

22. Haydock, D.A. et al., The efficacy of subcutaneous goretex implants in monitoring wound healing response in experimental protein deficiency, *Connect. Tissue Res.*, 17, 159, 1988.

23. Peacock, E.E., Jr., Effect of dietary proline and hydroxyproline on tensile strength of healing wounds, *Proc. Soc. Exp. Biol. Med.*, 105, 380, 1960.

24. Lindstedt, E. and Sandblom, P., Wound healing in man: tensile strength of healing wounds in some patient groups, *Ann. Surg.*, 181, 842, 1975.

25. Haydock, D.A. and Hill, G.L., Impaired wound healing in surgical patients with varying degrees of malnutrition, *J. Parenter. Enteral Nutr.*, 10, 550, 1986.

26. Breslow, R.A. et al., The importance of dietary protein in healing pressure ulcers, *J. Am. Geriatr. Soc.*, 41, 357, 1993.

27. Lewis, B., *Wound Healing: Alternatives in Management,* Davis Company, Philadelphia, 2002.

28. Williamson, M.B. and Fromm, H.J., The incorporation of sulfur amino acids into the proteins of regenerating wound tissue, *J. Biol. Chem.*, 212, 705, 1955.

29. Localio, S.A., Morgan, M.E., and Hintown, R., The biological chemistry of wound healing: the effect of di-methionine on healing of wounds in protein depleted animals, *Surg Gynecol. Obstet.*, 86, 582, 1948.

30. Cerra, F.B. et al., Branched chains support postoperative protein synthesis, *Surgery,* 92, 192, 1982.

31. Cerra, F.B. et al., Enteral feeding in sepsis: a prospective, randomized, double-blind trial, *Surgery,* 98, 632, 1985.

32. Sax, H.C., Talamini, M.A., and Fischer, J.E., Clinical use of branched-chain amino acids in liver disease, sepsis, trauma, and burns, *Arch. Surg.*, 121, 358, 1986.

33. McCauley, R. et al., Influence of branched chain amino acid infusions on wound healing, *Aust. N. Z. J. Surg.*, 60, 471, 1990.

34. MacKay, D. and Miller, A.L., Nutritional support for wound healing, *Altern. Med. Rev.*, 8, 359, 2003.

35. Bergstrom, N., Bennett, M.A., and Carlson, C.E., Pressure ulcer treatment. Quick reference guide for clinicians, *Clinical Practice Guidelines,* 15, 1994.

36. Long, C.L. et al., Contribution of skeletal muscle protein in elevated rates of whole body protein catabolism in trauma patients, *Am. J. Clin. Nutr.*, 34, 1087, 1981.

37. Wolfe, R.R., Herman Award Lecture, 1996: relation of metabolic studies to clinical nutrition — the example of burn injury, *Am. J. Clin. Nutr.*, 64, 800, 1996.

38. Young, V.R., 1987 McCollum Award Lecture. Kinetics of human amino acid metabolism: nutritional implications and some lessons, *Am. J. Clin. Nutr.*, 46, 709, 1987.

39. Sutton, R.A., Wong, N.L., and Dirks, J.H., Effects of metabolic acidosis and alkalosis on sodium and calcium transport in the dog kidney, *Kidney Int.*, 15, 520, 1979.

40. Kraut, J.A. et al., The effects of metabolic acidosis on bone formation and bone resorption in the rat, *Kidney Int.*, 30, 694, 1986.

41. Bushinsky, D.A. et al., Metabolic, but not respiratory, acidosis increases bone PGE(2) levels and calcium release, *Am. J. Physiol. Renal Physiol.*, 281, F1058, 2001.

42. Winthrop, A.L. et al., Injury severity, whole body protein turnover, and energy expenditure in pediatric trauma, *J. Pediatr. Surg.*, 22, 534, 1987.

43. Shi, H.P. et al., Effect of supplemental ornithine on wound healing, *J. Surg. Res.,* 106, 299, 2002.
44. De Bandt, J.P. et al., A randomized controlled trial of the influence of the mode of enteral ornithine -ketoglutarate administration in burn patients, *J. Nutr.,* 128, 563, 1998.
45. Donati, L. et al., Nutritional and clinical efficacy of ornithine -ketoglutarate in severe burn patients, *Clin. Nutr.,* 18, 307, 1999.
46. Danielsen, C.C. and Fogdestam, I., Delayed primary closure: collagen synthesis and content in healing rat skin incisions, *J. Surg. Res.,* 31, 210, 1981.
47. Jaksic, T. et al., Proline metabolism in adult male burned patients and healthy control subjects, *Am. J. Clin. Nutr.,* 54, 408, 1991.
48. Yu, Y.M. et al., Arginine and ornithine kinetics in severely burned patients: increased rate of arginine disposal, *Am. J. Physiol.,* 280, E509, 2001.
49. Fong, Y.M. et al., Skeletal muscle amino acid and myofibrillar protein mRNA response to thermal injury and infection, *Am. J. Physiol.,* 261, R536, 1991.
50. Mullen, J.L. et al., Prediction of operative morbidity by preoperative nutritional assessment, *Surg. Forum,* 30, 80, 1979.
51. Larsson, J., et al., Nitrogen requirements in severely injured patients, *Br. J. Surg.,* 77, 413, 1990.
52. Herndon, D.N. and Tompkins, R.G., Support of the metabolic response to burn injury, *Lancet,* 363, 1895, 2004.
53. Wolfe, R.R. et al., Response of protein and urea kinetics in burn patients to different levels of protein intake, *Ann. Surg.,* 197, 163, 1983.
54. Burdet, L. et al., Administration of growth hormone to underweight patients with chronic obstructive pulmonary disease. A prospective, randomized, controlled study, *Am. J. Respir. Crit. Care Med.,* 156, 1800, 1997.
55. Klein, C.J., Stanek, G.S., and Wiles, C.E., III, Overfeeding macronutrients to critically ill adults: metabolic complications, *J. Am. Diet. Assoc.,* 98, 795, 1998.
56. Hosch, M. et al., Ureagenesis: evidence for a lack of hepatic regulation of acid–base equilibrium in humans, *Am. J. Physiol. Renal Physiol.,* 286, F94, 2004.

5 Glutamine and Wound Healing

Mark B. Schoemann, C. Dustin Bechtold, Shefali Agarwal, and Christopher W. Lentz

CONTENTS

INTRODUCTION

Glutamine is the most abundant free amino acid in the human body. Although glutamine has been traditionally classified as a nonessential amino acid, decreased levels have been noted during periods of metabolic stress leading to its reclassification as a conditionally essential amino acid. Glutamine is a five-carbon amino acid with two amino moieties (Figure 5.1), and it accounts for 35 to 50% of all amino acid nitrogen transported in blood. It is produced primarily in the muscles from glutamate (Figure 5.2) and plays a key role in the transport of nitrogen between organs. Over the past several decades, research has revealed a plethora of important functions of glutamine in the human body (Table 5.1). It is a primary fuel for rapidly dividing cells, such as enterocytes, hepatocytes, and immune cells, as well as a nitrogen carrier. In addition to protecting the body against the toxic effects of ammonia, glutamine is the precursor to several important metabolic agents, including glutathione, arginine, taurine, and the building blocks of DNA and RNA.

Many studies have documented that glutamine levels are decreased when the body is physically and metabolically stressed, such as in patients with sepsis or traumatic injury. Researchers have actively sought the clinical significance of this decrease. It has been proven that glutamine is important for maintaining the barrier function of the intestines, promoting pancreatic growth, preventing hepatic steatosis, reducing ischemic reperfusion injury, and maintaining immune cell function. Based on this research, many have tried to elucidate whether glutamine supplementation in the catabolic state is beneficial to patients. Clinical trials have shown that supplementation with glutamine decreases infectious complications and length of hospital stay and in some patient populations reduces morbidity and mortality. However, there is currently much debate as to the optimal method of glutamine delivery and the amount needed to affect outcomes. A thorough background of glutamine metabolism in the normal metabolic state of the body is important before discussing the implications of glutamine deficiency and supplementatin.

TABLE 5.1
Important Functions of Glutamine

Gastrointestinal system	Energy source for enterocytes maintains mucosal integrity and barrier function of the gut
Immune system	Provides building blocks of DNA and RNA for rapidly dividing cells; energy source for macrophages, lymphocytes, and neutrophils; precursor to glutathione, a powerful antioxidant
Nervous system	Acts as a neurotransmitter
Hepatobiliary system	Transports ammonia from peripheral tissue to liver for conversion into urea; important for pancreatic growth and function
Renal system	Metabolized in the kidney to regulate acid–base homeostasis; substrate for gluconeogenesis in kidney

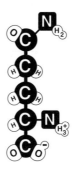

FIGURE 5.1 Molecular structure of glutamine.

METABOLISM IN THE WHOLE BODY

GLUTAMINE TRANSPORTS AMMONIA IN BLOOD

Free ammonia is toxic to the central nervous system and must be transported in a nontoxic form to the liver, where it can enter the urea cycle and eventually be excreted in the urine. The catabolism of proteins in muscle produces nitrogen that is then incorporated to form glutamine, a nontoxic transport form of ammonia [1]. It is estimated that 30 to 35% of amino acid nitrogen is transported in the plasma in the form of glutamine [2]. The formation of glutamine primarily takes place in peripheral muscle tissue from glutamate (Figure 5.3). However, glutamine metabolism in the liver and central nervous system serves as an important mechanism for decreasing ammonia levels. Once glutamine reaches the liver, it is ultimately converted from the transport form of ammonia to the disposal form of ammonia — urea. Thus, glutamine acts as a nitrogen "shuttle" or "buffer" by either accepting excess ammonia or liberating it to form other amino acids, nucleotides, or urea. The capacity of glutamine to perform these essential actions makes it the major nitrogen transporter between tissues of the human body [3].

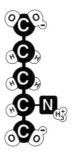

FIGURE 5.2 Molecular structure of glutamate.

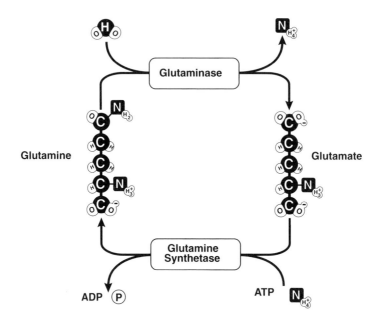

FIGURE 5.3 Interconversion of glutamate and glutamine. Glutamine is formed by the addition of an ammonia group to glutamate by the enzyme glutamine synthetase. Glutamate is formed by hydrolysis of glutamine by glutaminase.

INTERCELLULAR GLUTAMINE CYCLE OF THE LIVER

The liver is the principal location of nitrogen metabolism in the body, and it plays a fundamental role in glutamine homeostasis. The liver contains glutamine synthetase and glutaminase but is neither a net consumer nor a net producer of glutamine. Due to their distinct functions, these two enzymes are confined to different regions of the liver. Glutaminase and the urea cycle enzymes are concentrated in the periportal hepatocytes that surround the portal system as it branches throughout the liver. Glutamine enters the periportal cells and is hydrolyzed to contribute an ammonium ion for urea synthesis [4]. Glutamate formed in this process can either be metabolized into other amino acids or enter the route of gluconeogenesis. Glutamine synthetase is highly concentrated in the perivenous region of the liver, which drains the venous blood from the systemic circulation. This enzyme scavenges free ammonia in the plasma by joining it to glutamate to form glutamine [5]. Glutamine formed from this reaction is released into the blood, where it circulates back to the liver only to be taken up by the periportal cells that can process the nitrogen into urea for disposal. Therefore the liver plays a vital role in maintaining low blood ammonia levels by apprehending free ammonia molecules from the plasma as well as by producing urea. Glutamine and its associated enzymes are integral to both processes.

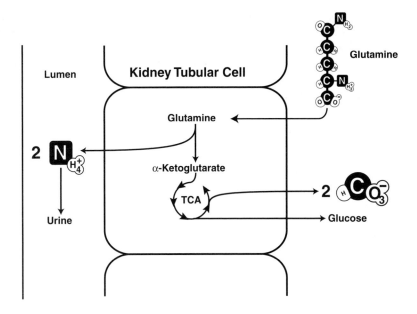

FIGURE 5.4 Glutamine is taken up by the proximal tubular cells of the kidney and metabolized yielding ammonium and bicarbonate. The ammonium is secreted into the lumen and lost in the urine. The bicarbonate moves into the plasma where it constitutes new bicarbonate.

GLUTAMINE PLAYS A CRITICAL ROLE IN ACID–BASE REGULATION

Regulation of acid–base balance, like that of nitrogen excretion, is shared by the liver and kidney, with glutamine playing a vital role. Complete catabolism of most amino acids derived from proteins yields carbon dioxide, water, and urea, which are neutral products. However, the breakdown of the positively charged amino acids arginine, lysine, and histidine and the sulfur-containing amino acids methionine and cysteine results in the net formation of protons (acid). Catabolism of the negatively charged amino acids glutamate and aspartate results in net utilization of protons but is only able to consume a portion of the protons produced by catabolism of the positively charged and sulfur-containing amino acids. In order for the body to remain in acid–base balance, the excess acid produced each day by the catabolism of proteins must be matched by an equivalent amount of a base. The kidney is able to produce this base in the form of bicarbonate by metabolizing glutamine, and thus maintaining acid–base neutrality. Glutamine taken up by the kidneys is deaminated by glutaminase to produce glutamate, which can then enter the tricarboxylic acid cycle after being metabolized into α-ketoglutarate. The metabolism of one molecule of glutamine by the kidney yields two bicarbonate molecules and two ammonium molecules (Figure 5.4). This can be represented as follows:

$$1 \text{ glutamine} \rightarrow 2HCO_3^- + 2NH_4^+$$

This is an entirely neutral reaction, but the ammonium produced is secreted into the lumen of the kidney tubules and taken away by the urine. The bicarbonate, on the other hand, enters the peritubular capillaries and corresponds to a net gain of base for the body. The protons produced by amino acid catabolism are thus balanced by the bicarbonate manufactured by glutamine metabolism in the kidney [6]. This renal metabolism of glutamine assumes even greater importance in metabolic acidosis, a condition associated with excessive acid production in the body. Certain pathologic conditions such as lactic acidosis, ketogenesis, or ingestion of certain chemicals can cause metabolic acidosis. Renal enzymes involved in glutamine metabolism are increased during times when the body is subjected to states of metabolic acidosis in order to generate more bicarbonate and neutralize the insult. The liver also contributes to neutralizing the blood during times of metabolic acidosis by decreasing the conversion of glutamine into urea. This increases the available pool of glutamine the kidney can metabolize into bicarbonate.

GLUCONEOGENESIS DURING A FASTING STATE REQUIRES GLUTAMINE FROM SKELETAL MUSCLE

Skeletal muscle tissue contains over 90% of the glutamine pool in the body and is the major site of glutamine synthesis. During the fasting or catabolic state, the body attempts to maintain plasma glucose levels in order to sustain glucose-requiring tissues such as the brain [1]. The breakdown of liver glycogen to glucose is an early response to starvation but is transient, as liver glycogen stores are depleted after 10 to 18 h of fasting. As glycogen stores decrease, gluconeogenesis in the liver and kidney intensifies, as these are the only two organs that contain the necessary gluconeogenesis enzyme glucose-6-phosphatase [7]. During the starvation period, alanine and glutamine are released after the breakdown of skeletal muscle and account for 40 to 70% of amino acids that are converted to glucose [8]. Alanine has long been considered the predominant amino acid substrate for gluconeogenesis, but recent evidence shows that glutamine makes a significant contribution. Furthermore, studies have shown that alanine and glutamine have particular inclinations toward one organ over the other. Alanine is predominantly metabolized by the liver into glucose, while glutamine is the preferred substrate in the kidney [9].

GLUTAMINE IS ESSENTIAL FOR CELLS OF THE IMMUNE SYSTEM

Although the immune system is composed of a diverse line of cells with different functions, they share a common goal of providing a cellular defense against infection. Until recently, little was known about the metabolism or preferred fuel source of these cells that include lymphocytes, macrophages, and neutrophils. Abundant evidence has shown that glutamine is the principal energy source for white blood cells of the immune system, and that they may utilize it at a rate greater than glucose [10]. Not only does glutamine serve as an energy source, but it also supplies the nitrogen to synthesize new purines and pyrimidines in lymphocytes [11]. These nucleotides are the building blocks of DNA and RNA that must be replicated in order for cell proliferation to occur. Tissue culture studies have demonstrated that failure to supplement culture media with glutamine severely limits the ability of lymphocytes to respond to mitogenic stimulation, which is probably related to its use as a precursor for nucleotide synthesis and as a source of energy [12]. In addition to providing energy and the ability to proliferate, glutamine has been shown to be involved in the specific functions of immune cells. Neutrophils, which engulf and digest foreign material, have been shown to increase phagocytic activity, increase superoxide production, and resist apoptosis when supplemented with glutamine [13]. Macrophages deprived of glutamine expressed less human leukocyte antigen DR, a critical gene product used by the macrophage for antigen presentation [14]. In trauma patients as well as surgery patients, human leukocyte antigen DR was increased with parenteral supplementation of glutamine [15,16].

METABOLISM OF GLUTAMINE IN OTHER ORGANS

The role of the lungs in maintaining glutamine homeostasis has only recently been appreciated. Similar to skeletal muscle, the lungs are glutamine donors with high levels of glutamine synthetase that release glutamine in response to endotoxin or glucocorticoid administration. Although the lung does not have the same tissue mass as skeletal muscle, it contains an equivalent concentration of glutamine synthetase and receives a greater proportion of the total circulation. Therefore, the lung is able to release a significant amount of glutamine and may increase glutamine output up to six times following major surgery, trauma, sepsis, starvation, or acidosis due to the upregulation of glutamine synthetase [17].

Glutamine is an important respiratory fuel for the exocrine and endocrine pancreas with arteriovenous differences in glutamine concentration indicative of glutamine extraction rates near 50%. Use of glutamine-enriched total parenteral nutrition (TPN) in rats before and after small bowel resection significantly increased pancreatic weight, DNA content, protein content, total trypsinogen, and lipase content [18]. Microscopic analysis of pancreatic sections demonstrated that exogenous glutamine resulted in pancreatic acinar hyperplasia. These investigators also demonstrated that glutamine supports pancreatic growth and function during elemental enteral feeding. Glutamine may also influence pancreatic endocrine function by enhancing β-cell secretion of insulin in response to glucose [19]. There is also evidence that glutamate dehydrogenase may have a regulatory role in the pancreatic β-cell, as individuals with a mutation in this enzyme have elevated insulin secretion [20].

Glutamate is the main neurotransmitter at excitatory synapses in the central nervous system, and γ-amino butyric acid (GABA) provides inhibitory signals [21]. Experiments have shown that glutamate and GABA are collected by astroglia in the synaptic space after nerve depolarization. Once contained within the astroglia, glutamate and GABA are ultimately converted to glutamine that is transported back into the neuron and modified to become glutamate again [22]. Researchers recently concluded that this glutamine–glutamate cycle in the brain "plays a central role in the normal functional energetics of the cerebral cortex" [23].

GLUTAMINE IS THE PRECURSOR TO PURINES AND PYRIMIDINES

Glutamine is partially oxidized by glutaminolysis in enterocytes and lymphocytes to supply energy and precursor molecules for the synthesis of purines and pyrimidines that are used by these rapidly dividing cells for the synthesis of RNA and DNA. As the nitrogen donor in the formation of carbamoyl phosphate, glutamine in conjunction with aspartic acid is required for the committed step in pyrimidine synthesis (formation of N-carbamoylaspartate). A transamination reaction involving glutamine is again used in the synthesis of the pyrimidine nucleotide cytosine triphosphate (CTP) from uridine triphosphate (UTP). In the purine biosynthetic pathway, glutamine contributes two amine groups in reactions leading to the synthesis of inosine monophosphate (IMP) and donates a third amine group in the conversion of IMP to guanosine monophosphate (GMP). Thus glutamine is an essential building block of DNA and RNA, which are required by the rapidly dividing cells of the intestine and immune system.

GLUTAMINE AND ITS RELATION TO GLUTATHIONE, A POWERFUL ANTIOXIDANT

Glutathione is a γ-glutamylcysteinylglycine tripeptide important in the detoxification of endogenously generated peroxides and exogenous chemical compounds. It is found in nearly all cells and is critical in stabilizing erythrocyte membranes, conjugating drugs to make them more water soluble, transporting amino acids across cell membranes, and acting as a cofactor for enzyme reactions. Glutamine is the precursor to glutamate (Figure 5.3), which is combined with cysteine and glycine in two separate reactions that both require adenosine triphosphate (ATP) [24]. Oxygen free radicals and peroxides are known to be harmful to the body on the molecular level. The glutathione formed from glutamine is the most important free radical scavenger in the body that can neutralize the oxidative threat [25]. Recent data suggest that glutamine is intimately involved in regulating glutathione levels, as shown in experiments in a human neuroblastoma cell line [26]. Furthermore, glutathione has been shown to preserve proteins in their reduced form, which ensures that certain enzymes function properly [27].

GLUTAMINE IS THE PREFERRED FUEL OF THE GUT

The intestines consume the largest amount of glutamine of any organ in the body, and it is their preferred fuel source. Glutamine can either be taken up by the intestinal epithelial cells (enterocytes) from the lumen or be delivered via the bloodstream. Once the glutamine has gone into the enterocyte, it is taken up by the mitochondria and converted into ATP via the following reactions:

$$\text{glutamine} \rightarrow \text{glutamate} \rightarrow \alpha\text{-ketoglutarate} \rightarrow \text{Krebs cycle} \rightarrow \text{ATP}$$

Because the enterocytes contain little glutamine synthetase and have an abundance of glutaminase, they are unable to synthesize glutamine from other molecules and must depend on a preformed supply of glutamine [3]. It will be shown later that glutamine is essential to maintain the integrity of the intestinal lining and prevent pathogens from violating it and entering surrounding tissues.

GLUTAMINE AND TAURINE

Taurine is a unique amino acid that possesses antioxidant as well as osmoregulatory properties. Inflammatory cells, especially neutrophils, contain an abundance of taurine in their cytosol. The major function of taurine is to travel with the neutrophils to wounded tissue and trap chlorinated oxidants and transform them into the nontoxic taurine chloramine form [28]. This has been shown to be important in maintaining the cell membrane and preventing self-destruction of the cell [29]. Glutamine is important in the regulation of taurine metabolism, as shown experimentally in rats fed a glutamine-enriched diet that increased taurine uptake in the kidneys. This increase in taurine concentration was also seen in trauma patients who were supplemented with glutamine [30]. Taurine is also important in maintaining intracellular osmolarity, as it can remain at high intracellular concentrations with minimal expenditure of energy and respond to osmotic changes rapidly [31]. It is believed that the decreased extracellular water retention seen with glutamine supplementation during a stressed state is mediated through taurine [32].

METABOLISM IN THE HEALING WOUND

Although glutamine is the most abundant free amino acid in the circulation, major physiologic stresses, such as surgery or sepsis, are sufficient to alter the balance significantly between net glutamine production and consumption. Animal studies by Kapadia et al. demonstrated that plasma and muscle glutamine levels may fall postoperatively by as much as 30 and 50% at 24 and 48 h, respectively [33]. Similarly, studies in patients undergoing major vascular operations showed that plasma glutamine concentrations diminished by 50% during the acute postoperative period [34]. This dramatic decline in circulating and muscle glutamine concentrations following major surgery exemplifies the increased demand for this amino acid by certain organ systems during stress.

LOCAL WOUND HEALING

Wound healing is a complex cascade of events that occur on the cellular and molecular level in response to injury. Platelets, polymorphonuclear (PMN) leukocytes, macrophages, and fibroblasts are recognized as the chief cell types of the immune system that respond at the site of injury in order to carry out their individual functions. As described previously, glutamine is an important fuel source for these rapidly dividing cells and is necessary for DNA and RNA replication prior to mitosis. There is evidence that there are considerable amounts of glutaminase activity in the skin of mice and rats that allow these tissues to utilize glutamine as an energy source [35]. These researchers were also able to demonstrate that glutaminase activity in the skin of the animals decreased as they aged.

In an acute wound, fibroblasts appear on day three at the start of the proliferative phase and produce the permanent wound matrix. Fibroblasts replace the transient fibronectin–fibrin framework with collagen, which is essential to increase the tensile strength of the wound over time. Research on the metabolism of these important wound healing cells revealed that α-ketoglutarate, a metabolite of glutamine, is taken up by these cells by an unmediated diffusion process [36]. Moreover, these cells are able to utilize glutamine as an energy source instead of glucose [37]. Although early research indicated that glutamine supplementation had no appreciable effect on local wound healing [38], more recent studies have shown it may be efficacious. Volunteers (average age 75.4 yr) had small polytetrafluoroethylene (PTFE) grafts implanted subcutaneously and were either supplemented with a combination of glutamine, arginine, and β-hydroxy-β-methylbutyrate (HMB) or with isonitrogenous nonessential amino acids. The grafts removed at 2 weeks from the supplemented patient group showed a more significant amount of collagen deposition than did the nonsupplemented group [39]. Because glutamine was given in combination with arginine and HMB, which have both been shown to increase collagen deposition, one cannot definitively conclude that glutamine promotes collagen deposition *in vivo*. However, in *in vitro* studies, it was shown that glutamine stimulates the synthesis of collagen in fibroblast cultures [40], and glutamine has a dose-dependent effect on collagen gene expression [41].

GASTROINTESTINAL TRACT

The cells lining the alimentary tract are particularly avid glutamine consumers, and utilization can increase markedly following surgery. Through animal studies, researchers have estimated that glutamine uptake by the canine gastrointestinal tract nearly doubles following surgery. This effect was subsequently shown to be related to the operative stress and not to a decrease in food intake [42]. Moreover, glutamine uptake by the gut is increased postoperatively despite reduced intestinal blood flow and diminished circulating plasma glutamine concentrations, suggesting that an active process for glutamine uptake independent of substrate delivery occurs. Glucocorticoid hormones elaborated in response to surgical stress have an integral role in regulating this uptake and determining the rate of consumption of glutamine by the gut. Administration of the glucocorticoid dexamethasone can reproduce the effects of laparotomy and more than double glutamine uptake in the canine gut through an increased extraction of the amino acid from the bloodstream [43]. Glutamine transported into the enterocyte is hydrolyzed by the enzyme glutaminase to generate glutamate and ammonia for a variety of cellular functions, including cellular respiration. Glucocorticoids also play an important regulatory role by increasing the intestinal mucosal glutaminase messenger RNA (mRNA) levels in a time-dependent manner [44]. It has been speculated that the increase in glutamine consumption by the gut during stress allows the gut to switch from an organ of glucose uptake to one of net release. This adaptation may increase available glucose for wound healing or for other tissues that are obligate glucose consumers. Furthermore, glutamine uptake in the gut supports alanine release for gluconeogenesis in the liver. Other mediators may also play a role in determining glutamine uptake and utilization in the gastrointestinal tract following surgical stress. The pancreatic hormone glucagon was also shown to increase intestinal glutamine uptake threefold as well as increase ammonia and decrease glutamine concentrations in the portal circulation [45].

The gut has received the most attention when evaluating the effects of glutamine supplementation. The importance of circulating glutamine in maintaining gut function and integrity was illustrated in a number of animal studies. In one study, the enzyme glutaminase was infused into several animal species to lower blood glutamine levels to nearly undetectable levels [46]. These animals rapidly developed diarrhea, mild villous atrophy, mucosal ulcerations, and intestinal necrosis. Likewise, Hwang et al. demonstrated that glutamine-enriched parenteral solutions increased jejunal mucosal weight and DNA content and significantly decreased the villous atrophy associated with the use of standard TPN [47]. Others have demonstrated the ability of glutamine-supplemented intravenous or enteral diets to increase villous height and mucosal nitrogen content and stimulate intestinal mucosal growth following starvation [48]. Furthermore, enteral or parenteral glutamine may offer some protection against aspirin-induced gastric ulcerations [49], peptic ulcer disease, and severe enteritis following chemotherapy and radiation therapy. Glutamine may also be useful in the treatment of infectious diarrhea, as indicated by Nath et al. who demonstrated that intestinal sodium absorption in diarrheogenic rabbits infected with *Escherichia coli* can be enhanced by administering enteral glutamine [50]. Frankel et al. showed that infusion of glutamine into the lumen of transplanted small intestine increased small bowel protein and glucose absorption [51].

Alverdy et al. initially reported that TPN promotes bacterial translocation in the rat intestine. However, when rats were infused with glutamine-enriched TPN, bacterial translocation was dramatically reduced. Glutamine-supplemented TPN was also associated with normalization of secretory immunoglobulin A levels compared to standard TPN [52]. Others have shown that glutamine-enriched TPN diminishes bacterial adherence to enterocytes while maintaining both B- and T-cell populations in the lamina propria of the terminal ileum [53]. Therefore the ability of glutamine to decrease bacterial translocation may be related to a combination of increased gut integrity and enhanced immune function.

LIVER AND PANCREAS

The flow of glutamine into and out of the liver in surgical patients varies widely depending on the clinical scenario. Physiologic concentrations of ammonia in the portal circulation can produce "feed-forward stimulation" of hepatic glutaminase, allowing the liver to increase glutamine consumption when glutamine is abundant. Similarly, during starvation proinflammatory cytokines and eicosanoids can increase glutamine transport and utilization in the liver [54,55]. However, during metabolic acidosis glutamine flow is directed away from the liver and is significantly increased in the kidney. Under these conditions hepatic ureagenesis is decreased but renal ammoniagenesis is increased to facilitate net bicarbonate gain in the body. Glucocorticoids and postoperative stress have also been shown to increase renal glutamine uptake. Because glucocorticoids, inflammatory cytokines, and acidosis may coincide with different levels in the surgical patient, the relative amounts of glutamine utilization by the liver and kidney can vary greatly between individuals.

Glutamine supports pancreatic growth and function during elemental enteral feeding as previously described. When isolated pancreatic islets were perfused with glutamine, the basal glucagon output was increased, and insulin production was diminished [56]. Alterations in the portal insulin-to-glucagon ratio can influence fatty infiltration of the liver. This observation was corroborated by the findings of Li et al., who showed that adult rats receiving standard TPN demonstrated panlobular vacuolation of hepatocytes on histology, while animals receiving glutamine-enriched TPN showed normal liver morphology [57]. These results suggested that in addition to supporting the numerous metabolic activities in the liver, nutritional glutamine may have a role in preventing hepatic steatosis.

IMMUNE SYSTEM

Glutamine is essential for optimal humoral and cell-mediated immune function, and tissue culture studies have demonstrated its requirement for *in vitro* lymphocyte function as described above. To examine the relation between glutamine depletion and lymphocyte and macrophage function *in vivo*, Parry-Billings et al. isolated lymphocytes from the blood of severely burned patients with profoundly low plasma glutamine levels [58]. Lymphocyte proliferation in response to antigenic stimulation *in vitro* was significantly limited under low media glutamine concentrations but increased as glutamine levels were restored to the normal plasma range. The implication of these studies is that the immunodeficiency which is so often encountered in the critically ill surgical patient may in part be related to decreased levels of glutamine. Furthermore, it suggests that at least part of this immunodeficiency may be amenable to therapy via glutamine-supplemented nutritional support.

Following surgical procedures or development of infection certain populations of immune cells, including neutrophils and macrophages, proliferate rapidly. Brand et al. demonstrated that glutamine utilization by proliferating thymocyte cells is tenfold greater than that by nonproliferating cells [59]. In addition, there is evidence that certain mediators, such as interleukin-1 (IL-1) and glucocorticoids, may augment lymphocyte glutaminase activity. Therefore it is reasonable to suggest that under traumatic stress conditions the immune system may increase its use of glutamine considerably.

SKELETAL MUSCLE

Not all organ systems increase glutamine consumption in response to surgical stress. Skeletal muscle and the lungs, the principal organs of glutamine production, increase their output of glutamine into circulation following surgical procedures or other physiologic stress. Dual regulatory mechanisms, including systemic release of glucocorticoids and regional factors such as upregulation of glutamine synthetase activity, finely control glutamine production and meet glutamine demand during stress.

The accelerated muscle glutamine release that occurs after surgical stress can be profound. Muhlbacher et al. demonstrated that following treatment with the glucocorticoid dexamethasone, glutamine efflux was increased fourfold from the hindquarter muscles in a canine model [60]. Over a period of 9 d, the steroid-treated dogs developed muscle glutamine depletion and a negative nitrogen balance. Similar results were described in animals during sepsis, starvation, acidosis, and burn injury

[10,60]. Although glutamine comprises more than 50% of the total muscle amino acid pool, this does not fully account for the quantity of glutamine released following stress. Instead, glutamine must be synthesized *de novo* in muscle cells from glutamate and ammonia in a process catalyzed by glutamine synthetase. This can be upregulated tenfold in response to a septic challenge or direct glucocorticoid administration [61].

Depletion of the glutamine stores in skeletal muscle following major surgery is a well-recognized phenomenon. A statistically significant correlation between survival and muscle glutamine concentration has been demonstrated in septic patients [62]. Glutamine infusion during the postoperative period can diminish the efflux of glutamine from the hind limbs in a canine model and can lead to increased protein synthesis [33]. The impact of exogenous glutamine on protein synthesis was greatest when intramuscular glutamine concentrations fell to the range typically encountered during critical illness. Parenteral glutamine can also significantly diminish the muscle atrophy characteristic of chronic glucocorticoid exposure [63]. Hammarqvist et al. demonstrated that glutamine-enriched TPN decreased the fall in muscle glutamine concentration in patients undergoing cholecystectomy, preserved the total muscle ribosome concentration, and significantly limited the cumulative nitrogen loss compared to a control group [64]. Although muscle function appears to be relatively preserved even during moderate to severe glutamine depletion, the effects of decreased glutamine have systemic ramifications for morbidity and mortality within the critically ill patient population.

LUNG

It was shown that the lung is an important source of glutamine during catabolic states. In addition to exportation, the lung is also a consumer of glutamine, particularly the endothelial surface. In a study examining the effects of glutamine infusion on lung weights after a bolus of endotoxin, researchers noted that there was more edema in endotoxin-treated animals that received a control amino acid infusion than in the glutamine-infused group [17]. Although the mechanism behind this phenomenon is not known, the role of glutamine in glutathione and taurine synthesis may be involved. It is possible that the lung may have increased ability to scavenge free radicals with glutathione and have increased osmoregulation via the activities of taurine. Additionally, glutamine supplementation significantly increased ATP levels and viability of pulmonary endothelial cells 5 h after hydrogen peroxide injury [65]. This suggests that glutamine may provide an important source of energy for the injured lung.

GLUTAMINE DEFICIENCY

The need for nutritional support in the critically ill patient has been well established over time through multiple studies in the setting of trauma or sepsis. The critically ill patient, regardless of the etiology of disease, lives in a catabolic state, which can at times be a prolonged process that eventually leads to malnutrition. The catabolic state is exemplified by loss of lean tissue and body mass and can also be seen after major surgery, chemotherapy, or radiation. Nutritional support may sometimes fail in preventing loss of lean body mass and in avoiding metabolic disorders, especially in the face of gastrointestinal failure and intolerance to enteral feeding [66]. Parenteral nutrition, therefore, becomes necessary when enteral nutrition is no longer a viable option. Providing nutrition intravenously was initially used as a means to provide the energy, protein, and micronutrients needed to avoid muscle wasting and immune system depression. Efforts are now being made to provide a mix of nutrients that will actually improve immune function in the face of critical illness [67]. There appears to be some evidence to suggest that *immunonutrition* can, in fact, reduce infectious complications and shorten hospital stays [68]. Although there has been significant investigative effort in this area, there is no full understanding or agreement regarding the optimal mix of nutrients needed to achieve this end. Furthermore, the exact composition and quantity of that nutrition are the source of much investigation and debate. While there is a fair amount of research available regarding the use of glutamine supplementation and outcomes for critically ill patients, there have been few investigations specifically examining the effects of glutamine on wound healing. Despite vast clinical research, there is no clear consensus regarding the role or benefit of glutamine supplementation in critically ill patients.

As described earlier, glutamine is the most abundant free amino acid in the body, with an array of important functions [69,70]. On account of this wealth of glutamine, there is no true defined deficiency state for glutamine in humans [71]. Despite the positive reports of glutamine supplementation in recent research, there are those who feel that glutamine is never decreased in the body to such a degree that it causes any derangements or is clinically relevant. Some feel that it is inappropriate to recommend glutamine for therapeutic use in any circumstance, and that the decrease in glutamine concentration found in catabolic states has no known clinical significance [72]. Others have shown that critically ill patients with low plasma glutamine levels have a higher mortality than those with normal levels, even when adjusted for the Acute Physiology and Chronic Health Evaluation (APACHE) II score [73]. Whether deficient levels of glutamine directly increase mortality or are a marker of critical illness is currently unknown.

First characterized as a nonessential amino acid because the body contains enzymes to produce it, glutamine is now often referred to as a conditionally essential amino acid [64,74]. This is to say that there are conditions in which glutamine becomes an essential amino acid. Some of these conditions include trauma, sepsis, major surgery, burns, bone marrow transplant, intense chemotherapy or radiation, or when patients with minimal energy and protein reserves, such as elderly patients and very low birth weight infants are stressed [71,75]. Although there is no true defined deficiency state for glutamine, there appear to be some negative consequences to decreased levels of plasma or total body glutamine, as mentioned earlier. Some of these include decreased immune cell proliferation, decreased T-cell activation, immune dysfunction, and decreased intestinal mucosa integrity [71,75,76].

In addition to the aforementioned consequences of decreased levels of glutamine, there are numerous studies that show that glutamine supplementation in those who are critically ill may be of benefit. These studies do not describe negative effects of glutamine deficiency, but rather the positive effects and benefits of supplementation.

One might conclude that the loss of such benefits may also be considered a negative effect of decreased glutamine in the critically ill patient.

Glutamine plays a major role in the physiology of the gut and is an important fuel source for the cells of the intestinal mucosa and gut-associated lymphoid tissue [77]. The relative lack of glutamine in catabolic patients has been postulated to cause a loss of integrity in the intestinal mucosa and decreased effectiveness of the gut-associated lymphoid tissue [71]. Glutamine has been shown to decrease the amount of gut atrophy that occurs during parenteral feeding and to decrease the permeability of the gut to chemicals while increasing DNA synthesis in enterocytes [75,77,78]. There have been some studies that suggest that increased gut permeability allows bacteria to translocate across the gut wall during parenteral feedings, and that glutamine supplementation of parenteral nutrition decreases the translocation of *Escherichia coli* [70,77].

Glutamine has been shown to be important for the function of immune cells involved in wound healing, but there has not been much in the basic science or clinical literature elucidating the effects of glutamine supplementation or deficiency on local wound healing. Glutamine is an important fuel for lymphocytes, macrophages, neutrophils, and natural killer cells [76,79]. Glutamine supplementation has been shown to improve lymphocyte function postoperatively and increase T cell DNA synthesis and cytokine production. It has also been shown to decrease the production of proinflammatory cytokines in the human intestinal mucosa, while increasing T-helper type 2 cytokines and reactive oxygen intermediaries from neutrophils, as well as improving phagocytosis [70,76,78,80]. Improved immune function from glutamine supplementation also results in fewer positive microbial cultures and a decreased number of clinical infections, including pneumonia, bacteremia, and sepsis [71,76,81]. Melis et al. hypothesized that glutamine deficiency during a stressed state can "make the patient more prone to infectious complications" [82].

The benefits of glutamine supplementation have been shown in primary investigations as well as in several meta-analyses. In 2002, Novak et al. critically evaluated many randomized trials of glutamine supplementation in surgery and intensive care unit (ICU) patients [75]. Their meta-analysis of glutamine trials in the literature revealed that glutamine supplementation had no effect on mortality of surgical patients but had a modest decline in mortality of critically ill patients. Both surgical patients and ICU patients were shown to have reduced complication rates when supplemented with glutamine. Reduced length of hospital stay was seen only in the surgical patient population and not the critically ill ICU patients. The route of administration, enteral or parenteral, was examined and shown to be statistically significant. Parenteral glutamine supplementation was shown to reduce morbidity and decrease length of hospital stay. Not included in this meta-analysis was a recent prospective randomized trial of parenteral glutamine supplementation in 144 ICU patients requiring TPN [66]. This study was able to show that survival at 6 months was improved in patients who received glutamine supplementation for more than 9 d. Six-month survival for the glutamine-supplemented group was 66.7% and that of the control group was 40% ($P = 0.03$).

Despite these findings, two large studies published recently failed to show that enteral glutamine supplementation had any effect on observed outcome. In a randomized controlled trial of enteral glutamine supplementation of 363 critically ill patients, no effect on 6-month mortality was observed [83]. No decrease in the incidence of nosocomial infections in 649 neonates given enteral glutamine supplementation was seen when compared to controls [84].

Most of the aforementioned benefits are seen when glutamine is given to a patient in a state of relative deficiency caused by total body stress. At some point, the body's need for supplemental glutamine will wane, and the potential for glutamine excess arises. As such, the question of safety in supplementation becomes important, as does the potential danger of glutamine excess.

GLUTAMINE EXCESS

Glutamine is abundant. There are mechanisms by which glutamine is transferred throughout the body based on the needs of the moment. Even with the body's innate ability to deal with large amounts of glutamine, one might theorize that a critical concentration could be reached that could cause harm. In the rodent, increased levels of body glutamine from exogenous sources results in increased expression of intestinal glutaminase and an increase in glutamine metabolism [72]. Whether a similar mechanism exists in humans is unclear. Nevertheless, it appears that the human body is well equipped to safely deal with any excess.

A review of available data concerning the safety of glutamine supplementation reveals that in most circumstances it is quite safe [85]. There are certain circumstances wherein glutamine has been the cause of untoward side effects. Oral glutamine may cause or worsen hepatic encephalopathy in patients with cirrhosis, possibly as a result of its conversion to glutamate and ammonia [72]. This may also explain the fact that it may be unsafe in patients with liver or kidney disease. However, there is some evidence to suggest that glutamine degradation to glutamate and ammonia does not produce neurotoxic effects in humans [85]. A case report details a patient who suffered mania and hypomania as a result of ingesting 4 g of glutamine per day, which could potentially be attributed to the fact that glutamine is a precursor for GABA, a neurotransmitter [86].

Elderly individuals, patients with Alzheimer's dementia, or Down syndrome showed increased glutamine toxicity in peripheral lymphocytes compared to controls [72]. Aside from these sporadic and somewhat anecdotal reports of toxicity, glutamine appears to be quite safe. Even with high intakes of glutamine, the concentrations of ammonia and glutamate are not greatly increased, and the plasma concentrations of other amino acids, hormones, and electrolytes are not altered [85].

When dealing with issues of safety and efficacy, it is important to address such parameters as the form of delivery and route of delivery, as well as dose amount, timing, and duration. Glutamine is stable as a dry solid, but after a short time in solution, it breaks down into toxic by-products, including pyroglutamate and ammonia [69,85]. Recently, delivery has been enhanced by the use of aseptic processing, air-permeable bags for solution, and dipeptide preparations such as alanine–glutamine and glycine–glutamine [87]. Practically speaking, the route of delivery for supplementation is likely to depend on the patient's clinical status and feeding needs.

RECOMMENDATIONS

The ideal dose of glutamine is not known. This is a consistent statement among many published articles on glutamine. A wide variety of doses were used in the many clinical trials of glutamine supplementation. One systematic review of glutamine supplementation chose to compare the effects of low-dose (< 0.2 g/kg/d) versus high-dose (> 0.2 g/kg/d) supplementation and found that high-dose glutamine was associated with reduction in mortality, complication rates, and length of hospital stay. Low-dose glutamine, on the other hand, had no observable treatment effect [75]. The literature specifically addressing safety indicates that doses up to 0.3 g/kg as a single oral dose or 0.57 g/kg/d given intravenously for 30 d are safe [85]. Typical dietary consumption of glutamine is less than 10 g, but 20 to 40 g/d may be needed in catabolic states [69]. There are some studies available where much more than 40 g/d were used, and although safety was not a measured endpoint, there were no adverse effects reported [85].

In the absence of a large study delineating the optimal treatment dose, it is difficult to make any recommendation concerning the ideal dosing of glutamine. Most studies showing a benefit used doses of 0.6 g/kg or less. In light of these facts and in the absence of high-quality evidence, an easy-to-remember dose of 0.5 g/kg/d seems a reasonable supplemental dose of glutamine.

FUTURE DIRECTIONS

Although glutamine is composed of merely 5 carbon atoms and 2 amino moieties, it has a multitude of important functions that have been elucidated through research over the past several decades. Glutamine is involved in diverse processes across different organ systems, including the gastrointestinal, central nervous, immune, and circulatory, to name a few. Wound healing is a complex series of events involving the different types of immune cells that cause inflammation, cell proliferation, and new tissue formation. Glutamine is important for all of these aspects, as it increases proliferation of inflammatory cells, enhances neutrophil phagocytic capability, and is involved in fibroblastic formation of collagen. However, more research needs to be done to clarify the direct effects of glutamine supplementation or deficiency on local wound healing. Clearly, glutamine is important to inflammatory cells metabolically, but whether a deficiency in glutamine causes delayed wound healing is unclear. Simple animal studies looking at wound tensile strength and wound histology over time in relation to glutamine levels would help answer this important question. Additionally, novel methods of glutamine delivery to wounded tissue could be developed that would eliminate the need for parenteral supplementation.

Other effects of glutamine, while lesser known and publicized, warrant further investigation. The relationship between glutamine and taurine, a potent osmoregulator during times of stress, needs further exploration. Taurine is reduced after surgery or during critical illness and may play an important role in the fluid shifts that are often seen in these states. How glutamine regulates taurine levels and how this can be manipulated for the benefit of the patient needs to be elucidated. Glutamine in the form of glutathione protects the body from oxidative stresses that can cause apoptosis, or programmed cell death. Ischemia/reperfusion injury is encountered in many disciplines of surgery. Revascularization of an extremity in vascular surgery, anastomosis of muscle flaps in plastic surgery, and transplantation of organs can all lead to ischemia/reperfusion injury. There are good basic science studies that have shown that glutamine has a definite function in increasing glutathione levels and decreasing oxidative stress. Application of this data in animal models of ischemia/reperfusion injury could help elucidate ways of increasing tissue flap and organ transplant viability.

There have been many clinical trials examining the supplementation of glutamine parenterally and enterally in the postsurgical as well as critically ill patient. The statistical quality and power of these clinical trials vary, as do their results. In some studies, supplemental glutamine was shown to be beneficial, while in others, it was not. Larger clinical studies that are adequately powered to show statistical significance are warranted. The exact amount and length of glutamine supplementation needed to achieve a benefit is not known. Dosing levels at which toxicity or adverse side effects occur are also not known. Research into dosing, bioavailability, and new methods of delivery could prove helpful in the future, as more basic science and clinical research on this most versatile amino acid comes to fruition.

REFERENCES

1. Champe, P.C. and R.A. Harvey, *Biochemistry. Lippincotts' Illustrated Reviews*, J.B. Lippincott, Philadelphia, 1994.
2. Krebs, H., Metabolism of amino acids. IV. The synthesis of glutamine from glutamic acid and ammonia and enzymatic hydrolysis of glutamine in animal tissues, *Biochem. J.*, 29, 1951–1969, 1935.
3. Miller, A.L., Therapeutic considerations of L-glutamine: a review of the literature, *Altern. Med. Rev.*, 4(4), 239–248, 1999.
4. Haussinger, D., Nitrogen metabolism in liver: structural and functional organization and physiological relevance, *Biochem. J.*, 267(2), 281–290, 1990.
5. Haussinger, D., Liver glutamine metabolism, *J. Parenter. Enteral Nutr.*, 14(4 Suppl.), 56S–62S, 1990.
6. Vander, A.J., *Renal Physiology*, 5th ed., McGraw-Hill, New York, 1995.
7. Murray, R.K. et al., *Harper's Biochemistry*, Appleton & Lange, Norwalk, CT, 1988.
8. Nurjhan, N. et al., Glutamine: a major gluconeogenic precursor and vehicle for interorgan carbon transport in man, *J. Clin. Invest.*, 95(1), 272–277, 1995.
9. Stumvoll, M. et al., Human kidney and liver gluconeogenesis: evidence for organ substrate selectivity, *Am. J. Physiol.*, 274(5 Pt 1), E817–E826, 1998.
10. Ardawi, M.S. and E.A. Newsholme, Glutamine metabolism in lymphocytes of the rat, *Biochem. J.*, 212(3), 835–842, 1983.
11. Newsholme, P., Why is L-glutamine metabolism important to cells of the immune system in health, postinjury, surgery or infection? *J. Nutr.*, 131(9 Suppl.), 2515S–2522S; discussion 2523S–2524S, 2001.
12. Taudou, G., J. Wiart, and J. Panijel, Influence of amino acid deficiency and tRNA aminoacylation on DNA synthesis and DNA polymerase activity during the secondary immune response *in vitro*, *Mol. Immunol.*, 20(3), 255–261, 1983.

13. Furukawa, S. et al., Supplemental glutamine augments phagocytosis and reactive oxygen intermediate production by neutrophils and monocytes from postoperative patients *in vitro*, *Nutrition*, 16(5), 323–329, 2000.

14. Spittler, A. et al., Influence of glutamine on the phenotype and function of human monocytes, *Blood*, 86(4), 1564–1569, 1995.

15. Boelens, P.G. et al., Glutamine-enriched enteral nutrition increases *in vitro* interferon-production but does not influence the *in vivo* specific antibody response to KLH after severe trauma. A prospective, double blind, randomized clinical study, *Clin. Nutr.*, 23(3), 391–400, 2004.

16. Spittler, A. et al., Postoperative glycyl-glutamine infusion reduces immunosuppression: partial prevention of the surgery induced decrease in HLA-DR expression on monocytes, *Clin. Nutr.*, 20(1), 37–42, 2001.

17. Plumley, D.A. et al., Accelerated lung amino acid release in hyperdynamic septic surgical patients, *Arch. Surg.*, 125(1), 57–61, 1990.

18. Helton, W.S. et al., Effects of glutamine-enriched parenteral nutrition on the exocrine pancreas, *J. Parenter. Enteral Nutr.*, 14(4), 344–352, 1990.

19. Gao, Z.Y. et al., Glucose regulation of glutaminolysis and its role in insulin secretion, *Diabetes*, 48(8), 1535–1542, 1999.

20. Yorifuji, T. et al., Hyperinsulinism-hyperammonemia syndrome caused by mutant glutamate dehydrogenase accompanied by novel enzyme kinetics, *Hum. Genet.*, 104(6), 476–479, 1999.

21. Fontana, G. et al., AMPA-evoked acetylcholine release from cultured spinal cord motoneurons and its inhibition by GABA and glycine. *Neuroscience*, 106(1), 183–191, 2001.

22. Martinez-Hernandez, A., K.P. Bell, and M.D. Norenberg, Glutamine synthetase: glial localization in brain, *Science*, 195(4284), 1356–1358, 1977.

23. Behar, K.L. and D.L. Rothman, *In vivo* nuclear magnetic resonance studies of glutamate γ-aminobutyric acid-glutamine cycling in rodent and human cortex: the central role of glutamine, *J. Nutr.*, 131(9 Suppl.), 2498S–2504S; discussion 2523S–2524S, 2001.

24. Zubay, G.L., *Biochemistry*, 4th ed., Wm. C. Brown, Dubuque, IA, 1998.

25. Beutler, E., Nutritional and metabolic aspects of glutathione, *Annu. Rev. Nutr.*, 9, 287–302, 1989.

26. Soh, H. et al., Glutamine regulates amino acid transport and glutathione levels in a human neuroblastoma cell line, *Pediatr. Surg. Int.*, 21(1), 29–33, 2005.

27. Meister, A., Glutathione deficiency produced by inhibition of its synthesis, and its reversal; applications in research and therapy, *Pharmacol. Ther.*, 51(2), 155–194, 1991.

28. Marcinkiewicz, J. et al., Taurine chloramine, a product of activated neutrophils, inhibits *in vitro* the generation of nitric oxide and other macrophage inflammatory mediators, *J. Leukoc. Biol.*, 58(6), 667–674, 1995.

29. Koyama, I. et al., The protective effect of taurine on the biomembrane against damage produced by the oxygen radical, *Adv. Exp. Med. Biol.*, 315, 355–359, 1992.

30. Boelens, P.G. et al., Plasma taurine concentrations increase after enteral glutamine supplementation in trauma patients and stressed rats, *Am. J. Clin. Nutr.*, 77(1), 250–256, 2003.

31. Huxtable, R.J., Physiological actions of taurine, *Physiol. Rev.*, 72(1), 101–163, 1992.

32. Scheltinga, M.R. et al., Glutamine-enriched intravenous feedings attenuate extracellular fluid expansion after a standard stress, *Ann. Surg.*, 214(4), 385–393; discussion 393–395, 1991.

33. Kapadia, C.R. et al., Maintenance of skeletal muscle intracellular glutamine during standard surgical trauma, *J. Parenter. Enteral Nutr.,* 9(5), 583–589, 1985.

34. Greig, J.E. et al., Inter-relationships between glutamine and other biochemical and immunological changes after major vascular surgery, *Br. J. Biomed. Sci.,* 53(2), 116–121, 1996.

35. Keast, D., T. Nguyen, and E.A. Newsholme, Maximal activities of glutaminase, citrate synthase, hexokinase, phosphofructokinase and lactate dehydrogenase in skin of rats and mice at different ages, *FEBS Lett.,* 247(1), 132–134, 1989.

36. Aussel, C. et al., α-Ketoglutarate uptake in human fibroblasts, *Cell. Biol. Int.,* 20(5), 359–363, 1996.

37. Zielke, H.R. et al., Growth of human diploid fibroblasts in the absence of glucose utilization, *Proc. Natl. Acad. Sci. U.S.A.,* 73(11), 4110–4114, 1976.

38. McCauley, R. et al., Effects of glutamine infusion on colonic anastomotic strength in the rat, *J. Parenter. Enteral Nutr.,* 5(4), 437–439, 1991.

39. Williams, J.Z., N. Abumrad, and A. Barbul, Effect of a specialized amino acid mixture on human collagen deposition, *Ann. Surg.,* 236(3), 369–374; discussion 374–375, 2002.

40. Bellon, G. et al., Effects of preformed proline and proline amino acid precursors (including glutamine) on collagen synthesis in human fibroblast cultures, *Biochim. Biophys. Acta,* 930(1), 39–47, 1987.

41. Bellon, G. et al., Glutamine increases collagen gene transcription in cultured human fibroblasts, *Biochim. Biophys. Acta,* 1268(3), 311–323, 1995.

42. Souba, W.W. et al., Postoperative alterations in interorgan glutamine exchange in enterectomized dogs, *J. Surg. Res.,* 42(2), 117–125, 1987.

43. Souba, W.W., R.J. Smith, and D.W. Wilmore, Effects of glucocorticoids on glutamine metabolism in visceral organs, *Metabolism,* 34(5), 450–456, 1985.

44. Dudrick, P.S. et al., Dexamethasone stimulation of glutaminase expression in mesenteric lymph nodes, *Am. J. Surg.,* 165(1), 34–39, 1993.

45. Battezzati, A. et al., Glucagon increases glutamine uptake without affecting glutamine release in humans, *Metabolism,* 47(6), 713–723, 1998.

46. Baskerville, A., P. Hambleton, and J.E. Benbough, Pathological features of glutaminase toxicity, *Br. J. Exp. Pathol.,* 61(2), 132–138, 1980.

47. O'Dwyer, S.T. et al., Maintenance of small bowel mucosa with glutamine-enriched parenteral nutrition, *J. Parenter. Enteral Nutr.,* 13(6), 579–585, 1989.

48. Barber, A.E. et al., Harry M. Vars award. Glutamine or fiber supplementation of a defined formula diet: impact on bacterial translocation, tissue composition, and response to endotoxin, *J. Parenter. Enteral Nutr.,* 14(4), 335–343, 1990.

49. Okabe, S. et al., Inhibitory effect of L-glutamine on gastric irritation and back diffusion of gastric acid in response to aspirin in the rat, *Am. J. Dig. Dis.,* 20(7), 626–631, 1975.

50. Nath, S.K. et al., [15N]- and [14C]glutamine fluxes across rabbit ileum in experimental bacterial diarrhea, *Am. J. Physiol.,* 262(2 Pt. 1), G312–G318, 1992.

51. Frankel, W.L. et al., Glutamine enhancement of structure and function in transplanted small intestine in the rat, *J. Parenter. Enteral Nutr.,* 17(1), 47–55, 1993.

52. Alverdy, J.A. et al., The effect of glutamine-enriched TPN on gut immune cellularity, *J. Surg. Res.,* 52(1), 34–38, 1992.

53. Burke, D.J. et al., Glutamine-supplemented total parenteral nutrition improves gut immune function, *Arch. Surg.,* 124(12), 1396–1399, 1989.

54. Fischer, C.P. et al., Hepatic uptake of glutamine and other amino acids during infection and inflammation, *Shock,* 3(5), 315–322, 1995.

55. Low, S.Y. et al., Transport of L-glutamine and L-glutamate across sinusoidal membranes of rat liver. Effects of starvation, diabetes and corticosteroid treatment, *Biochem. J.*, 284(Pt. 2), 333–340, 1992.

56. Opara, E., Characterization of glutamine regulated pancreatic islet hormone release, *Surg. Forum*, 48, 297, 1990.

57. Li, S.J. et al., Addition of L-glutamine to total parenteral nutrition and its effects on portal insulin and glucagon and the development of hepatic steatosis in rats, *J. Surg. Res.*, 48(5), 421–426, 1990.

58. Parry-Billings, M. et al., Does glutamine contribute to immunosuppression after major burns? *Lancet*, 336(8714), 523–525, 1990.

59. Brand, K., Glutamine and glucose metabolism during thymocyte proliferation. Pathways of glutamine and glutamate metabolism, *Biochem. J.*, 228(2), 353–361, 1985.

60. Muhlbacher, F. et al., Effects of glucocorticoids on glutamine metabolism in skeletal muscle, *Am. J. Physiol.*, 247(1 Pt. 1), E75–E83, 1984.

61. Lukaszewicz, G.C., W.W. Souba, and S.F. Abcouwer, Induction of muscle glutamine synthetase gene expression during endotoxemia is adrenal gland dependent, *Shock*, 7(5), 332–338, 1997.

62. Roth, E., Metabolic disorders in severe abdominal sepsis: glutamine deficiency in skeletal muscle, *Clin. Nutr.*, 1(25), 25–41, 1982.

63. Hickson, R.C., S.M. Czerwinski, and L.E. Wegrzyn, Glutamine prevents downregulation of myosin heavy chain synthesis and muscle atrophy from glucocorticoids, *Am. J. Physiol.*, 268(4 Pt. 1), E730–E734, 1995.

64. Hammarqvist, F. et al., Addition of glutamine to total parenteral nutrition after elective abdominal surgery spares free glutamine in muscle, counteracts the fall in muscle protein synthesis, and improves nitrogen balance, *Ann. Surg.*, 209(4), 455–461, 1989.

65. Hinshaw, D.B. and J.M. Burger, Protective effect of glutamine on endothelial cell ATP in oxidant injury, *J. Surg. Res.*, 49(3), 222–227, 1990.

66. Goeters, C. et al., Parenteral L-alanyl-L-glutamine improves 6-month outcome in critically ill patients, *Crit. Care Med.*, 30(9), 2032–2037, 2002.

67. McCowen, K.C. and B.R. Bistrian, Immunonutrition: problematic or problem solving? *Am. J. Clin. Nutr.*, 77(4), 764–770, 2003.

68. Heyland, D.K. et al., Should immunonutrition become routine in critically ill patients? A systematic review of the evidence, *JAMA*, 286(8), 944–953, 2001.

69. Hall, J.C., K. Heel, and R. McCauley, Glutamine, *Br. J. Surg.*, 83(3), 305–312, 1996.

70. Neu, J., V. DeMarco, and N. Li, Glutamine: clinical applications and mechanisms of action, *Curr. Opin. Clin. Nutr. Metab. Care*, 5(1), 69–75, 2002.

71. Boelens, P.G. et al., Glutamine alimentation in catabolic state, *J. Nutr.*, 131(9 Suppl.), 2569S–2577S; discussion 2590S, 2001.

72. Buchman, A.L., Glutamine: commercially essential or conditionally essential? A critical appraisal of the human data, *Am. J. Clin. Nutr.*, 74(1), 25–32, 2001.

73. Oudemans-van Straaten, H.M. et al., Plasma glutamine depletion and patient outcome in acute ICU admissions, *Intensive Care Med.*, 27(1), 84–90, 2001.

74. Lacey, J.M. and D.W. Wilmore, Is glutamine a conditionally essential amino acid? *Nutr. Rev.*, 48(8), 297–309, 1990.

75. Novak, F. et al., Glutamine supplementation in serious illness: a systematic review of the evidence, *Crit. Care Med.*, 30(9), 2022–2029, 2002.

76. De Bandt, J.P. and L.A. Cynober, Amino acids with anabolic properties, *Curr. Opin. Clin. Nutr. Metab. Care*, 1(3), 263–272, 1998.

77. Scheppach, W. et al., Effect of L-glutamine and *n*-butyrate on the restitution of rat colonic mucosa after acid induced injury, *Gut*, 38(6), 878–885, 1996.

78. Wilmore, D.W., The effect of glutamine supplementation in patients following elective surgery and accidental injury, *J. Nutr.*, 131(9 Suppl.), 2543S–2549S; discussion 23550S–2551S, 2001.

79. Newsholme, P. et al., Glutamine metabolism by lymphocytes, macrophages, and neutrophils: its importance in health and disease, *J. Nutr. Biochem.*, 10(6), 316–324, 1999.

80. Morlion, B.J. et al., Total parenteral nutrition with glutamine dipeptide after major abdominal surgery: a randomized, double-blind, controlled study, *Ann. Surg.*, 227(2), 302–308, 1998.

81. Houdijk, A.P. et al., Randomised trial of glutamine-enriched enteral nutrition on infectious morbidity in patients with multiple trauma, *Lancet*, 352(9130), 772–776, 1998.

82. Melis, G.C. et al., Glutamine: recent developments in research on the clinical significance of glutamine, *Curr. Opin. Clin. Nutr. Metab. Care*, 7(1), 59–70, 2004.

83. Hall, J.C. et al., A prospective randomized trial of enteral glutamine in critical illness, *Intensive Care Med.*, 29(10), 1710–1716, 2003.

84. Vaughn, P. et al., Enteral glutamine supplementation and morbidity in low birth weight infants, *J. Pediatr.*, 142(6), 662–668, 2003.

85. Garlick, P.J., Assessment of the safety of glutamine and other amino acids, *J. Nutr.*, 131(9 Suppl.), 2556S–2561S, 2001.

86. Mebane, A.H., L-Glutamine and mania, *Am. J. Psychiatry*, 141(10), 1302–1303, 1984.

87. Newsholme, E. and G. Hardy, Supplementation of diets with nutritional pharmaceuticals, *Nutrition*, 13(9), 837–839, 1997.

SELECTED READINGS

Buchman, A.L., Glutamine: commercially essential or conditionally essential? A critical appraisal of the human data, *Am. J. Clin. Nutr.*, 74(1), 25–32, 2001.

Hall, J.C., K. Heel, and R. McCauley, Glutamine, *Br. J. Surg.*, 83(3), 305–312, 1996.

Melis, G.C. et al., Glutamine: recent developments in research on the clinical significance of glutamine, *Curr. Opin. Clin. Nutr. Metab. Care*, 7(1), 59–70, 2004.

Newsholme, P. et al., Glutamine metabolism by lymphocytes, macrophages, and neutrophils: its importance in health and disease, *J. Nutr. Biochem.*, 10(6), 316–324, 1999.

Novak, F. et al., Glutamine supplementation in serious illness: a systematic review of the evidence, *Crit. Care Med.*, 30(9), 2022–2029, 2002.

6 Arginine and Wound Healing

Vanita Ahuja, Majida Rizk, and Adrian Barbul

CONTENTS

Arginine was first isolated from lupin seedlings in 1886 and was thereafter identified as a component of animal proteins. Arginase, the enzyme that hydrolyzes arginine to ornithine and urea was identified in liver in 1904. Later, the discovery of the urea cycle by Krebs and Henseleit in 1932 elucidated the role of arginine in physiology and metabolic pathway.[1] The dietary essentiality of arginine was discovered in 1950 when Rose found that young growing rats demonstrated more rapid growth when receiving dietary arginine. The role of arginine in wound healing was demonstrated first in animals placed on an arginine-deficient diet. Arginine supplementation has been shown to enhance collagen synthesis and wound strength. Rats fed an arginine-deficient diet after minor trauma had increased postoperative weight loss and increased mortality when compared with rats fed a similar defined diet containing arginine. Though several pathways have been studied, the exact mechanism of action of arginine on wound healing and collagen metabolism is not known.

ARGININE METABOLISM

Arginine, a dibasic amino acid, is considered to be a dietary conditionally dispensable amino acid. Arginine is synthesized endogenously in the kidney from gut-derived citrulline. The small intestine converts dietary amino acids to citrulline. The quantities of arginine produced normally are sufficient to maintain muscle and connective tissue mass. However, endogenous synthesis of arginine is insufficient to meet the heightened demands that increased protein turnover requires during period of stress.

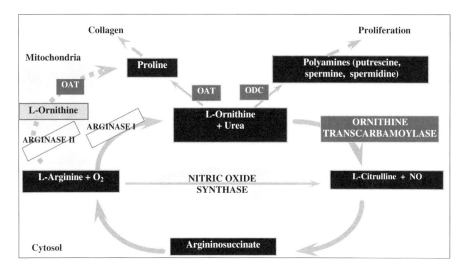

ODC = ornithine decarboxylase
OAT = ornithine aminotransferase

FIGURE 6.1 Arginine metabolism.

In such situations, arginine becomes indispensable for optimal growth and maintenance of positive nitrogen balance.

The major synthesis pathway involves the intestinal–renal axis in which the small intestine releases citrulline into the blood circulation and is then extracted by the kidney for conversion into arginine. It is released into the bloodstream for uptake by tissues for protein synthesis. The hepatic arginine pathway contributes the lowest arginine amount, because the liver does not express large amounts of the cationic transporter for the basic amino acid arginine. Therefore, most of the portal venous arginine and citrulline enters the systemic circulation and serves as substrate for extrahepatic tissues. The intestinal absorption of arginine occurs via a transport system shared with lysine, ornithine, and cysteine. Arginine, ornithine, and lysine also share a common uptake and transport system in the brain, leukocytes, erythrocytes, fibroblasts, and leukocytes.[2]

Arginine catabolism occurs in a wound via two separate enzymatic pathways — nitric oxide synthase isoforms and the two arginase isoforms. Arginine plays a key role within the urea cycle, the major pathway for ammonia detoxification (Figure 6.1). There are two distinct isoenzymes of mammalian arginase, which are encoded by separate genes. Type I arginase, a cytosolic enzyme, is highly expressed in liver as a component of the urea cycle and is also present in wound-derived fibroblasts. Type II arginase is a mitochondrial enzyme expressed at lower levels in the kidney, brain, small intestine, mammary gland, and macrophages. Any condition that increases demand for ammonia detoxification is likely to increase arginine requirements. Inherited defects in the hepatic type I arginase are partially compensated for by elevated expression of type II arginase in the kidney, resulting in a less severe clinical disorder.

Arginine has been shown to be the unique substrate for the production of the highly reactive radical nitric oxide (NO) molecule. This important pathway has been shown to be present in many tissues and cells, including endothelium, brain, inflammatory cells (lymphocytes, macrophages, neutrophils, mast cells), platelets, and hepatocytes. NO is pharmacologically and chemically identical to endothelial-derived relaxant factor (EDRF), a biological effector molecule. In addition to its role in vasodilation, NO is a putative neurotransmitter and cytotoxic effector molecule. NO is formed by the oxidation of one of the two identical terminal guanidino groups of L-arginine by the enzyme NO synthase (NOS), a dioxygenase, of which there are at least two identified isoforms. Both isoforms of NOS have been identified as flavoproteins, each containing flavine adenine dinucleotide and flavine adenine mononucleotide, and both are inhibited by diphenyleneiodonium, a flavoprotein inhibitor. Neuronal NOS and endothelial NOS, collectively referred to as cytosolic NOS (cNOS), are expressed constitutively and are activated by Ca^{2+}/calmodulin. Inducible NOS is calcium dependent and is expressed in response to inflammatory cytokines and endotoxins, including interleukin-1, tumor necrosis factor-α, γ-interferon, and lipopolysaccharide.

There are strong regulatory mechanisms between the different metabolic pathways. L-hydroxyarginine and nitrite, the intermediate end products, respectively, of the NO pathway, are both strong arginase inhibitors. Furthermore, urea, an end product of arginase activity, inhibits NO formation. Each pathway is stimulated by a well-defined set of cytokines that then downregulates the alternate pathway (e.g., transforming growth factor [TGF]-β stimulates arginase but inhibits inducible nitric oxide synthetase [iNOS]).[3,4]

ARGININE AND WOUND HEALING METABOLISM

Arginine is considered an essential amino acid under periods of severe stress. In 1976 Seifter, Barbul, Rettura, and Levenson first studied the role of arginine in injured animals. This was based on the rationale that a growing animal requires more arginine than a mature animal. In the growing animal, much of the arginine is used for the synthesis of connective tissue proteins. In the injured animal, an increase in arginine would be expected to synthesize reparative connective tissue. When subjected to minor trauma, such as dorsal skin incision and closure, rats have shown increased postoperative weight loss and increased mortality compared to rats fed a similar defined diet containing arginine. Furthermore, the arginine deficiency results in decreased wound breaking strength and wound collagen accumulation. Subsequent experiments showed that rats fed a chow diet, not deficient in arginine, and additionally supplemented with 1% arginine also have enhanced wound breaking strength and collagen synthesis when compared to chow-fed controls (Figure 6.2). Similar findings were noted in parenterally fed rats given an amino acid mixture containing high doses (7.5 g/l) of arginine in rats. This effect was observed in elderly rats fed a diet supplemented with a combination of both arginine and glycine. It was noted that these rats had an enhanced rate of wound collagen deposition when compared to controls.[5]

Two studies have been done so far on the effect of arginine supplementation on collagen accumulation in healthy human subjects (Figure 6.3). A micromodel was

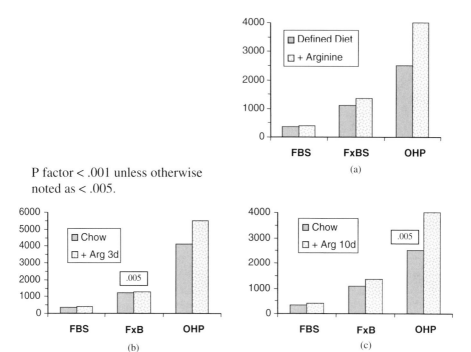

P factor < .001 unless otherwise
noted as < .005.

FIGURE 6.2 Effect of arginine deficiency (a) and arginine supplementation (b,c) on wound fresh breaking strength (FBS), g; formalin-fixed breaking strength (FxBS), g; and hydroxy-proline accumulation (OHP), μg/100 mg sponge. Note that the *P* factor < 0.001 unless otherwise noted as < 0.005.

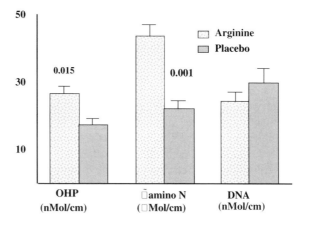

FIGURE 6.3 Effect of arginine on wound healing parameters in healthy elderly human volunteers.

described in which the collagen accumulation occurs in a subcutaneously placed 5 cm segment of polytetrafluoroethylene (PTFE) tubing to study the human fibroblastic response. In the first study, young healthy human volunteers (25 to 35 yr) were found to have a significant increase in wound collagen deposition following oral supplementation with either 30 g of arginine aspartate (17 g of free arginine) or 30 g of arginine HCL (24.8 g of free arginine) daily for 14 d. In a subsequent study of healthy elderly humans (67 to 82 yr), daily supplements of 30 g of arginine aspartate for 14 d resulted in significantly enhanced collagen and total protein deposition at the wound site when compared to placebo controls. This study evaluated the wound response using the PTFE catheters and examined epithelialization on a split thickness wound created on the upper thigh of each subject. The catheters in this study were analyzed for -amino nitrogen content (assessment of total protein content), DNA accumulation (index of cellular infiltration), and hydroxyproline content. There was no enhanced DNA present in the wounds of the arginine-supplemented subjects, suggesting that the effect of arginine is not mediated by an inflammatory mode of action. There was no observed effect in the rate of epithelialization of a superficial skin defect, suggesting that the predominant effect of arginine on wound healing is to enhance wound collagen deposition.[6–8]

There are several theories on the mechanism of the beneficial effect of arginine on wound healing. Arginine comprises less than 5% of the collagen molecule, and it is possible that supplemental arginine is a necessary substrate for collagen synthesis at the wound site. This may be possible through the direct use of arginine as substrate for the pathway arginine- > ornithine- > glutamic semialdehyde- > proline. Studies have shown that increased deposition of collagen early in the wound healing process correlates with an increase in wound strength. Arginine levels are undetectable within the wound during the late phases when fibroplasia predominates. However, studies done by Albina showed that although ornithine levels are higher in wound plasma, the rate of conversion of ornithine to proline is quite low. Therefore, this would make the arginine-to-proline mechanism very unlikely.[9]

It was shown that NO plays a more dominant role in wound healing (Figure 6.4). Arginine is catabolized to NO specifically through iNOS with ultimate production of citrulline. Previous studies have shown that iNOS is upregulated following tissue injury, and that systemic administration of NOS inhibitors, such as S-methyl isothouronium, impairs wound tensile strength and collagen deposition in a dose-dependent manner. The iNOS is synthesized in the early phase of wound healing by inflammatory cells, mainly macrophages.[10] NO inhibition has been shown to significantly impair wound healing of cutaneous incisional wounds and colonic anastamosis in rodents.[11] *In vitro* studies have noted increased collagen synthesis in association with exogenous NO administration in cultured dermal fibroblasts. Supranormal collagen deposition has been noted after transfection of iNOS DNA into wounds. Conversely, mice lacking the iNOS gene (iNOS knockout mice) have delayed closure of excisional wounds, an impairment that is corrected by adenoviral transfer of the iNOS gene to the wound bed. The loss of a functional iNOS gene negates the beneficial effect of arginine in wound healing, while supplemental dietary arginine enhances wound healing in normal mice.[12] NO synthesis is also decreased in the wound milieu

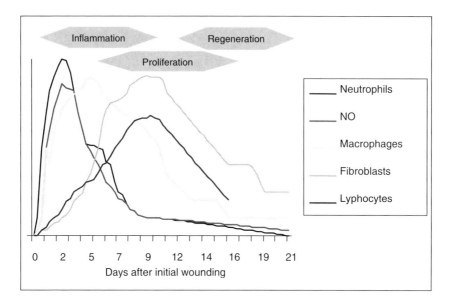

FIGURE 6.4 Phases of wound healing and generation of wound nitric oxide (NO).

of diabetics, and arginine supplementation restored healing by normalizing the NO pathway without affecting the arginase activity.[13] This suggests that the metabolism of arginine via the NO pathway is one mechanism responsible for arginine enhancing wound healing (Figure 6.5).

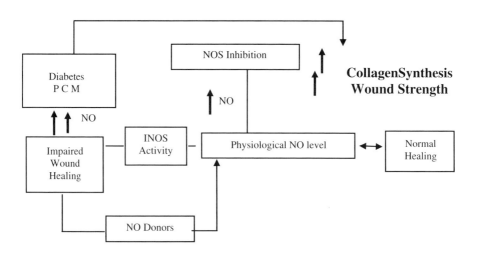

FIGURE 6.5 Nitric oxide and wound healing.

ARGININE AND IMMUNE FUNCTION

Arginine given in large doses has a unique effect on T-cell function. T lymphocytes are essential for wounding, and the depletion of arginine significantly impairs the wound healing response. Arginine acts as a thymotropic agent and stimulates *in vitro* and *in vivo* T-cell response. Arginine also reduces the inhibitory effect of injury and wounding on T-cell function. Supplemental dietary arginine increases thymic weight in uninjured rats and minimizes the thymic involution that occurs with injury. The gain in thymic weight is due to significant increases in the lymphocyte content of the thymic glands. In healthy humans, arginine enhances the mitogenic activity of peripheral blood lymphocytes and greatly reduces posttraumatic impairment in lymphocyte blastogenesis.[14]

The trophic effect that arginine exerts on the thymus results in improved host immunity. Saito et al. showed that diets containing 2% arginine of the total nonprotein calories increased survival and improved delayed hypersensitivity in a third-degree 30% body surface burn model in guinea pigs. In a study of severely burned children, it was noted that plasma arginine had a high correlation with a number of parameters, indicating resistance to infection, such as total protein, albumin, transferrin, and C_3 levels. The exact mechanism of the arginine thymotropic effect is not known. It has been postulated that the thymic effects may be related to the pituitary secretagogue activity, because hypophysectomized rats fail to attain an adequate immune response, which can be reversed by giving them prolactin or growth hormone (Table 6.1).[15,16]

ARGININE AND SEPSIS

Sepsis impairs the intestinal absorption of amino acids by affecting the transporters. Analysis of the transport kinetics suggests that the decreased transport capacity is caused by a reduction in the number or affinity of the transporter proteins.

TABLE 6.1
Immune Effects of Arginine

Action	Animals	Humans
Mitogenic response of lymphocytes		
- Health	Yes	Yes
- Injury or stress	Yes	Yes
Allograft rejection	Yes	ND[a]
Number of T cells, mitogenic reactivity, and delayed-type hypersensitivity responses in immunocomprised host	Yes[b]	Yes[c]
Antitumor cytotoxicity *in vitro*	Yes	Yes
Antitumor response *in vivo*	Yes	ND
Response to sepsis	Yes	ND

[a]Not done.
[b]Athymic nude animals.
[c]HIV infected.

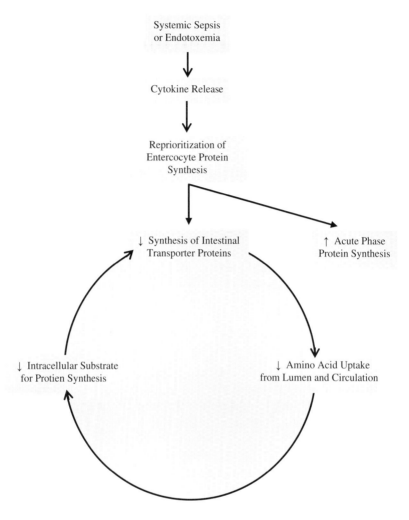

FIGURE 6.6 Implications of impaired intestinal amino acid absorption. From Gardiner, K. and Barbul, A. Intestinal amino acid absorption during sepsis. *J. Parent. Enternal Nutr.* 17, 280, 1993.

Experimental sepsis, induced by either cecal ligation and puncture or intraperitoneal injection of lipopolysaccharide, showed a significant decrease in intestinal absorption of amino acids. Furthermore, the utilization of arginine may be decreased, and its biosynthesis may be impaired during sepsis as suggested by the significantly decreased plasma arginine levels in septic patients (Figure 6.6).[17–19]

Enteral feeding in comparison with parenteral feeding has been shown to improve outcome in burned children and in adults after trauma. It also has been demonstrated that enteral feeding improves survival in animals after hemorrhage and sepsis. A reversal of the alteration in T-cell function associated with trauma or surgery has been demonstrated in patients fed enteral diets rich in arginine. Additionally, moderately stressed intensive care unit patients given an enteral arginine-rich diet show enhancement of T-cell blastogenesis. This suggests that enteral feeding, to supply the amino acid nutrients, may impart a benefit during septic illness.[20–22]

ARGININE CLINICAL RECOMMENDATION

Plasma arginine concentration in human adults ranges from 0.04 to 0.1 mM. A daily arginine requirement was calculated to be approximately 5 to 6 g/d. Clinically, arginine given alone or in complete nutritional support has been shown to reduce nitrogen loss in postoperative patients. Thus, elective surgical patients given 30 g/d of arginine hydrochloride intravenously for the first 3 d postcholecystectomy had a 60% reduction in urinary nitrogen excretion. Postoperative patients after major abdominal surgery who received immediate enteral feedings supplemented with 25 g of arginine had a mean positive nitrogen balance when compared to glycine-supplemented controls. Healthy elderly (67–82 yr) human volunteers demonstrate increased nitrogen retention, enhanced collagen, and total protein deposition at the wound site following supplementation with 30 g of arginine aspartate (17 g of free arginine) for 2 weeks. A diet that contains 9% protein as arginine was found to be important in the healing of burn wounds, reducing the infection rate and hospital length of stay.[23–25]

Arginine supplementation at an approximate dose of 500 mg/kg/d given to rodents either enterally or parenterally enhanced thymic size, lymphocyte content, and lymphocyte mitogenesis in response to mitogens and alloantigens. Arginine is required *in vitro* for optimal lymphocyte mitogenic responses and lymphokine production and for induction of cytotoxic T cell and natural killer cell function. Maximum mitogenic stimulation and lymphokine production occur at an arginine concentration of 0.04 mM, and further increase does not result in enhanced responses. Maximal natural killer and cytotoxic T-lymphocyte generation and activation *in vitro* is observed at an arginine concentration between 0.04 and 0.1 mM.[26]

A relative deficiency of arginine can occur in the presence of excessive ammonia, excessive lysine, growth, pregnancy, trauma, or protein deficiency and malnutrition. Approximately twice as much ornithine and four times as much citrulline are needed to achieve the same degree of protection against hyperammonemia as that provided by arginine. Ammonia excess may occur even in the presence of a normal liver when amino acids lacking arginine are infused. The toxicity associated with excess ammonia was reversed by a diet infused with arginine. The hereditary urea cycle enzyme deficiencies that affect the formation of ornithine are argininosuccinate synthetase (ASS) deficiency and argininosuccinate lyase (ASL) deficiency. These cause citullinemia and argininosuccinate acidemia, respectively. A diet rich in arginine can improve patients with ASS and ASL deficiency.[27]

The LD_{50}% (intraperitoneal, after 24 h starvation) for arginine in rats is 18 mM/kg (3.8 g/kg), which makes arginine in a class of compounds with very low toxicity for normally nourished animals. A dose of 0.5 g/kg up to 30 g total given intravenously over 20 to 30 min in humans being studied for pituitary function causes no untoward reaction. The use of arginine in this clinical context is generally safe. A single case of anaphylaxes reaction with intravenous arginine was reported. Human subjects given 30 g of arginine daily for 1 week have no side effects except for mild gastrointestinal discomfort. There are reported cases of severe hyperkalemia in patients with renal and hepatic failure. Arginine infusion was shown to lead to hypophosphatemia in normal subjects and in patients with insulin-dependent diabetes. Overall, patients can tolerate high doses of arginine (30 to 60 g/d), but those who are hepatic or renal insufficient should be carefully monitored for electrolyte levels.[28]

FUTURE RECOMMENDATIONS

As can be seen, arginine possesses numerous pharmacologic actions that have great potential benefit in clinical practice. Although the animal experimental data are compelling, there is a need for continued clinical study in order to better define the role of arginine in the care of patients. Previous studies have been limited to small volunteer groups, and no study exists on the dosage and its efficacy of arginine in humans during periods of stress. Though arginine is considered relatively safe at high dosages, there is no study on the minimum effective dose in human clinical practice. Recently, it was shown that impaired healing of diabetic wounds can be partially corrected by arginine supplementation, and this effect is accompanied by enhanced wound nitric oxide synthesis. Further studies of this finding need to be done in clinical practice. Finally, the exact mechanism of arginine and wound healing needs to be further elucidated, especially the role of nitric oxide in healing.[29]

REFERENCES

1. Wu, G. and Morris, S.M., Arginine metabolism: nitric oxide and beyond, *Biochem. J.*, 336, 1–17, 1998.
2. Morris, S.M., Arginine synthesis, metabolism, and transport: regulators of nitric oxide synthesis, in *Cellular and Molecular Biology of Nitric Oxide*, Laskin, J.D. and Laskin, D.L., Eds., Marcel Dekker, New York, 1999, pp. 57–85.
3. Barbul, A., Arginine: biochemistry, physiology, and therapeutic implications, *J. Parenter. Enteral Nutr.*, 10, 227–238, 1986.
4. Witte, M.B. and Barbul, A., Role of nitric oxide in wound repair, *Am. J. Surg.*, 183, 406–410, 2002.
5. Barbul, A., Rettura, G., Levenson, S.M., et al., Arginine: a thymotropic and wound healing promoting agent, *Surg. Forum*, 28, 101–103, 1977.
6. Barbul, A., Lazarou, S.A., Efron, D.T., et al., Arginine enhances wound healing and lymphocyte immune responses in humans, *Surgery*, 108, 331–337, 1990.
7. Hurson, M., Regan, M.C., Kirk, S.J., et al., Metabolic effects of arginine in a healthy elderly population, *J. Parenter. Enteral. Nutr.*, 19, 227–230, 1994.
8. Williams, J.Z., Abumrad, N., and Barbul, A., Effect of a specialized amino acid mixture on human collagen deposition, *Ann. Surg.*, 236, 369–375, 2002.
9. Albina, J.E., Mills, C.D., et al., Arginine metabolism in wounds, *Am. J. Phys.*, 254, 459–467, 1988.
10. Lee, R.H., Efron, D.T., Tantry, U., et al., Nitric oxide in the wound healing: a time course study, *J. Surg. Res.*, 101, 104–108, 2001.

11. Efron, D.T., Thornton, F.J., et al., Expression and function of inducible nitric oxide synthase during rat colon anastomotic healing, *J. Gastrointest. Surg.*, 3, 592–601, 1999.

12. Shi, H.P., Efron, D.T., Most, D., et al., Supplemental dietary arginine enhances wound healing in normal but not inducible nitric oxide synthase knockout mice, *Surgery*, 128, 374–378, 2000.

13. Witte, M.B., Thornton, F.J., Tantry, U., et al., L-Arginine supplementation enhances diabetic wound healing: involvement of the nitric oxide synthase and arginase pathway, *Metabolism*, 51, 1269–1273, 2002.

14. Kirk, S.J., Regan, M.C., Wassenberg, H.L., et al., Arginine enhances T-cell responses in athymic nude mice, *J. Parenter. Enteral Nutr.*, 16, 429–431, 1992.

15. Barbul, A., Wassenberg, H.L., Seifter, E., et al., Immunostimulatory effects of arginine in normal and injured rats, *J. Surg. Res.*, 29, 228–235, 1980.

16. Barbul, A., Supplemental arginine, wound healing and thymus: arginine–pituitary interaction, *Surg. Forum*, 29, 93–95, 1978.

17. Gardiner, K.R., Gardiner, R.E., and Barbul, A., Reduced intestinal absorption of arginine during sepsis, *Crit. Care Med.*, 23, 1227–1231, 1995.

18. Sodeyama, M., Garfiner, K.R., Regan, M.C., et al., Sepsis impairs amino acid absorption, *Am. J. Surg.*, 165, 150–154, 1993.

19. Gardiner, K.R., Ahrendt, G.M., Gardiner, R.E., et al., Failure of intestinal amino acid absorptive mechanisms in sepsis, *J. Am. Coll. Surg.*, 181, 431–436, 1995.

20. Gardiner, K. and Barbul, A., Intestinal amino acid absorption during sepsis, *J. Parent. Enteral Nutr.*, 17, 277–283, 1993.

21. Kiyama, T., Witte, M.B., Thornton, F.J., et al., The route of nutrition support affects the early phase of wound healing, *J. Parent. Enteral Nutr.*, 22, 276–279, 1998.

22. Kiyama, T., Efron, D.T., Tantry, U., et al., Trauma and wound healing: role of the route of nutritional support, *J. Surg. Invest.*, 2, 483–489, 2001.

23. Barbul, A., Fishel, R.S., Shimazu, S., et al., Intravenous hyperalimentation with high arginine levels improves wound healing and immune function, *J. Surg. Res.*, 38, 328–334, 1985.

24. De-souza, D.A. and Greene, L.J., Pharmacological nutrition after burn injury, *J. Nutr.*, 128, 797–803, 1998.

25. Barbul, A., Asserkrug, H.L., Penbarthy, L.T., et al., Optimal levels of arginine in maintenance intravenous hyperalimentation, *J. Parenter. Enteral Nutr.*, 8, 281–284, 1983.

26. Barbul, A., Sisto, D.A., Wasserkrug, H.L., et al., Nitrogen sparing and immune mechanisms of arginine: differential dose-dependent responses during postinjury intravenous hyperalimentation, *Curr. Surg.*, 40, 114–116, 1983.

27. Zieve, L., Conditional deficiencies of ornithine or arginine, *J. Am. Coll. Nutr.*, 5, 167–176, 1986.

28. Kirk, S.J. and Barbul, A., Arginine and immunity, in *Encyclopedia of Immunology*, Roitt, I.M. and Delves, P.J., Eds., Academic Press, San Diego, 1992, pp. 160–161.

29. Witte, M.B., Thornton, F.J., Tantry, U., et al., L-arginine supplementation enhances diabetic wound healing: involvement of the nitric oxide synthase and arginine pathways, *Metabolism*, 51, 1269–1272, 2002.

7 B Vitamins and Wound Healing

George U. Liepa, Carol Ireton-Jones,
Hemendra Basu, and Charles R. Baxter

CONTENTS

WATER-SOLUBLE B VITAMINS: WHAT IMPACT DO THEY HAVE ON WOUND HEALING?

B vitamins are organic molecules that must be supplied in foods, because they cannot be produced in the body. They have a multitude of functions in wound healing; however, they are best known for their coenzymatic roles in energy and protein metabolism as well as immune functions. The primary way to classify vitamins is by their level of solubility in water. The water-soluble vitamins include the following B vitamins: vitamin B$_1$ (thiamin), vitamin B$_2$ (riboflavin), vitamin B$_3$ (nicotinic acid or nicotinamide), biotin, vitamin B_5 (pantothenic acid), vitamin B_6 (pyridoxine, pyridoxal, pyridoxamine), folate (folacin, folic acid, pteroyl glutamic acid), and vitamin B_{12} (cobalamin). Each vitamin will be referred to by its most common name throughout this chapter.

Recommended intakes of the B vitamins will be identified as either recommended dietary allowance (RDA) or adequate intake (AI) as defined by the U.S. Department of Agriculture (USDA).[1] The RDA represents the average daily intake of a nutrient which meets the requirements of approximately 98% of all healthy people and is listed related to age and gender. The estimated average requirement is calculated from scientific evidence. When there is not enough scientific evidence about a nutrient to determine a specific estimated average requirement for an RDA, an AI is estimated. While the AI is based on current scientific research, further research is needed to determine a more exact amount of the specific nutrient. The AI is also designed to meet the needs of all healthy children and adults.[1]

Although the role of nutrition in the various phases of wound healing is well recognized, the action of each of the B vitamins in this regard is still being defined. It is clear that the B vitamins have specific metabolic functions, and that they interact with one another in order to ensure that wound-related energy metabolism and tissue synthesis occur appropriately. Studies have shown that B vitamins play initial coenzymatic roles during the inflammatory phase and during the removal of dead tissue and bacteria. B vitamins also have critical roles in the proliferative and remodeling phases of wound healing in that they participate in the synthesis and interlinking of collagen and, therefore, the synthesis of new tissues and blood vessels. During the third or final phase of wound healing, myofibroblasts are dependent on B vitamins when they pull the edges of wounds inward and continue to strengthen the scar for up to 2 yrs.[2] During all phases of wound healing, substantial amounts of energy (kcals) are required for the construction of compounds that are necessary for tissue rebuilding and are inherently dependent on an adequate supply of B vitamins. Multiple vitamin preparations given either intravenously or orally have B vitamins included, and these are routinely given to patients as part of an overall multivitamin regimen. DiBiasse and Wilmore[3] recommended that uncomplicated critically ill patients should be provided with significantly greater amounts of all eight B vitamins as part of their normal care (Table 7.1).

In this chapter, background material about each of the B vitamins including information about normal absorption, metabolism, functions, deficiencies, toxicities, and recommended intakes will be presented. Specific wound-related research data regarding vitamins B_1, B_2, B_5, and B_6 will also be provided.

THIAMINE (VITAMIN B₁)

Thiamine plays a critical role in energy metabolism. It is highly soluble in water and stable to both heat and oxidation at pH < 5.0. The structural formula of thiamine is shown in Figure 7.1.

Because of its structure, thiamine can form ester linkages with various acid groups, allowing for the formation of its active forms (thiamine pyrophosphate [TPP],

TABLE 7.1
Suggested B Vitamin Intakes for Uncomplicated Critically Ill Patients as Compared to Recommended Dietary Allowances (RDA) for Healthy Men and Women

Vitamin	Critically Ill	RDA (men)	RDA (women)
Vitamin B_1	10 mg/day	1.5 mg/day	1.1 mg/day
Vitamin B_2	10 mg/day	1.7 mg/day	1.3 mg/day
Niacin	200 mg/day	19.0 mg/day	15.0 mg/day
Vitamin B_6	20 mg/day	2.0 mg/day	1.6 mg/day
Pantothenic acid	100 mg/day	5.0–7.0 mg/day	same as men
Vitamin B_{12}	20 μgm/day	2.0 μgm/day	2.0 μgm/day
Biotin	5 mg/day	30.0–100.0 μgm/day	same as men
Folic acid	2 mg/day	200 μgm/day	180 μgm/day

thiamine monophosphate [TMP], and thiamine triphosphate [TTP]). There are three enzymes that are known to participate in the formation of these phosphate esters:

1. Thiamine pyrophosphokinase catalyzes the formation of TPP from thiamine and adenosine triphosphate (ATP).
2. TPP-ATP phosphoryl transferase catalyzes the formation of TTP from TPP and ATP.
3. Thiamine pyrophosphatase hydrolyzes TPP to form TMP.

The percentages of the three active forms of thiamine found in the body are 80% TPP, 10% TTP, and 10% TMP and thiamine. Higher concentrations are found in the skeletal muscle (50%), heart, liver, kidneys, and brain.[3]

The absorption of thiamine takes place in the upper part of the small intestine (i.e., duodenum). Oral thiamine is well absorbed and rapidly converted to its phosphorylated forms. It was shown that when the upper section of the small intestine is removed due to ulcers or injury, thiamine absorption is significantly affected by alkaline pH found in the lower intestinal tract. After absorption, thiamine is carried by the hepatic portal system to the liver. In normal adults, 20 to 30% of thiamine in the plasma is protein bound in the form of TPP. The biological

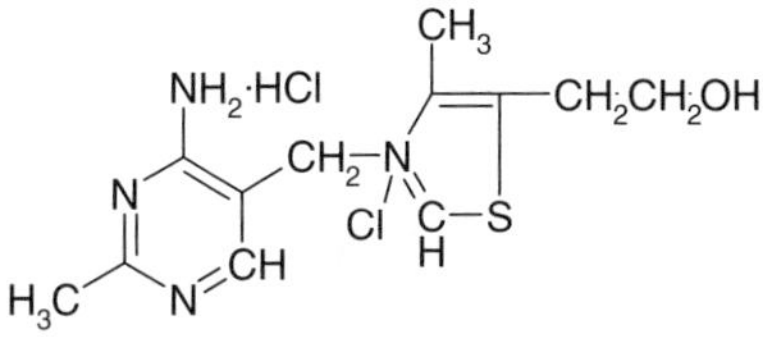

FIGURE 7.1 Vitamin B_1 (thiamine).

half-life of ^{14}C-thiamine in the body is 9 to 18 d.[4] Because thiamine is not stored in large amounts in any tissue, a continuous supply from the diet is necessary.

Thiamine deficiency in animals and humans affects the cardiovascular, muscular, nervous, and gastrointestinal systems, with end results including cardiac failure, muscular weakness, peripheral and central neuropathy, and gastrointestinal malfunction. This broad-based impact is primarily due to the fact that thiamine is required for the conversion of glucose to pyruvate with the help of the coenzyme NAD (nicotinamide adenine dinucleotide). Thiamine pyrophosphate plays a vital role in the energy metabolism of the cells by first converting pyruvate to acetyl coenzyme and CO_2 and also promoting the conversion of a five-carbon compound of tricarboxylic acid (TCA) to a four-carbon compound. It is clear that the main metabolic function of thiamine is in oxidative decarboxylation. Clinically, thiamine deficiency has been shown to cause beriberi, heart disease and, in alcoholics, Wernicke-Korsakoff syndrome. Polyneuropathy is a common problem with this deficiency, because failure of energy metabolism predominantly affects neurons and their functions in selected areas of the central nervous system.

Thiamine deficiency is more common in the elderly. It is also noted to occur in alcoholics. It has been postulated that thiamine deficiency that is induced by excess alcohol intake or liver disease may affect levels of apoenzyme transketolase or its cofactor binding and, thus, prevent the formation of TPP. However, it has been observed that in well-nourished alcoholics, sufficient amounts of thiamine are maintained in the organs, and there is no abnormality in the maintenance of appropriate concentrations of phosphorylated species of thiamine. Acute thiamine deficiency was recently reported in foreign workers who complained of weakness and lower limb edema. One worker died of refractory metabolic acidosis and shock.[5] Thiamine deficiency is also more common in subjects taking diuretics, because thiamine is readily excreted in the urine.[6]

Various biochemical tests are available to detect thiamine deficiency. These include urinary thiamine excretion, thiamine concentrations in cerebral spinal fluid (CSF), erythrocyte transketolase activity (ETKA) and thiamine pyrophosphate effect (TPPE) on ETKA. Presently, there are no known data that indicate that thiamine has toxic effects when large amounts are consumed in the diet or via long-term supplementation.

Thiamine is present in a variety of animal and vegetable food products; however, the best sources are yeast, lean pork, and legumes. A number of compounds are known to be thiamine antagonists or antithiamine factors. These include alcohols, polyphenols, flavonoids, and thiaminase (a heat-labile enzyme found in certain foods).[7] Alcohol has been shown to inhibit intestinal ATP-ase, which is involved in thiamine absorption.[8] The RDA for thiamine in the United States is 0.5 mg/1000 kcal/day.[8]

THIAMINE AND WOUND HEALING

Although most of the research regarding thiamine deficiency has focused on the role it plays in the TCA cycle and ATP synthesis, some work has analyzed its role in wound healing. In a study done by Ostrovskii and Nikitin[9] using hypovitaminotic white mice as experimental models, thiamine deficiency was induced by feeding a thiamine-deficient diet for 30 d or by supplying animals with a thiamine antagonist (oxythiamine) for the same period of time. When this type of deficiency was produced in mice and then followed by mechanical trauma, a delay in necrotic mass resorption was noted 2 to 3 d after the trauma. An inhibition in the reparative process was also recorded. This effect on both resorption and repair was shown to be associated with a decrease in macrocytic activity. Macrocyte cytoplasm was shown to have a decreased volume fraction of both lysosomes and phagosomes. Differentiation of fibroblasts was also delayed in these animals. It was proposed that these alterations in macrophages played a major role in delayed wound healing.

Thiamine's impact on wound repair has also been studied using rat models. Alvarez and Gilbreath[10] showed that inadequate thiamine intake also leads to a decrease in the tensile strength of wounds in thiamine-deficient animals. The focus of this study was on the breaking strength of excised wounds, the isometric shrink tension of skin, and the lysyl oxidase activity of both normal and repairing skin. Lysyl oxidase was analyzed, because it controls one of the initial steps in the cross-linking of elastin and collagen. Three groups of rats were fed either a thiamine-deficient diet or a thiamine-deficient diet that was supplemented with either 1 or 3 mg of thiamine HCl. Deficiency was established via measurement of urinary thiamine concentrations, and at this time, the animals were wounded. Ten days later, significant differences were noted in both isometric shrink tension and breaking strength of all three groups. Lysyl oxidase activity was significantly different between control animals and those provided with 1 mg of thiamine HCL.

RIBOFLAVIN (VITAMIN B$_2$)

Riboflavin plays a critical role in protein metabolism and is a key component of the oxidative phosphorylation enzyme system that is intimately involved in the production of cellular energy. Its chemical structure is shown in Figure 7.2.

Riboflavin is primarily absorbed in the proximal small intestine, and uptake is facilitated by bile salts. Transport in the blood is accomplished via attachment to protein complexes (i.e., albumin). Very little riboflavin is stored in the body, and therefore, urinary excretion of metabolites (7- and 8-hydroxymethylflavins; i.e., 7-α-hydroxyriboflavin) reflects dietary intake.

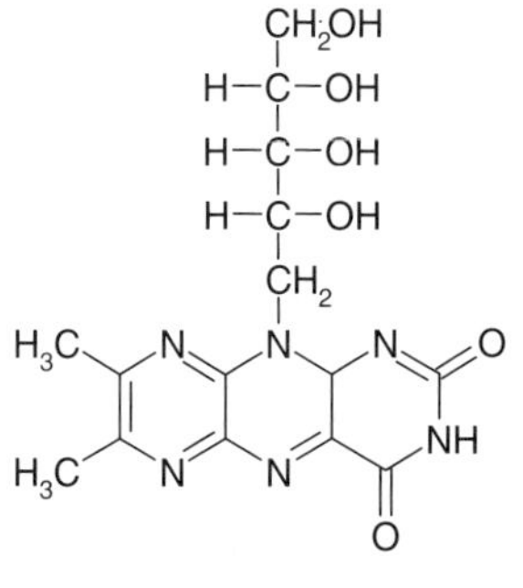

FIGURE 7.2 Vitamin B$_2$ (riboflavin).

The coenzyme forms of riboflavin are flavin mononucleotide (FMN) and flavin adenine dinucleotide (FAD). Riboflavin is converted to its coenzyme forms within the cellular cytoplasm of most tissues, but particularly in the small intestine, liver, heart, and kidney. In this process, FMN forms of riboflavin are complexed with specific active enzymes to form several functional flavoproteins, but most of it is further converted to FAD. Thus, the biosynthesis of flavo-coenzymes is tightly regulated and dependent on riboflavin status. Thyroxine and triiodothyroxine stimulate FMN and FAD synthesis in mammalian systems. Riboflavin has been shown to participate in oxidation-reduction reactions in numerous metabolic pathways and in energy production via the respiratory chain. A variety of chemical reactions are catalyzed by flavoproteins.[4]

When a riboflavin deficiency occurs, its symptoms include sore throat, cheilosis, angular stomatitis, glossitis, seborrheic dermatitis, and normocytic, normochromic anemia. Riboflavin deficiencies have rarely been reported. Riboflavin toxicities are almost never reported; however, electroencephalographic abnormalities have been mentioned as a rare side effect of excessive riboflavin intake.[4]

Riboflavin is present in a variety of foods. Some of the best sources are eggs, lean meats, milk, broccoli, and enriched breads and cereals. The RDA for riboflavin in adolescent and adult males is 1.3 mg/d, whereas in adolescent females, it is 1.0 mg/d, and in adult females it is 1.1 mg/d.[8]

RIBOFLAVIN AND WOUND HEALING

Riboflavin has an impact on wound healing through the general role it plays in hypermetabolic tissues with electron transport and protein/amino acid metabolism as well as its more specific function in tissue repair, and so forth. Specific roles in this process have been established via small animal (rat) research. Research done in the laboratories of Lakshmi et al.[11,12] has shown that riboflavin is involved in all of the phases of the wound repair process. In their initial studies,[10] rat models were used to examine the relationship between riboflavin deficiency and the healing of both excision and incision wounds. When riboflavin-deficient animals were compared to controls or fasted animals, the period for epithelialization of excision wounds was 4 to 5 d longer in riboflavin-deficient animals compared to weight-matched ad libitum-fed control animals. Riboflavin deficiency as well as food restriction was shown to slow the rate of wound contraction, with riboflavin deficiency having the greater impact of the two treatments. The tensile strength of incision wounds was also reduced 42% in deficient animals when compared to ad libitum-fed controls and 63% compared to weight-matched controls. Total collagen content of incision wounds was also shown to decrease by 25%. Food restriction had similar effects but of lower magnitude. Data suggested that the alteration of collagen content and maturity was responsible for the lower tensile strength in the incision wounds of the riboflavin-deficient rats. This data supported earlier studies by Bosse and Axelrod[13] in which riboflavin deficiency was associated with delayed epithelialization of wounds and by Prasad et al.[14,15] in which riboflavin-deficient rats were shown, both quantitatively and qualitatively, to have impaired collagen synthesis and cross-linking. The proposed mechanism for this impaired cross-linking of collagen involves riboflavin's role as a carbonyl cofactor for lysyl oxidase activity and the role this enzyme plays in the cross-linking process.[16,17]

In a subsequent study, Lakshmi et al.[11] studied the inflammatory response in riboflavin-deficient rats. In this study, the animals, after having their paws injured, showed a 54% and 52% reduction in critical enzyme activity (nicotinamide adenine dinucleotide phosphate [NADPH] oxidase and superoxide dismutase, respectively) in leukocytes elicited from the peritoneal cavity. Food restriction did not seem to affect this leukocyte enzyme activity. It was concluded that riboflavin deficiency did not enhance inflammation in this model.

The impact that riboflavin has on incisional wound healing has also been studied indirectly by Elbanna et al.[18] Thirty-eight surgical patients were monitored for wound healing. The patients were split into two groups with 22 in the control group and 16 in the experimental group. The control subjects were provided with the same meals that other surgical patients received. Experimental subjects were monitored in regards to their diet using a 24 h diet recall system for the 3 d prior to and after surgery. Diets were then modified to optimize nutritional support. Preoperative diet analysis data were used to determine appropriate modifications in nutrition support. Those patients who were found to need preoperative repletion received calories and proteins at levels that were 30 to 50% above maintenance, and minerals, vitamins, and fluids for normal recovery were provided. A wound healing checklist was used to establish recovery. The experimental group had a significantly better score for wound healing than did the control group and the group also had a shorter hospital stay. In the postoperative stage, the dietary intake of riboflavin, as well as protein, iron, calcium, and vitamin A was better than in the control population.

High riboflavin intake is not known to have toxic effects on humans. Some research has shown that when riboflavin and chromium are combined in cell cultures, there is an increase in DNA strand breaks.[19]

NIACIN (VITAMIN B₃)

Niacin is the term that is commonly used for nicotinamide and nicotinic acid. It is best known for its role as a component of two active coenzymes NAD and nicotinamide adenine dinucleotide phosphate (NADP) that play key roles in energy metabolism. The structure of niacin is shown in Figure 7.3. This vitamin can also be made in the body from tryptophan, a relatively common amino acid.

Niacin absorption occurs readily in the intestine. Approximately 25% of niacin is carried through the blood bound to protein. Niacin is easily absorbed by adipocytes; however, it is poorly stored in the body, and excess amounts are generally excreted in the urine as niacin and nicotinamide metabolites.

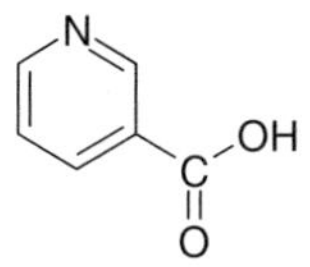

FIGURE 7.3 Vitamin B₃ (niacin).

Niacin functions primarily as a constituent of key nucleotide-containing enzymes that play critical roles in oxidation-reduction reactions as well as ATP synthesis and adenosine diphosphate (ADP)-ribose transfer reactions. NAD is converted into NADP in the mammalian liver. NADP can also be converted to NAD. NAD plays a critical role in catabolic reactions, where it transfers the potential free energy stored in micronutrients, such as carbohydrates, lipids, and proteins, to NADH, which is then used to form ATP, the primary energy currency of the cell. NADP-dependent enzymes are preferentially involved in anabolic reactions, such as the synthesis of fatty acids and cholesterol.

Another key role played by NAD is in DNA repair. By serving as an ingredient in the formation of a DNA polymerase (poly [ADP ribose] polymerase, PARP) it plays a critical role in DNA maintenance. It has been suggested that proper repair of DNA damage would require functional PARP and abundant NAD. The current hypothesis is that if a small amount of DNA damage occurs, PARP activity can repair it, whereas, if more DNA damage occurs, a functional PARP would trigger apoptosis (cell death) probably via NAD depletion.

Increased niacin intake has been proposed to be of benefit for a wide variety of disorders, including diabetes, atherosclerosis, arthritis, and cataracts. High doses of niacin have been used to prevent the development of atherosclerosis and to reduce recurrent complications, such as heart attacks and peripheral vascular disease. Niacin is commonly used to lower elevated low-density lipoprotein (LDL) cholesterol and triglyceride levels in the blood and is more effective in increasing high-density lipoprotein (HDL) levels than other cholesterol-lowering medications. Researchers also found that the combination of niacin and the cholesterol-lowering drug Simvastatin (Merck and Company, Whitehouse Station, New Jersey) may slow the progression of heart disease, reducing risk of a heart attack, and even death.[20] Although niacin has been shown to boost HDL cholesterol and decrease triglyceride and LDL cholesterol concentrations, there has been some concern that it may raise blood glucose concentrations. In a recent study involving 125 diabetics and 343 controls, it was shown that high doses of niacin (roughly 3000 mg/d) increased blood glucose concentrations in both groups, but hemoglobin A1C concentration (considered a better measure of blood glucose overtime) actually decreased in the diabetics over a 60 week follow-up period.[21]

It was also suggested in some preliminary studies that an active form of niacin (niacinamide) may improve symptoms of arthritis, including increased joint mobility and a reduced need for anti-inflammatory medications. Researchers[22] speculate that dietary niacin may aid in cartilage repair (damage to joint cartilage causes arthritis) and suggest that it may be used safely along with nonsteroidal anti-inflammatory medications to reduce inflammation. It was also suggested that long-term use (at least 3 yr) may slow the progression of arthritis. Niacin, along with other nutrients, is also important for the maintenance of normal vision and the prevention of cataracts.[23] Severe niacin (nicotinic acid)/tryptophan deficiency has historically been associated with the development of pellagra. This disease has four primary symptoms that are often referred to as the 4 "D"s (diarrhea, dermatitis, dementia, and death).

The Food and Nutrition Board has set the tolerable upper intake level (UL) of niacin at 35 mg/d because of high intakes being associated with flushing of the face, arms, and chest. This limit is not meant to apply to patients under a physician's care who are being treated for hypercholesterolemia.[8]

The best source of niacin is milk. Other sources are organ meats, whole grains, and some vegetables. The 1998 RDAs for niacin for men and women were 16 and 14 mg of NE (niacin equivalents)/d, respectively.[8] American women and men consume an average of 700 mg and 1100 mg of tryptophan, respectively, per day, which represents 16 and 24 NE for women and men, respectively.

NIACIN AND WOUND HEALING

Niacin's specific role in wound healing has not been established. It is clear that the B vitamins work together to ensure normal energy metabolism and cell division. Niacin is a key player in both of these essential steps of tissue repair.

BIOTIN

Biotin (see Figure 7.4) acts as an energy metabolism coenzyme and is necessary for a maintaining a variety of normal functions in the body. Biotin is primarily absorbed from the small intestine; however, it has also been shown to be absorbed via the colon after it is synthesized by enteric flora. Biotin plays an important role in cells as a carbon dioxide carrier, and it has been shown to deliver a carbon molecule that is used in the formation of three-carbon pyruvate and eventually acetyl CoA. This process is vital for keeping the TCA cycle functioning. Biotin also plays critical roles in gluconeogenesis, fatty acid synthesis, and fatty acid and amino acids breakdown. Hymes and Wolf[24] proposed that biotin, by binding to histones, may also play a role in DNA replication and transcription.

Biotin is needed for normal growth and the maintenance of healthy hair, skin, nerves, bone marrow, and sex glands. Biotin deficiency symptoms include hair loss and the development of a scaly rash around the mouth, eyes, nose, and genital area. Depression and lethargy as well as numbness and tingling in the extremities have also been observed. Most recently, biotin deficiency has been associated with non-insulin-dependent diabetes mellitus. When these subjects are provided with biotin, there is a significant decrease in fasting blood glucose concentrations. It was proposed that biotin may increase glucose conversion to fatty acids and also may increase insulin secretion.[25]

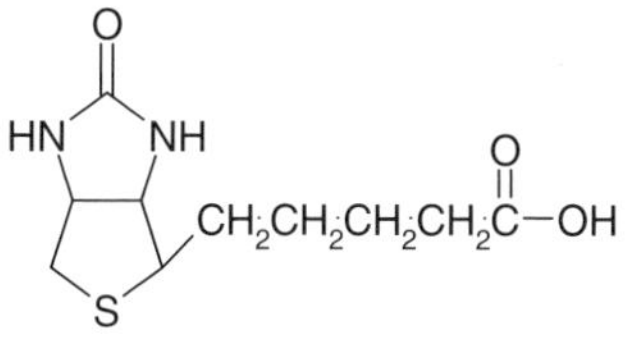

FIGURE 7.4 Biotin.

The Institute of Medicine did not establish a tolerable upper level of intake for biotin, because it is not known to be toxic.[8] One case report of a negative reaction (development of eosinophilic pleuropericardial effusion) was noted for an elderly woman who consumed large quantities of biotin (10 mg/d) and pantothenic acid (300 mg/d) for 2 months.[26]

Recommendations for daily intake have not been established, but the estimated safe and adequate intake for Americans has been determined to be between 30 to 100 µg/d and for Canadians 1.5 µg/kg body weight/d.[8] Good food sources of biotin include cooked eggs, cooked liver, whole grain products, and fish. Certain drugs interact with biotin and would alter the amounts needed in the diet. Specific families of drugs include some anticonvulsants, which impact on both absorption and excretion, and antibiotics that destroy bacteria in the gastrointestinal tract that normally produce biotin.

BIOTIN AND WOUND HEALING

Biotin's pivotal role in converting glucose to ATP makes it extremely important in the wound healing process. Research has not been done to establish the specific impact that biotin has on wound recovery.

PANTOTHENIC ACID (VITAMIN B$_5$)

Pantothenic acid is an important cofactor of CoA and is essential for the completion of biologic acetylation reactions, as illustrated by the formation of sulfonamide in the liver and choline in the brain. The structure of pantothenic acid is shown in Figure 7.5.

Pantothenic acid is ingested in its CoA form and is then hydrolyzed in the intestine to pantothenic acid, which is then absorbed into the bloodstream. Pantothenate containing CoA is essential for the maintenance of the respiratory TCA cycle, fatty acid synthesis, and the degradation of a variety of other compounds. All of the enzymes required for CoA synthesis are present in cell cytoplasm. Mitochondria are the final site of CoA synthesis, because 95% of CoA is found in mitochondria, and CoA does not cross the mitochondria membranes. Multiple hydrolytic steps liberate pantothenic acid from CoA and allow for it to eventually be excreted in the urine. Pantothenic acid has also been shown to be required for the synthesis of key amino acids (methionine, leucine, and arginine).[3]

Pantothenic acid deficiencies are rare in humans, because this vitamin is found in so many sources of our diet. Severe malnutrition leads to pantothenic acid deficiency with symptoms that include painful burning sensations in the feet and

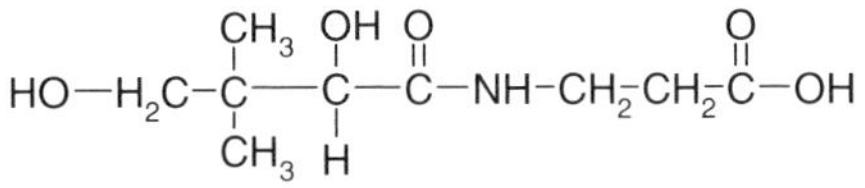

$$HO-H_2C-\underset{\underset{CH_3}{|}}{\overset{\overset{CH_3}{|}}{C}}-\underset{\underset{H}{|}}{\overset{\overset{OH}{|}}{C}}-\overset{O}{\overset{||}{C}}-NH-CH_2CH_2C-OH$$

FIGURE 7.5 Vitamin B$_5$ (pantothenic acid).

numbness in the toes. When pantothenic acid antagonists are provided along with a pantothenic acid deficient diet, headaches, fatigue, and insomnia have been noted.

The Food and Nutrition Board of the Institute of Medicine did not establish a tolerable upper level of intake (UL) for pantothenic acid, because it is well tolerated in large amounts and has no known toxic effects in humans.[8] Very high intakes of calcium D-pantothenate have been shown to result in diarrhea.[27]

Because inadequate data are available to set an RDA for pantothenic acid, the Food and Nutrition Board of the Institute of Medicine has set an AI of 5 mg/d for male and female adolescents as well as adults.[8] Sources of this vitamin include liver, egg yolk, yogurt, avocados, milk, sweet potatoes, broccoli, and cooked chicken.

PANTOTHENIC ACID AND WOUND HEALING

In a number of animal studies, oral pantothenic acid or topically applied panthenol was shown to accelerate the closure of skin wounds.[28–31] Most of the mechanistic research done in this area involves looking at the impact pantothenic acid has on fibroblast function and concomitant wound closure and scar formation. Substantial amounts of work have also focused on how pantothenic acid enhances both collagen synthesis and collagen cross-linking and the role this vitamin plays in altering trace elements that have an impact on wound healing.

Because fibroblasts play such an important role in collagen formation, pantothenic acid has also been studied in regard to its effect on fibroblast migration, proliferation, and protein synthesis.[32] In a fibroblast culture study conducted by Weimann and Hermann,[33] it was observed that human dermal fibroblast migration into a wounded area was dose-dependently stimulated by calcium (Ca) D-pantothenate. The number of fibroblasts that migrated across the edge of the wound in their study when Ca D-pantothenate was not present was 32 ± 7 cells/mm. When 100 mg/ml of Ca D-pantothenate was present in the medium, this increased to 76 ± 2 cells/mm. Moreover, the mean migration distance/cell increased from 0.23 ± 0.05 mm to 0.33 ± 0.02 mm. The mean fibroblast migration speed increased from 10.5 mm/h when there was no Ca D-pantothenate to 15 mm/h when it was present. It was concluded in this study that Ca D-pantothenate accelerated the wound healing process by increasing the number of migrating cells, their distance, and their speed. Cell division and protein synthesis both were increased with the addition of Ca D-pantothenate to the culture.

In a study by Lacroix et al.,[34] pantothenic acid's impact on protein metabolism in foreskin fibroblast cultures was determined. In these cultures, the addition of pantothenic acid led to a significant increase in cell proliferation and in 3H-thymidine incorporation. It was also noted that pantothenic acid stimulated intracellular protein synthesis but did not induce a release of proteins into the culture medium. In a separate but similar study,[32] it was shown that pantothenic acid increased the basal incorporation of ^{14}C-proline into precipitated material, and that the release of intracellular protein into the medium increased. The authors concluded that pantothenic acid might be of use in postsurgical therapy and wound healing for improvement of fibroblast activity as it is related to protein metabolism.

Studies have also been done with subjects who have had tattoos removed to determine the impact pantothenic acid has on the actual strength of scar tissue.[35] In this study, 18 of 49 patients were supplemented for 21 d with both pantothenic acid (0.2 g/d) and vitamin C (1.0 g/d) prior to the removal of tattoos by successive resection. Hydroxyproline and trace element concentrations were measured in both skin and scar tissue. Fibroblast counts and mechanical properties of the scar tissue were also established. In the patients who received supplements, it was shown that the concentration of iron (Fe) in the skin increased, whereas manganese decreased; in scar tissue, Fe, copper (Cu), and manganese (Mn) decreased, and magnesium (Mg) increased. This type of mineral analysis is considered to be of importance, because ferrous Fe "overload" has been shown to have a negative effect on the wound healing process and to cause an increase in toxic hydroxyl radicals at the site of injury,[36] with the concomitant development of a "poor" scar, whereas supplemental Cu improves collagen synthesis and seems to be involved in the cross-linking of collagen molecules.[37] More specifically, lysyl oxidase has been shown to be involved in the cross-linking of collagen and elastin and requires a carbonyl cofactor in addition to Cu.[17,38,39] It was also suggested that pyridoxal may act as the carbonyl cofactor. Cu was also shown to increase the activity of radical scavenging enzymes.[40] Zinc (Zn) was shown to be a cofactor for more than 200 metalloenzymes that are involved in cellular growth as well as protein and collagen synthesis. When riboflavin is supplemented, Zn increases in scars, leading to a decrease in bacterial growth and an improvement in the inflammatory process of skin wound healing. In the present study, mechanical properties of scars in group A were correlated to the status of Fe, Cu, and Zn, with Zn and Cu both shown to be increased at the wound site. The authors proposed that this was of benefit, because both trace elements are known to improve collagen cross-linking[41,42] as well as increase the activity of free radical scavenging enzymes.[40] It was proposed that Fe might impair wound healing by catalyzing the production of toxic radicals.[36] Results of this study suggested that benefits associated with ascorbic acid and pantothenic acid supplementation could be due to the variations in the trace element concentrations, as they are associated with the immunological response as well as the mechanical properties of scars.

Another study that focused on the mechanical properties of scars was done by Aprahamian et al.[41] In this study, rabbits were provided with pantothenic acid supplements prior to having two colonic segments removed and then having continuity restored. Control animals received placebos prior to surgery. On the third postoperative day, the animals were killed, and the anastomoses were removed. Mechanical properties of both normal colon and anastomoses were determined using bursting pressure tests and tabulating the number of burst anastomoses. Other tests performed included fibroblast counts, hydroxyproline concentrations, and trace element content microanalysis for Mg, P, sulfur (S), sodium (Na), Fe, Cu, Zn, and manganese (Mn). Pantothenic acid decreased the number of burst anastomoses and restored normal Zn levels at the anastomotic site. Pantothenic acid supplementation also increased Fe, Cu, and Mn concentrations, all of which are intimately involved in collagen formation. It was clear that pantothenic acid enhanced colonic wound healing.

PYRIDOXINE (VITAMIN B₆)

Vitamin B_6 plays a critical role in protein metabolism and occurs in three forms in the body as pyridoxine, pyridoxal, and pyridoxamine. All three forms of vitamin B_6 are relatively stable in an acidic medium but are not heat stable under alkaline conditions. The active coenzyme forms are pyridoxal 5′-phosphate (PLP) and pyridoxamine-5′-phosphate (PMP) (see Figure 7.6).

All forms of vitamin B_6 are absorbed in the upper part of the small intestine. They are phosphorylated within the mucosal cells to form PLP and PMP. PLP can be oxidized further to form other metabolites that are excreted in the urine. Vitamin B_6 is stored in muscle tissues.

PLP plays an important role in amino acid metabolism. It has the ability to transfer amino groups from compounds by removing an amino acid from one component and adding to another. This allows the body to synthesize nonessential amino acids when amino groups become available. The ability of PLP to add and remove amino groups makes it invaluable for protein and urea metabolism. Vitamin B_6 is transferred in the blood both in plasma and in red blood cells. PLP and PMP can both be bound to albumin, with PLP binding more tightly, or to hemoglobin in the red blood cell. The liver is the primary organ responsible for the metabolism of vitamin B_6 metabolites. As a result, the liver supplies the active form of PLP to the blood as well as to other tissues. The three nonphosphorylated forms of vitamin B_6 are converted to their respective phosphorylated forms by pyridoxine kinase, with Zn and ATP as cofactors. PMP and pyridoxine can then be converted to PLP by flavin mononucleotide (FMN) oxidase.

It was shown in both animal and human studies that a low intake of vitamin B_6 causes impaired immune function due to decreased interleukin-2 production and lymphocyte proliferation. It was also demonstrated that PLP inhibits the binding of steroid receptors to DNA and may, therefore, impact on endocrine-mediated diseases. It was suggested that reactions between physiologic concentrations of PLP and receptors for estrogen, androgen, progesterone, and glucocorticoids depend on the vitamin B_6 status of an individual.

A number of vitamin B_6 antagonists have been identified, including certain food additives, oral contraceptives, and alcohol.[43] When alcohol is broken down in the body, acetaldehyde is produced, and acetaldehyde knocks PLP loose from its enzyme, which is broken down and then excreted. Thus, alcohol abuse causes a loss of vitamin B_6 from the body. Some drugs have been shown to be vitamin B_6 antagonists, including cycloserine, ethionarnide, furfural, hydralazine, isoniazid,

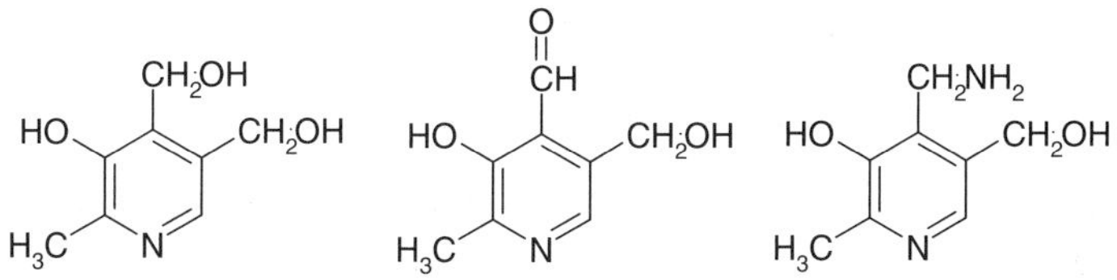

FIGURE 7.6 Vitamin B_6 (pyridoxine).

isonicotinic acid, L-dopa, penicillamin, pyrazinamide, theophylline, and thiosemi-carbizones.[44] Another drug that acts as a vitamin B_6 antagonist is INH (isonicotinic acid hydrazide), a potent inhibitor of the growth of the tuberculosis bacterium. INH binds and inactivates the vitamin, inducing a vitamin B_6 deficiency. In a number of disease states, it has been shown that apparent alterations of vitamin B_6 metabolism can cause concomitant alterations in tryptophan metabolism. These alterations have been observed in patients with asthma, diabetes, breast and bladder cancers, renal disease, coronary heart disease, and sickle cell anemia.

High-protein diets have been shown to alter vitamin B_6 requirements, because vitamin B_6 coenzymes play important roles in amino acid metabolism. The RDA for vitamin B_6 is 1.3 mg/d for adolescent and adult males up to the age of 50 and 1.7 mg/d for those age 51 and older. For women, the requirements are 1.2 mg/d for adolescents, 1.3 mg/d for adults until they reach the age of 50, and 1.5 mg/d for those who are age 51 yr and older.[8] When vitamin B_6 is deficient in the diet, symptoms include weakness, irritability, and insomnia. Advanced symptoms include growth failure, impaired motor function, and convulsions.

Vitamin B_6 toxicity can arise if one routinely takes large doses of it over a lengthy period of time. This process may cause irreversible sensory neuropathy and nerve damage. Intakes of 200 mg/d or less show no evidence of damage; however, levels of 500 to 1000 mg/d have been associated with sensory damage.[45]

Excellent food sources include fortified cereal, baked potatoes (with skin), meats, fish, poultry, and green vegetables. The RDA for vitamin B_6 in adolescent and adult males under the age of 50 yr is 1.3 mg/d, whereas for older adults, it is 1.7 mg/d. The RDA for females is 1.2, 1.3, and 1.5 mg/d, respectively, for adolescents, adults under the age of 51 yr, and adults over the age of 51 yr.[8]

VITAMIN B_6 AND WOUND HEALING

Vitamin B_6 has been studied in regards to its role in inflammatory response. In rat studies by Lakshmi et al.,[12] it was reported that pyridoxine deficiency led to increases in thiobarbituric acid reactive substance levels (30% and 43%, respectively) in the edematous paw and wounded skin. This is significant, because thiobarbituric acid concentrations are good indicators of lipid peroxidation. It was concluded that inflammation is enhanced when these animals are pyridoxine deficient.

It was also shown that vitamin B_6 deficiency causes marked diminution in the glucose 6-phosphate dehydrogenase (G6PD) activity in the periosteal region of bone formation and in the developing callous. This causes a significant delay in the maturation of the callus. Deficiencies also caused changes in the bones that are suggestive of imbalance in the coupling between osteoblasts and osteoclasts. These results suggest that vitamin B_6 status is important in the healing of fractures of bones.

FOLACIN (VITAMIN B_9)

Folic acid, or folate, consists of a pteridine base that is attached to one molecule each of P-aminobenzoic acid (PABA) and glutamic acid. Folacin is the generic term used for folic acid and related substances that act like folic acid. The structure is shown in Figure 7.7.

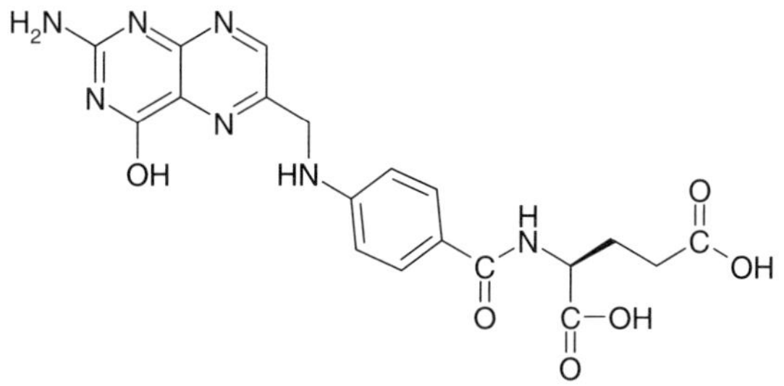

FIGURE 7.7 Vitamin B₉ (folacin).

Folic acid has been shown to be involved in the transfer of one-carbon units, as well as in the metabolism of both nucleic acids and amino acids. Because of this, symptoms of deficiencies include anemia as well as an increase in serum homocysteine concentrations.

Folate derivatives in the diet are cleaved by specific intestinal enzymes to prepare monoglutamyl folate (MGF) for absorption. Most MGF is reduced to tetrahydrofolate (THF) in the intestinal cells by the enzyme folate reductase. This enzyme uses NADPH as a donor of reducing equivalents. Tetrahydrofolate polyglutamates are the functional coenzymes in tissues. The folate coenzymes participate in reactions by carrying one-carbon compounds from one molecule to another. Thus, glycine can be converted to a three-carbon amino acid, serine, with the help of folate coenzymes. This action helps convert vitamin B_{12} to one of its active coenzyme forms and helps synthesize the DNA required for all rapidly growing cells. Enzymes on the intestinal cell surface, while hydrolyzing polyglutamate to monoglutamate, attach a methyl group. Special transport systems then help to deliver monoglutamate to the liver and other body cells. Folate is only stored in polyglutamate forms. When the need arises, it is converted back to monoglutamate and released. Excess folate is disposed of by the liver into bile fluid and stored in the gallbladder until it is released into the small intestine. An important role served by methyl THF is the methylation of homocysteine to methionine. Methylcobalamin serves as a cofactor along with vitamin B_{12}. If these vitamins are missing, folate becomes trapped inside cells in its methyl form, unavailable to support DNA synthesis and cell growth.

Because folate is repeatedly reabsorbed, any injury to gastrointestinal tract cells causes an interference with absorption, and folate is lost from the body. The cells lining the gastrointestinal tract are the most rapidly renewed cells in the body, so not only will the folate be lost, but also other nutrients will not be absorbed.

Folate deficiency impairs both cell division and protein synthesis. Deficiencies of this vitamin are found most often in older people whose primary symptom is megaloblastic anemia. Another symptom is an increase in homocysteine concentrations. Deficiencies can also occur in patients who have cancer, skin-destroying diseases, and severe burns. Of all the vitamins, folate is most vulnerable to interactions with drugs, because some drugs have chemical structures similar to the vitamin.

High intake of folate from foods has not been shown to have negative side effects. The Food and Nutrition Board of the Institute of Medicine recommends that adults limit their intake of vitamin B_{12} to 1 mg/d in the treatment of megaloblastic anemia, and take care to ensure that the vitamin B_{12} deficiency does not mask a folate deficiency.[8] This is critical, because misdiagnosis can result in irreversible neurological damage.

The RDA for folate in dietary folate equivalents (DFEs) is 400 mcg/d in both male and female adolescents and adults.[8] Because animals cannot synthesize PABA or attach glutamic acid to pteroic acid, folate must be obtained from the diet. Common sources of folate are green leafy vegetables, fortified breakfast cereal, orange juice, and cooked pasta and rice.[8]

No adverse effects have been associated with excessive intake of folate from food sources.

FOLIC ACID AND WOUND HEALING

Although specific studies have not been done in which folate needs are established in wound healing, the fact that this vitamin is required for the synthesis of DNA and for the methylation of DNA, as well as the metabolism of a number of important amino acids that are involved in the homocysteine/methionine pathway make it a critical vitamin for both before and after wound healing.

VITAMIN B_{12} (COBALAMIN)

Vitamin B_{12} (cobalamin; see Figure 7.8) is synthesized exclusively by microorganisms. Although vitamin B_{12} is absent from plants, it is synthesized by bacteria and is stored by the liver in animals as methyl cobalamin, adenosyl cobalamin, and hydroxyl cobalamin. Intrinsic factor (a highly specific glycoprotein in gastric secretions) is necessary for absorption of vitamin B_{12}. After absorption, the vitamin is bound by a plasma protein (transcobalamin II) that transports it to various tissues. It is also stored in the liver in this form. The active coenzyme forms of vitamin B_{12} are methyl cobalamin and deoxyadenosyl cobalamin. In the blood, free cobalamin is released into the cytosol of cells as hydroxycobalamin. It is then either converted in the cytosol to methyl cobalamin or it enters mitochondria where it is converted to 5-deoxyadenosyl cobalamin. The methyl group bound to cobalamin is eventually transferred to homocysteine to form methionine, and the remaining cobalamin then removes the methyl group from N^5-methyl tetrahydrofolate to form tetrahydrofolate (THF). Thus, in this metabolic process, methionine is stored, and THF is available to participate in purine, pyrimidine, and nucleic acid synthesis.[46]

A deficiency of vitamin B_{12} leads to the development of megaloblastic anemia. This deficiency can be caused by pernicious anemia, a condition in which an autoimmune inflammation occurs in the stomach that leads to a breakdown in the cells lining the stomach. Because the final result is a decrease in acid production, vitamin B_{12} cannot be released from food. Treatment of pernicious anemia requires vitamin B_{12} injections or high-dose supplementation. Approximately 2% of all adults over 60 yr of age have pernicious anemia.[7] True vegetarians are at risk of vitamin B_{12} deficiency, because this vitamin is found only in foods of animal origin.

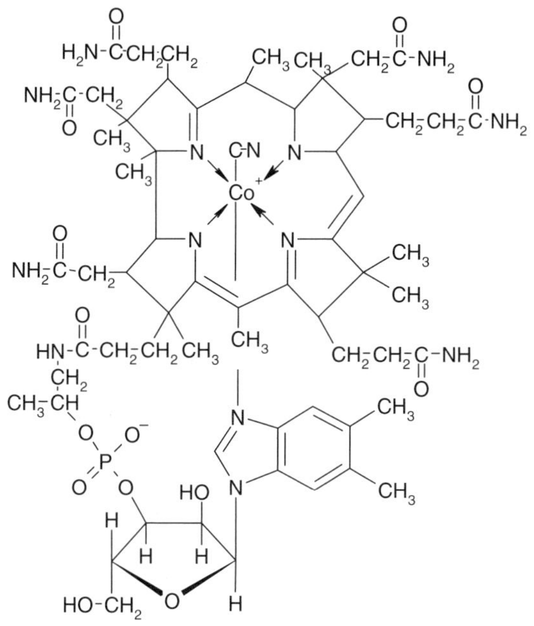

FIGURE 7.8 Vitamin B$_{12}$ (cobalamin).

A deficiency of this vitamin causes impairment in the methionine synthase reaction. Anemia is the result of impaired DNA synthesis, thus preventing cell division and formation of the nucleus of new erythrocytes, with consequent accumulation in the bone marrow of megaloblastic red blood cells.

A number of drugs have been shown to decrease absorption, including gastric acid inhibitors (Tagamet [GlaxoSmithKline], Pepcid [Merck and Co., Inc.], and Zantac [Warner Lambert Co.]) and proton pump inhibitors (omeprazole and lansoprazole).[47] Other drugs that inhibit absorption of vitamin B$_{12}$ include cholestyramine (cholesterol binding agent), neomycin (antibiotic), and colchicine (gout treatment). A drug used in the treatment of adult onset diabetes (Metformin [Mylan Laboratories]) requires use with calcium-containing foods in order to allow for vitamin B$_{12}$ absorption.[48]

The RDA for vitamin B$_{12}$ is 2.4 mcg/d for adolescent and adult males and females.[8] Food sources are found only in animal products such as cooked beef, salmon, and milk.

No toxic effects have been associated with intake of vitamin B$_{12}$.

VITAMIN B$_{12}$ AND WOUND HEALING

Although specific studies have not been done that illustrate a direct relationship between vitamin B$_{12}$ and wound healing, it is clear that its fundamental roles in the maintenance of red blood cells make it an important component of nutrition support before and after the wound was sustained.

B-VITAMIN INTAKE

It is critical that B vitamins be included in the diet in adequate amounts as specified by the RDA or AI. B vitamins work in concert with each other, for example, if vitamin B_{12} deficiency is suspected, folate status should also be checked. People who are especially at risk of B-vitamin deficiency are those who have a history of alcoholism or those who have had a nutrient-deficient diet, such as older people or those who are poor or malnourished due to disease or malabsorption. If deficiencies are found, these should be corrected with supplemental B vitamins either individually or as a multiple vitamin.

When an oral diet is inadequate, B vitamins can be provided as a supplement in a multivitamin form that can be swallowed, or it can be provided in a liquid form. Most commercially available enteral (tube feeding) formulas have adequate amounts of B vitamins at a minimal level of formula intake. Higher levels of formula based on increased caloric needs should not pose a problem with toxicity for B vitamins.[49,50] Patients who receive parenteral nutrition as their sole source or major source of nutrition support should be receiving an intravenous multivitamin product with adequate amounts of B vitamins. Individual B vitamins are also available in various forms to accommodate the absorptive capacity of the patient with wounds. If a nutrient deficiency is suspected and confirmed, supplementation will be necessary to bring the level to within normal limits.

Wound healing is dependent on B vitamins in a variety of ways. Both laboratory and clinical research indicate that the B vitamins are involved in all three phases of wound development. Studies have shown that B vitamins play a part in necrotic resorption, immunological response to infection, and the actual repair of wounds. These data also show that specific aspects of the recovery process are improved, such as fibroblast function and collagen synthesis and cross-linking. B vitamins should be provided in amounts that meet the RDA or AI and supplemented when deficient in order to assure that their functions in wound healing can be accomplished.

FUTURE DIRECTIONS FOR RESEARCH

B vitamins have been treated as the neglected stepchild in the field of "nutrition and wound healing." It is clear that this family of vitamins plays a monumental role in wound healing in both the tissue repair process and in the optimization of immune function. Unfortunately, some of these vitamins (niacin, biotin, folacin, and vitamin B_{12}) have not been individually studied in regard to their specific roles in the healing process. In general, more work needs to be done to establish specific roles for the B vitamins in wound healing and to determine how they interact with each other to allow for a successful outcome in the healing process.

REFERENCES

1. Dietary Reference Intakes (RFI) and Recommended Dietary Allowances (RDA), Food and Nutrition Information Center, www.nal.usda.gov/fnic/etext/000105.html.
2. Leininger, S.M., The role of nutrition in wound healing, *Crit. Care Nursing Q.*, 25 (1), 13, 2002.

3. DeBiasse, M.A. and Wilmore, D.W., What is optimal nutrition support?, *New Horizons*, 2 (20), 122, 1994.

4. Shils, M.E. et al., Thiamin, in *Modern Nutrition in Health and Disease*, 9th ed., Shils, M.E., Olson, J.A., Shike, M., and Ross, A.C., Eds., Lippincott Williams & Wilkins, Baltimore, MD, 1999, chap. 21.

5. Klein, M., Weksler, N., and Gurman, G.M., Fatal metabolic acidosis caused by thiamine deficiency, *J. Emerg. Med.*, 26 (3), 301, 2004.

6. Suter, P.M., Vergessene metaboishe Nebenwirkungen der Diuretika: Lipid-Glucose- und Vitamin B_1 (thiamine) metabolism [Forgotten metabolic side effects of diuretics: lipids, glucose and vitamin B_1 (thiamine) metabolism, *Schweiz. Rundsch. Med. Prax.*, 93 (20), 857, 2004.

7. World Health Organization, Thiamine Deficiency and Its Prevention and Control in Major Emergencies (WHO Monograph Series No. 13), Geneva, 1999.

8. Dietary Reference Intakes for Thiamin, Riboflavin, Niacin, Vitamin B_6, Folate, Vitamin B_{12}, Pantothenic Acid, Biotin, and Choline, Institute of Medicine (IOM), National Academies Press, Washington, DC, 1998.

9. Ostrovskii, A.A. and Nikitin, V.S., Morphological characteristics of cellular elements in the focus of posttraumatic inflammation in thiamine deficiency, *Vopr Pitan (Voprosy Pitaniia)* Sept.–Oct., 5, 57, 1987.

10. Alvarez, O.M. and Gilbreath, R.L., Effect of dietary thiamine on intermolecular collagen cross linking during wound repair: a mechanical and biochemical assessment, *J. Trauma*, 22 (1), 20, 1987.

11. Lakshmi, R., Lakshmi, A.V., and Barnji, M.S., Skin wound healing in riboflavin deficiency, *Biochem. Med. Metab. Biol.*, 42 (3), 185, 1989.

12. Lakshmi, R. et al., Effect of riboflavin or pyridoxine deficiency on inflammatory response, *Indian J. Biochem. Biophys.*, 28 (5–6), 481, 1991.

13. Bosse, M.D. and Axelrod, A.E., Nutrition, in *Fundamentals of Wound Management in Surgery,* Levenston, S.M., Seifter, E., and Vanwinkle, W., Eds., Appleton-Century Crofts, South Plainfield, NJ, 1977, p. 37.

14. Prasad, R., Lakshmi, A.V., and Bamji, M.S., Impaired collagen maturity in vitamins B-2 and B-6 deficiency: probable molecular basis of skin lesions, *Biochem. Med.*, 30 (3), 333, 1983.

15. Prasad, R., Lakshmi, A.V., and Bamji, M.S., Metabolism of 3 H-proline in riboflavin deficiency, *Ann. Nutr. Metab.*, 30, 300, 1986.

16. Williamson, P.R. and Kagan, H.M., Alpha-proton abstraction and carbanion formation in the mechanism of action of lysyl oxidase, *J. Biol. Chem.*, 262 (17), 8196, 1987.

17. Levene, C.I., O'Shea, M.P., and Carrington, M.J., Protein lysine 6-oxidase (lysyl oxidase) cofactor: methoxatin (PQQ) or pyridoxal? *Int. J. Biochem.*, 20 (12), 1451, 1988.

18. Elbanna, H.M., Tolba, K.G., and Darwish, O.A., Dietary management of surgical patients: effects on incisional wounds, 2 (2), 243, 1996.

19. Sugiyama, M., Role of physiological antioxidants in chromium (VI) induced cellular injury, *Free Rad. Biol. Med.*, 12 (5), 397, 1992.

20. Brown, B.G. et al., Simvastatin and niacin, antioxidant vitamins, or the combination for the prevention of coronary disease, *N. Engl. J. Med.*, 345 (22), 1583, 2001.

21. Garg, A., Lipid-lowering therapy and macrovascular disease in diabetes mellitus, *Diabetes*, 41 (Suppl. 2), 111, 1992.

22. Jonas, W.B., Rapoza, C.P., and Blair, W.F., The effect of niacinamide on osteoarthritis: a pilot study, *Inflamm. Res.*, 45 (7), 330, 1996.

23. Jacques, P.F. et al., Long-term nutrient intake and early age related nuclear lens opacities, *Arch. Ophthalmol.*, 119 (7), 1009, 2001.

24. Hymes, J. and Wolf, B., Human biotinadase isn't just for recycling biotin, *J. Nutr.*, 129 (2S Suppl.), 485-s, 1999.

25. Romero-Navarro, G. et al., Biotin regulation of pancreatic glucokinase and insulin in primary cultural rat islets and in biotin-deficient rats, *Endocrinology*, 140 (10), 4594, 1999.

26. Debourdeau, P.M. et al., Life-threatening eosinophilic pleuropericardial effusion related to vitamins B_5 and H, *Ann. Pharmacother.*, 35 (4), 424, 2001.

27. Flodin, N., *Pharmacology of Micronutrients*, Alan R. Liss, New York, 1988.

28. Casadio, S. et al., On the healing properties of esters of D-pantothenol with terpene acids, with particular reference to D-pantothenyl trifarnesylacetate, *Arzneim. Forsch.*, 17 (9), 1122, 1967.

29. Weiser, H. and Erlemann, G., Acceleration of superficial wound healing by panthenol zinc oxide, *Cosmetics Toiletries*, 103 (1010), 79, 1988.

30. Neidermeir, S., Animal experiment studies on the problem of treating corneal lesions, *Klin. Monatsbl. Augenheilkd.*, 190, 28, 1987.

31. Hosemann, W. et al., Normal wound healing of the paranasal sinuses: clinical and experimental investigations, *Eur. Arch. Otorhinolaryngol.*, 248 (7), 390, 1991.

32. Lacroix, B., Didier, E., and Grenier, J.F., Role of pantothenic and ascorbic acid in wound healing processes: *in vitro* study on fibroblasts, *J. Vitam. Nutr. Res.*, 58 (4), 407, 1988.

33. Weimann, B.J. and Hermann, D., Studies on wound healing: effects of calcium D-pantothenate on the migration, proliferation and protein synthesis of human dermal fibroblasts in culture, *Int. J. Vit. Nutr. Res.*, 69 (2), 113, 1999.

34. Lacroix, B., Didier, E., and Grenier, J.F., Effects of pantothenic acid on fibroblastic cell cultures, *Res. Exp. Med.*, 188, 391, 1988.

35. Vaxman, F. et al., Effect of pantothenic acid and ascorbic acid supplementation on human skin wound healing process. A double-blind, prospective and randomized trial, *Eur. Surg. Res.*, 27 (3), 158, 1995.

36. Ackermann, Z. et al., Overload of iron in the skin of patients with varicose ulcers, *Archv. Detmatol.*, 124 (9), 1376, 1988.

37. Levenson, S.M. and Seifter, E., Dysnutrition, wound healing and resistance to infection, *Clin. Plast. Surg.*, 4 (3), 375, 1977.

38. Williamson, P.R. and Kagan, H.M., Reaction pathway of bovine aortic lysyl oxidase, *J. Biol. Chem.*, 261 (20), 9477, 1986.

39. Ruberg, R.L., Role of nutrition in wound healing, *Surg. Clin. North Am.*, 64 (4), 705, 1984.

40. Carville, D.G.M. and Strain, J.J., The effect of a low copper diet on blood cholesterol and enzymatic antioxidant and defense mechanisms in male and female rats, *Int. J. Vitam. Nutr. Res.*, 58 (4), 456, 1988.

41. Aprahamian, M. et al., Effects of supplemental pantothenic acid on wound healing: experimental study in rabbit, *Am. J. Clin. Nutr.*, 41 (3), 578, 1985.

42. Levenson, S.M. and Seifter, E., Dysnutrition, wound healing and resistance to infection, *Clin. Plast. Surg.*, 4, 375, 1977.

43. Rucker, R.B., Murray, J., and Riggins, R.S., Nutritional copper deficiency and penicillamine administration: some effects on bone collagen and arterial elastin crosslinking, *Adv. Exp. Med. Biol.*, 86B, 619, 1977.

44. Osiecki, H., *The Physician's Handbook of Clinical Nutrition*, 5th ed., Bioconcepts publishing, Kelvin Grove, Queensland, Australia, 1998.

45. Bender, D.A., Non-nutritional uses of vitamin B_6, *Br. J. Nutr.*, 81 (1), 7, 1999.

46. Shils, M.E. et al., Cobalamin, in *Modern Nutrition in Health and Disease*, 9th ed., Shils, M.E., Olson, J.A., Shike, M., and Ross, A.C., Eds., Baltimore, MD, Lippincott Williams & Wilkins, 1999, chap. 27.

47. Kasper, H., Vitamin absorption in the elderly, *Int. J. Vitam. Nutr. Res.*, 69 (3), 169, 1999.

48. Herbert, V., Vitamin B_{12}, in *Present Knowledge in Nutrition*, 7th ed., Ziegler, E.E. and Filer, L.J., Eds., ILSI Press, Washington D.C., 1996, pp. 191–205.

49. National Advisory Group on Standards and Practice Guidelines for Parenteral Nutrition Formulations, *J. Parenter. Enteral Nutri.*, 22, 49–66, 1998.

50. Parenteral multivitamin products: drugs for human use; drug efficacy study implementation; amendment (21 CFR 5.70), *Federal Register*, April 20, 2000; 65, 77, pp. 21200–21201.

8 Vitamin C and Wound Healing

Hideharu Tanaka and Joseph A. Molnar

CONTENTS

BACKGROUND

Scurvy, the disease we now associate with ascorbic acid deficiency, was described by the ancient Egyptians as early as 3000 B.C.[1] The ancient Greeks and Romans later referred to a "plague" that was almost certainly scurvy.[2] Lack of understanding of the importance of vitamin C and its sources continued to have an effect on the general population of these cultures as well as on the military. In 1536, Jacques Cartier, while in Newfoundland, had numerous crew members suffering with the disease. The wisdom of local Native Americans allowed successful treatment with an extract of the arborvitae tree. In that same century, Sir Richard Hawkins recommended the use of oranges and lemons to prevent the disease in British sailors.[2]

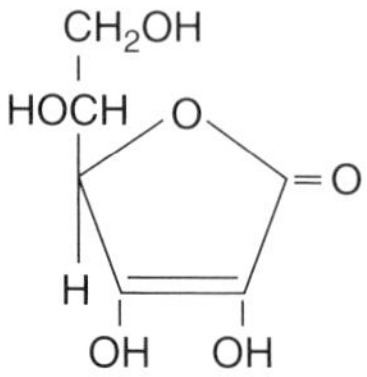

FIGURE 8.1 Vitamin C, also known by the chemical name of L-ascorbic acid, has the chemical formula C6H8O6.

Nonetheless, the Scottish naval surgeon James Lind working two centuries later is often credited with the first description that citrus fruit can cure scurvy.[1-4] This was prompted by the disastrous voyage of George A. Anson, whose circumnavigation of the globe resulted in the death of over half of his sailors from scurvy. The subsequent classic experiments of Lind in 1747 proved the efficacy of lemon juice to prevent the disease. The wide acceptance of the recommendation to provide a lemon juice and later a lime juice ration aboard ship led to the "limey" nickname for the British sailors. Capt. James Cook compulsively employed these measures as well as others to successfully demonstrate that prolonged sea voyages need not result in scurvy. These successes continued to be ignored by some, leading to rampant scurvy among soldiers of the American Civil War and even to the tragic demise of Robert Scott's South Pole expedition in 1912.

It was not until the 20th century that the chemical nature of the active ingredient of these food sources was understood. It became apparent that only certain species, such as man and the guinea pig, needed this factor that could either prevent or cure scurvy. Working independently, Szent-Gyorgyi and King identified this antiscorbutic factor. Identified as hexuronic acid, it was later named ascorbic acid by Szent-Gyorgyi, who was awarded the Nobel Prize for his work in 1937.[1-4]

Vitamin C, or chemically, L-ascorbic acid, has the chemical formula C6H8O6 (Figure 8.1). It is derived from D-glucuronic acid conversion to D-gluconic acid and then to L-glulonolactone and finally to ascorbic acid in animals. In animals such as man, nonhuman primates, capybaras, Indian fruit bats, bulbuls, swallows, trout, salmon, locusts, and guinea pigs, it is the inability to complete this last step in the synthesis process that requires vitamin C to be provided in the diet.[1,5,6] It is available in a wide variety of fresh fruits and vegetables. However, due to its relative chemical instability, vitamin C is less available in preserved foods. Thus, the hospitalized patient on a limited diet, a sailor at sea, or a geriatric patient on a minimal income is at greater risk of deficiency than the individual on a mixed fresh diet.

ASCORBIC ACID DEFICIENCY

Ascorbic acid deficiency is characterized by hemorrhage, hematological alterations, impaired wound healing, depressed immune functions, and psychological disturbance.[1-4,7] The deficiency state of scurvy and its effect on wound healing is probably best described by George Anson, a British commodore in the 1740s, who wrote "a most extraordinary circumstance (occurred) . . . the scars of old wounds, healed for

TABLE 8.1
Manifestations of Scurvy

Constitutional	Cutaneous
Fatigue, listlessness; decreased exercise tolerance; depression, uncooperative	Dry, rough skin; pale skin; follicular hyperkeratosis; hemorrhagic lesions; capillary fragility, petechiae; edema, especially legs; subungual hemorrhages; alopecia; poor wound healing or breakdown of old wounds; acne
Oral	**Musculoskeletal**
Gingivitis, halitosis, easy bleeding of gums	Polymyalgia, polyarthralgias, hemarthroses, back pain, osteoporosis
Ophthalmologic	**Cardiorespiratory**
Conjunctival varicosities, retinal hemorrhages, retrobulbar hemorrhages, optic atrophy, dryness, photophobia	Dyspnea, congestive heart failure, syncope, chest pain, sudden death
Gastrointestinal	**Hematologic**
Anorexia, submucosal hemorrhage	Anemia, leukopenia

Source: Levine, M., Katz, A., and Padayatty, S. Chapter 31, in *Modern Nutrition in Health and Disease*, Shils, Shike, Ross, Caballero, and Cousins, Eds., Lippincott Williams & Wilkens, Philadelphia, 2006, p. 520. Reprinted by permission.

many years were forced open again . . ."[3,8] As discussed in detail below and in Chapter 1, deficiency of ascorbic acid has profound effects on wound healing, primarily through its effect on collagen synthesis. However, independent effects on the immune system — presumably through its effects on the function of phagocytes, T-lymphocyte proliferation, production of interferon, its antioxidant activity, and gene expression of monocyte adhesion molecules — also play a role.[1,4,9–11] Due to the crucial importance of the immune response in the inflammatory phase of wound healing, it is not surprising that deficiency of ascorbate would have devastating effects on wound healing. The multitude of findings of vitamin C deficiency are described in Table 8.1. The diversity of findings with ascorbate deficiency indicates the diverse functions of this vitamin for many chemical processes and organs of the body.

BIOCHEMICAL FUNCTIONS OF ASCORBIC ACID

VITAMIN C AS AN ENZYMATIC COFACTOR

One of the major functions of ascorbic acid, like most vitamins, is as a cofactor in enzymatic reaction, where it serves as an electron donor. As will be seen below, this ability to function as a reducing agent also allows it to have a powerful effect on the metabolism of oxygen free radicals in a nonenzymatic fashion. At least eight different mammalian enzyme systems use ascorbic acid as a cofactor (Table 8.2).[1,12,13] While it is the function as a cofactor in collagen metabolism that is most relevant to scurvy and the process of wound healing, it is likely that the effects on carnitine biosynthesis and

TABLE 8.2
Numerous Activities of Vitamin C

	Cofactor for Enzymes	
Known Roles	**Enzyme**	**Function of Enzyme (Reference)**
	Mammalian	
	Dopamine ß-monooxygenase	Norepinephrinebiosynthesis
	Peptidyl-glycerine α-amidating monooxygenase	Amidation of peptide hormones
	Prolyl 4-hydroxylase	Collagen hydroxylation
	Prolyl 3-hydroxylase	
	Trimethyllysine hydroxylase	Carnitine biosynthesis
	Γ-Butyrobetaine hydroxylase	
	4-hydroxyphenylpyruvate dioxygenase	Tyrosine metabolism
	Fungi	
	Deoxyuridine 1´-hydroxylase	Reutilization pathways for pyrimidines or the deoxyribose moiety of deoxynucleosides
	Thyamine 7-hydroxylase	
	Pyridine deoxyribonucleoside 2´ hydroxylase	

	Reducing Agent	
Site		**Action**
Small intestine		Promote iron absorption

	Antioxidant	
Postulated Roles		**Action**
Cells		Regulate gene expression and mRNA translation, prevent oxidant to intracellular proteins
Plasma		Quench aqueous peroxyl radicals and lipid peroxidation products
Stomach		Prevent formation of N-nitroso compounds

	Pro-Oxidant	
Target		**Effect**
DNA		DNA damage
Lipid hydroperoxidase		Decomposition of lipid peroxidase leading to DNA damage
Ascorbyl radical targets		Cell damage

Source: From Levine, M., Katz, A., and Padayatty, S., in *Modern Nutrition in Health and Disease*, Shils, Shike, Ross, Caballero, and Cousins, Eds., Lippincott Williams & Wilkins, Philadelphia, 2006, chap. 31, p. 511. Adapted from Padayatty, S.J., Daruwala, R., Wang, Y. et al., in *Handbook of Antioxidants*, 2nd ed., Marcel Dekker, New York, 2002, pp. 117–145. With permission.

tyrosine metabolism also play a role.[14,15] Deficiency of ascorbate and the effects on hormone and neurotransmitter production could also play a less obvious role, as it may have an effect on the ability of the organism to respond to the metabolic stress of injury.

Ascorbic acid is necessary for the posttranslational hydroxylation of proline and lysine residues in procollagen, which is necessary for its release from the ribosome and subsequent conversion to collagen[13] (see also Chapter 1 and Chapter 4) (Figure 8.2). In the course of this reaction, ascorbic acid is reversibly oxidized to dehydroascorbic acid (DHASA). Hydroxyproline stabilizes the collagen triple-helix structure by hydrogen bonding. Hydroxylysine is essential for mature collagen cross-links that provide progressive tensile strength in the healing wound as well as in other tissues, such as skin, tendon, bone, vessel walls, and ligaments. Collagen types I and III are the major proteins of the healing wound and provide the majority of the tensile strength of that wound once healed. However, in addition to types I and III, there are numerous other collagen types, such as type IV collagen found in basement membrane and type II found in cartilage.[16] Collagen also has an essential function in the extracellular matrix of all organs of the body as well as in the healing of all wounds invading below the epidermis. All of these collagen types require the same hydroxylation reactions for normal structure and function. Were this not enough, ascorbate is also

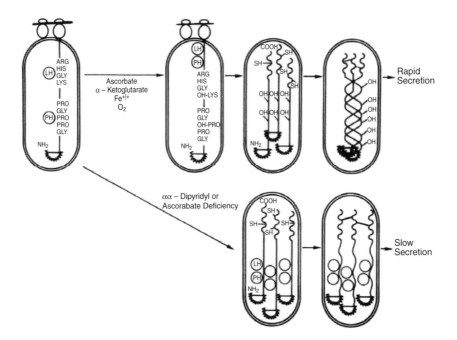

FIGURE 8.2 Posttransitional hydroxylation of procollagen. Inadequately hydroxylated procollagen will either be slowly secreted from the cell or intracellularly degraded, emphasizing the importance of the cofactors for the hydroxylation reaction. (PH, LH: prolyl and lysyl hydroxylases.) (Peterkofshy, B., Ascorbate requirements for hydroxylation and secretion of procollagen: relationship to inhibition of collagen synthesis in scurvy, *Am. J. Clin. Nutr.,* 54, 11365, 1991. With permission.)

necessary in the hydroxylation reactions of other molecules with collagenous domains such as elastin and complement.[17] It is not surprising that deficiency of collagen caused by ascorbate deficiency may have diffuse and severe manifestations.

Ascorbic acid deficiency causes abnormal collagen fibers and alterations of the extracellular matrix that manifest as cutaneous lesions, poor adhesion of endothelium cells, and decreased tensile strength of fibrous connective tissues, accounting for many of the manifestations in Table 8.1. It also explains the early descriptions of scurvy in sailors that included the breakdown of previously healed wounds. Clearly, ascorbate is not only essential for strong closure of the healing wound but also to maintain that closure for the rest of the life of the injured organism during the normal process of protein turnover (see also Chapter 4).

VITAMIN C AS A FREE RADICAL SCAVENGER

Because the human body has adopted as its basic energy production the highly effective aerobic metabolic pathways, it constantly exposes itself to the "toxin" called oxygen. All nutrients may, in some cases, be harmful to the human body, especially when in excess quantities. While oxygen is essential for our survival, it also may be harmful to the body when in the form of free radicals. An oxygen radical is defined as an oxygen molecule with an unpaired electron in its outer orbital. Generally, these radicals are thought to provide an on-site defense system. On the other hand, it is also known that these same free radicals may attack the body (Figure 8.3).

The major pathway of oxygen metabolism occurring in man involves the tetravalent reduction of molecular oxygen by the cytochrome oxidase system in the mitochondria. However, 1 to 2% of the oxygen substrate may "leak" from the system to become metabolized by univalent reduction, producing various oxygen radicals.[18] In addition, oxygen radicals can be produced by radiation, chemical agents, and various enzymatic systems, including xanthine oxidase and NADPH oxidase[19,20] (Figure 8.3 and Figure 8.4).

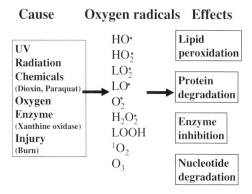

FIGURE 8.3 Free radicals are produced in response to a variety of "causes," resulting in a variety of biochemically defined oxygen radicals that have a multitude of "effects" on lipids, proteins, and nucleotides. "L" represents lipid. Although these molecules are part of the body's defense system, they can also cause damage to the host.

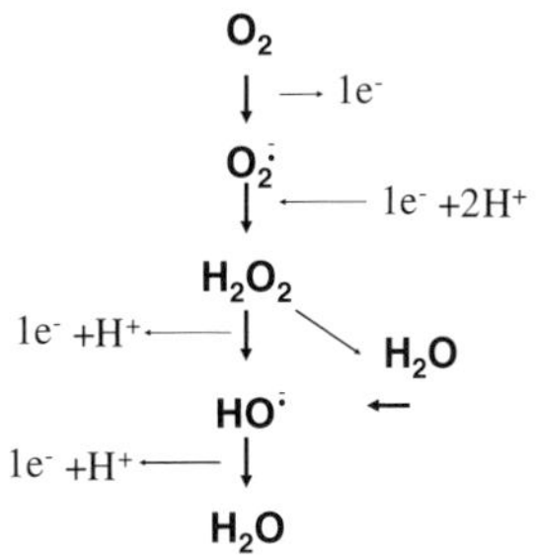

$$O_2$$
$$\downarrow \; \longleftarrow 1e^-$$
$$O_2^{\cdot -}$$
$$\downarrow \longleftarrow 1e^- + 2H^+$$
$$H_2O_2$$
$$1e^- + H^+ \longrightarrow \downarrow \;\; \searrow \;\; H_2O$$
$$HO^{\cdot}$$
$$1e^- + H^+ \longrightarrow \downarrow \;\; \longleftarrow$$
$$H_2O$$

FIGURE 8.4 Under normal situations, 98% of oxygen reduction is catalyzed by the cytochrome oxidase system in mitochondria. (From Angel, M.F., *Plast. Reconstruc. Surg.*, 79, 990, 1987. With permission.)

Typically, oxygen radicals are short lived, and their effects are limited to a radius of a few microns. However, reaction with polyunsaturated fatty acids in the cell membranes generates more stable lipid peroxides that may exert their damage at a distance from the original site. Furthermore, polyunsaturated fatty acids and their phospholipid esters are readily oxidized by a chain reaction mechanism. Once an initiating lipid radical is generated, it attacks another lipid to form a second lipid radical; thus, this lipid peroxidation cycle is propagated[21] (Figure 8.5; see also Chapter 3).

Two types of defense systems protect aerobic organisms from oxygen radicals. One system includes the preventative antioxidants, such as catalase and peroxidase, which decompose substrates without the generation of oxygen radicals (Table 8.3).

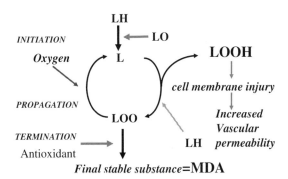

FIGURE 8.5 Lipid peroxidation in cell membrane. By reaction with polyunsaturated fatty acids in the cell membranes, more stable lipid peroxides are generated, which may exert their damage at a distance from the original site. Furthermore, polyunsaturated fatty acids and their phospholipid esters are readily oxidized by a chain reaction mechanism. Once an initiating lipid radical is generated, it attacks another lipid to form a second lipid radical; thus, this lipid peroxidation cycle is propagated. (See also Niki, E. et al., *J. Biol. Chem.*, 259, 4177, 1984.) The final stable substance, malondialdehyde (MDA) is often used as a way to study free radical metabolism. (L = lipid.) (From Niki, E., *Ann. N.Y. Acad. Sci.*, 498: 186, 1987. With permission.)

TABLE 8.3
Protective Mechanisms against Oxygen Radicals*

Preventative Antioxidant	Mechanism
Vitamin C	Scavenger
Superoxide dismutase (SOD)	Enzymatic
Glutathione (GSH) peroxidase	Enzymatic
Peroxidase	Enzymatic
Transferrin	Iron requiring
Ceruloplasmin	Copper requiring
Allopurinol	Iron requiring
Chain-Breaking Antioxidant	**Mechanism**
Vitamin E	Terminates lipid peroxidation
Vitamin C	Terminates lipid peroxidation
Glutathione (GSH)	Regenerates vitamin E from its radical
Coenzyme Q	Regenerates vitamin E from its radical

*The systems that protect us against oxygen radicals may be categorized as preventable or chain breaking — vitamin C functions in both categories

The other system includes chain-breaking antioxidants, such as uric acid, ubiquinone, bilirubin, vitamin C, vitamin E, cysteine, and glutathione (GSH). These terminate the chain reaction of the lipid peroxidation reaction by scavenging oxygen-free radical reactions within and outside of the cell. It is thought that the decreased tissue concentration of vitamin C under invasive situations, such as burn injury, shock, and multiple trauma, is largely due to vitamin C consumption in these processes[21] (Figure 8.6).

Because vitamin C is water soluble, it is an aqueous phase antioxidant. It may function as a preventive antioxidant by scavenging oxygen radicals, such as superoxide (O_2^-), hydroxyl radical (OH^-) and singlet oxygen (O_2).[22–24] Along with vitamin E, it also has a chain-breakage-type antioxidizing effect, terminating oxygen radical reaction within and outside of cell membranes.[21] Vitamin C can interact with and remove the oxygen radicals from the vitamin E free radicals and, thus, regenerate vitamin E (Figure 8.6). Other reducing compounds, such as cysteine and glutathione, also reduce the vitamin E radicals but at a slower rate than that of vitamin C (Figure 8.7). One

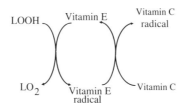

FIGURE 8.6 Interrelationship of vitamin E and vitamin C. Lipid-free radicals may be reduced by vitamin E. The vitamin E radical may subsequently be regenerated by vitamin C in the cell membrane (L = lipid).

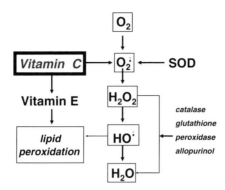

FIGURE 8.7 Vitamin C and vitamin E interactions. Vitamin C can interact with and remove the oxygen radicals from the vitamin E free radicals and, thus, regenerate vitamin E (see also Figure 8.6). Other reducing compounds, such as cysteine and glutathione, and enzyme systems also reduce the vitamin E radicals but at a slower rate than that of vitamin C. (From Niki, E., *Ann. N.Y. Acad. Sci.*, 498, 186, 1987. Reprinted by permission.)

may speculate that an adequate amount of ascorbate in the extracellular fluid continuously scavenges oxygen radicals that are spilled into the extracellular fluid. Thus, vitamin C protects both the capillary endothelium and the circulating cells, such as erythrocytes and leukocytes, from oxygen injury. As a result, it is thought to be the major plasma antioxidant in the human body.[1,25,26]

Understanding how the free radical scavenging property of vitamin C may aid in wound healing requires a review of the basic process of wound healing and inference from a variety of clinical situations (Chapter 1). During the inflammatory stage of wound healing, and to a lesser degree throughout the healing process, inflammatory cells and other processes in the healing wound produce free radicals, presumably for their bacterial killing properties. Unfortunately, in some cases, this process may exceed its usefulness and cause local "collateral damage" to the host. In addition, in situations of metabolic stress, such as burns and trauma, systemic inflammatory response syndrome (SIRS) may ensue, leading to a systemic excess of oxygen free radicals. In this situation, the metabolic response to injury may initiate cascades of tissue and organ damage throughout the body (Chapter 11). Clearly, control of the inflammatory response in this situation may be life saving.[27,28]

ASCORBIC ACID REQUIREMENTS

In addition to its function in collagen production, ascorbic acid enhances neutrophil function, increases angiogenesis, and functions as a powerful antioxidant.[26] Thus, while most discussions of vitamin C and wound healing concentrate on its pivotal function in the accumulation and cross-linking of collagen, the other functions of ascorbate must not be ignored. To address the amount of ascorbate that must be included in the diet for wound healing, the function one is attempting to support must be considered, as the dietary requirements may be different for these different functions, as seen below.

Oral ascorbate is readily absorbed by the bowel by an energy requiring a Na$^+$-dependent transport system.[1,11] It passes through the portal circulation to circulate in the plasma unbound as ascorbic acid. Little or no other species are found in the blood.[29] Circulating ascorbate is readily filtered through glomeruli and reabsorbed in the proximal collecting tubule.[30] After saturation of these resorptive mechanisms, ascorbic acid is excreted in the urine. Regulation of concentrations of ascorbate in the body appears to be achieved at multiple levels, including a noninducible active absorption in the bowel and by saturatable renal absorption.[11,27,31] This would indicate that although it is difficult if not impossible to develop progressively high tissue or plasma levels of ascorbate with oral intake in an individual with normal kidney function, these protective mechanisms would not be active in individuals receiving intravenous ascorbate or in a patient with renal failure (Figure 8.8).

In most tissues of the body, ascorbate is accumulated against a concentration gradient in millimolar concentrations. The concentration in human tissues varies from 5 to 15 mg/100 mg in the kidney to 30 to 50 mg/100 mg in the adrenal or pituitary gland.[1,10] It is unclear why cells accumulate ascorbate, but this must be related to the metabolic function of tissues that need ascorbate as either cofactors for enzymatic reactions or as a mechanism to control harmful free radicals. In

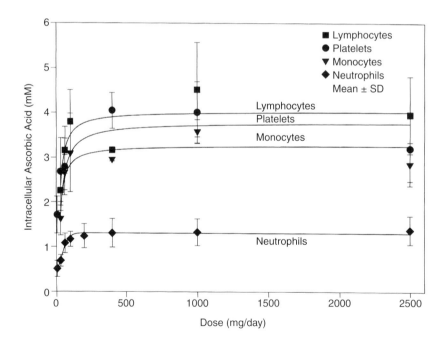

FIGURE 8.8 Functioning doses of intracellular vitamin C in circulating cells. The concentration of intracellular vitamin C plateaus at relatively low levels of vitamin C intakes indicate that most of the higher doses are secreted in the urine. (From Levine, M., Katz, A., and Padayatty, S., in *Modern Nutrition in Health and Disease*, Lippincott Williams & Wilkins, Philidelphia, 2006, chap. 31, p. 517. With permission. From Levine, M., Wang, Y., Padayatty, S.J., et al., *Proc. Natl. Acad. Sci. U.S.A.*, 98, 9842–9846, 2001, with permission of the National Academy of Sciences, Washington, D.C.)

addition, it is clear from this that assessments of vitamin C nutrition based on plasma levels alone may be erroneous, as plasma levels may not reflect tissue levels. Most investigators use concentrations of circulating cells as an acceptable index of ascorbate nutrition, but many studies still report plasma levels.[1,11,27]

Dietary reference intakes for ascorbate for the general population are found in Table 8.4. The results were based on neutrophil vitamin C concentrations, putative

TABLE 8.4
Dietary Intake Values for Vitamin C[a]

Life Stage	Gender	Age (y)	EAR	RDA	AI	UL
Infants		0–6			40[b]	
(months)		7–12			50	
Children	Boys and	1–3	13	15		400
	girls	4–8	22	25		650
	Boys	9–13	39	45		1,200
		14–18	63	75		1,800
	Girls	9–13	39	45		1,200
		14–18	56	65		1,800
Adults	Men	19–30	75	90		2,000
		31–50	75	90		
		51–70	75	90		
		> 70	75	90		
	Women	19–30	60	75		
		31–50	60	75		
		51–70	60	75		
		> 70	60	75		
Pregnancy		14–18	66	80		1,800
		19–30	70	85		2,000
		31–50	70	85		
Lactation		14–18	96	115		1,800
		19–30	100	120		2,000
		31–50	100	120		
Smokers	Men	> 19	110	130c		
	Women	> 19	95	115c		

AI, adequate intake; EAR, estimated average requirement; RDA, recommended dietary allowance; UL, tolerable upper intake level.

[a]Dietary reference intake values for vitamin C in milligrams, by life stage and gender.

[b]It is not possible to establish ULs for infants and children, for whom the source of vitamin C intake should be infant formula and food only.

[c]Whereas EARs were stated for smokers, RDAs for smokers were not explicitly documented. We calculated RDAs for smokers based on stated EAR × 1.2.

From Levine, M., Katz, A., and Padayatty, S. in *Modern Nutrition in Health and Disease*, Shils, M.E., Shike, M., Ross, A.C., Cabellero, B., and Cousins, R.J., Eds., Lippincott Williams & Wilkins, Philadelphia, 2006, Chap. 31, p. 522. With permission.

antioxidant functions, and urinary vitamin C secretion.[32] While estimated average requirements (EARs) were determined to be 75 mg/d for men and 60 mg/d for women, the recommended dietary allowances (RDAs) were 90 and 75 mg/d, respectively.

Although these numbers are useful for the general population, there are numerous circumstances in which these values are not applicable. According to Agency for Health Care Policy and Research (AHCPR) guidelines, ill patients may need ten times the RDAs for water-soluble vitamins when specific deficiencies are diagnosed. This means a RDA of 750 mg/d for women and 900 mg/day for men.[33] Certain populations are more likely to be deficient in ascorbic acid, including the elderly, alcoholics, drug abusers, and individuals with general proteinñcalorie malnutrition[34] In these situations, vitamin C deficiency is associated with prolonged hospitalization and more severe manifestation of illnesses.[35]

In mammals, ascorbic acid is necessary for a normal response to physiological stressors, with the need for ascorbic acid increasing during times of injury or stress.[36] Studies have shown that even the physiological stress of intense exercise generates an increased utilization of ascorbate.[37] Wounds, including trauma, burn, and major surgery, are also perceived as physiological stressors that have been correlated with a decrease in plasma ascorbic acid.[38,39] Thus, the acute stress experienced by patients undergoing trauma or surgery may unmask marginal vitamin C deficiencies, leading to deficiency symptoms. In the paragraphs that follow, we will explore the requirements for vitamin C in illness and in injury, looking at the two major functions of this vitamin as an enzymatic cofactor and as an antioxidant.

WOUND HEALING AND ASCORBIC ACID AS AN ENZYMATIC COFACTOR

Although it is clear that chronic lack of vitamin C results in breakdown of previously healed wounds, it is also clear that inadequate intake leads to deficient healing of the wound. In 1933, Wolbach et al. found that scorbutic guinea pigs failed to make intercellular substances; this failure was reversed when ascorbic acid was provided.[40] Subsequent studies in a variety of wounds involving primarily skin, fascia, or models involving polyvinyl alcohol sponges demonstrated decreased tensile strength and collagen production as well as altered angiogenesis.[4,25,41] Ascorbate supplementation was reported to decrease elastin messenger RNA (mRNA) stability, while collagen type I mRNA was stabilized to a much greater extent.[42] Kaplan et al. also reported that ascorbate and hydroxyproline content of the wound increased over the first 5 d. The tensile strength and ascorbic acid level of the wound also increased significantly on day seven, while hydroxyproline levels decreased. These studies suggest that effects other than an alteration of hydroxylation may explain some of the alteration in wound healing with vitamin C deficiency.[42]

Some studies have been clouded by the fact that animals taking in decreased ascorbic acid have secondary decreased intake of other nutrients, leading to proteinñcalorie malnutrition. This results in a general decrease in collagen synthesis independent of the hydroxylase cofactor activity of ascorbate.[4]

Not only do scorbutic animals heal poorly, but also animals on a marginal vitamin C diet can become scorbutic, as demonstrated in a study with femur fractures in guinea pigs.[43] During time of injury, there appears to be a decreased urinary excretion of ascorbate, decreased plasma concentrations, and a redistribution of ascorbate in soft tissues and wounds.[4,44] Levenson demonstrated that when guinea pigs on an adequate ascorbate diet were wounded, they healed normally with appropriate fibroplasia and collagen without hemorrhage. When similar wounds were made in animals on the same diet with third-degree burns, there was fibroplasias, but with hemorrhage, increased ground substance, and decreased collagen production. Supplementing the animals with vitamin C prevented these abnormalities in wound healing.[45] In a similar fashion, patients in an otherwise healthy state but with marginal ascorbic acid intake may become ascorbic acid deficient with injury. This is not unlike the intake of other nutrients, where the demand is increased with injury.

The total body pool of ascorbic acid of young healthy males is 2.3 g; this may be maintained with intakes of 20 to 30 mg/d.[1,32,33,46] It takes months of low intake to have an effect on wound healing. Crandon reported in a human case study that, although plasma levels of ascorbate were undetectable after 40 d of no vitamin C intake, wound healing was not affected until 180 d without ascorbic acid intake.[7] This is consistent with the understanding that wound healing ranks high in the body's metabolic priorities.

Two randomized clinical trials evaluated the effect of vitamin C supplementation on pressure ulcer healing. Taylor et al. in a prospective randomized clinical trial compared patients with pressure ulcers receiving either a placebo or 500 mg/d of vitamin C.[47] At 1 month, the treatment group had a larger reduction in wound size (84%) versus controls (43%). Reit et al. conducted a similar study in which the control group received 20 mg/d of vitamin C and the treatment group 1 g/d in divided doses.[48] The comparison was between patients on a minimal intake to avoid deficiency versus patients with an intake 50 times the presumed minimal intake. Eighty-eight patients from 11 hospitals were involved in the study. Unlike Taylor et al., no significant difference resulted in the quantitative or qualitative healing between the two groups. These disparate studies give no definitive answer on the proper intake of vitamin C for pressure ulcer healing.

Other studies have evaluated the effect of ascorbate administration in patients undergoing elective surgery. In women undergoing abdominal surgery, Shukla gave 500 mg/d of vitamin C, controlling other ascorbate intake.[49] Despite this intake, plasma vitamin C levels dropped from 2.6 to 1.5 mg, suggesting that a higher intake would be necessary to maintain constant plasma levels. Although this study looked only at plasma levels, Irvin et al. looked at ascorbate levels in plasma leukocytes in perioperative patients.[50] A 42% reduction in levels was found by the third postoperative day, suggesting that in perioperative patients, both plasma and tissue concentrations decrease after surgery. Bartlett et al. studied the effects of either 100 mg or 1100 mg of vitamin C intake in a patient with a thigh wound.[51] Supplementation with 1100 mg produced a three- to sixfold increase in connective tissue.

Ringsdorf et al. looked at an experimental model of oral gingival healing by following the rate of healing of a punch biopsy.[52] Supplementation of the diet with 1000 mg of vitamin C per day resulted in a 40% decrease in the time to healing. Increasing the dose to 2000 mg per day resulted in a 50% decrease in the time to healing, even in these otherwise healthy dental students.

Afifi et al. evaluated the effect of vitamin C administration to patients with thalassemia leg ulcers in a double-blind crossover study.[53] Patients were given 3000 mg of vitamin C per day or a placebo for an 8-week period. Seven of 14 leg ulcers completely healed in the treatment group vs. only 4 of 12 that partially healed in the control group. When the patients crossed over in the next 8 weeks, 4 additional patients healed in the first group, and 9 of 12 of the ulcers healed in the other group. This study indicates not only an important effect of vitamin C on the healing rate of the wounds, but also that loading the patients with ascorbate continues to aid healing for a period of time after discontinuing the intake.

Supplementation of vitamin C has also been evaluated in larger injuries, such as burns and trauma (see Chapter 11). The dynamics of metabolism and fluids and the heterogeneity of these patients make determination of appropriate vitamin supplementation problematic. For example, wound healing endpoints would be difficult, because the nature of the wounds would be heterogeneous and the comorbidities variable. As a result, studies looking at plasma levels or leukocyte levels of vitamin C are often published. In patients receiving high-volume fluid resuscitation, it would be expected that water-soluble vitamins such as ascorbate will have increased losses in the urine. In addition, consumption of ascorbate will be increased in large wounds. Long et al. demonstrated that plasma levels of ascorbate in 12 critically ill trauma patients were decreased to 0.11 ± 0.03 mg/dl on 300 mg/d and only reached low normal plasma levels (0.32 ± 0.08) on 1000 mg/d, reaching 1.2 ± 0.03 on 3000 mg/d.[27] They suggested that at least 3000 mg be given to such patients. Nonetheless, in burn patients it has been suggested to provide 500 to 1500 mg/d of vitamin C.

Although it is often assumed that these studies are determining the proper ascorbate administration to optimize collagen synthesis, this may not be accurate. Clearly, any of the numerous activities of vitamin C listed in Table 8.2 could be involved. The numerous functions of ascorbate include effects on the immune response and antibacterial activity that may also play a role, as well as interactions with other nutrients.[54] The programmed sequences of the cellular and molecular processes occurring during wound repair are also dependent on immune function. Infection resulting from impaired immunity is one of the most commonly encountered and clinically significant impediments to wound healing.[55] In addition, altered cellular immunity and dysregulation of cytokines can impair wound healing.[56] Ascorbic acid has been shown to improve immune function in humans.[57,58] Human volunteers who ingested 2 to 3 g of ascorbate daily for several weeks exhibited enhanced neutrophil motility to chemotactic stimulus and stimulation of lymphocyte transformation.[59]

In the following section, we will explore the effects of ascorbate on free radical metabolism and the implications for metabolic support of the patient with a healing wound.

CLINICAL APPLICATION OF VITAMIN C AS A FREE RADICAL SCAVENGER

As discussed above, oxygen free radicals may cause cell injury through cellular membrane lipid peroxidation and degradation of nucleic acids, leading to increased membrane permeability and cell lysis. Delay in wound healing of older rats may result at least partially from increased free radical damage. Eighteen-month-old wounded male rats were compared to 3- to 4-month-old rats pre-wound and 7 d post-wound.

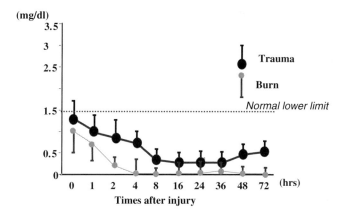

FIGURE 8.9 Serum vitamin C levels in burn and trauma patients. Vitamin C levels decrease in the serum of burn and trauma patients in the early hours after injury. Although much of this may be the result of urinary excretion, the early drop in vitamin C is due to vitamin C consumption in metabolic processes and compartmentalization to areas of greater need. (From Tanaka, H. et al., *Arch. Surg.,* 135, 326, 2000. With permission.)

The normal skin of aged and young rats showed no difference in ascorbic acid content. However, a 59% decrease in ascorbic acid content was observed in wound tissues of aged animals compared to its content in young adult wounds.[60]

Several investigators have reported that the ascorbic acid level significantly decreased in critically ill patients, and those with trauma and burns, suggesting the consumption of vitamin C[61,62] (Figure 8.9). Miyagatani et al. reported that high levels of ascorbic acid (133 mg/kg/h) result in an 80% survival of septic rats compared to 50% without high-dose ascorbic acid supplementation.[63] They also noted increased levels of hepatic glutathione, the principal intracellular free radical scavenger, in the rat administered high-dose ascorbic acid, suggesting that vitamin C replenishes the scavenging activity of glutathione.

LUNG INJURY AND ARDS (ADULT RESPIRATORY DISTRESS SYNDROME)

Adult respiratory distress syndrome (ARDS) is a pulmonary response to a variety of hypermetabolic life-threatening processes, such as trauma and sepsis. The inflammatory response of the lung in ARDS appears to be mediated, at least in part, by oxygen free radicals, suggesting that supplementing with free radical scavengers could help this disease process. Nathens reported that supplemental tocopherol (vitamin E) 3000 IU and 3000 mg intravenous ascorbic acid during 28 d of an intensive care unit (ICU) stay could attenuate alveolar inflammatory response, decrease the multiple organ failure score, and lessen ICU length of stay.[64] Ascorbate may play a role in the prevention of lung oxidant injury, not only as an oxidant scavenger but also as an inhibitor of PMN (polymorphonuclear) leukocyte influx to the pulmonary tissue.[65,66]

PARAQUAT INTOXICATION

Paraquat (an ingredient of Gramoxone) is a potent producer of oxygen radical injury resulting in organ failure. The effects of the ascorbic acid administered after paraquat intoxication (LD_{50} of Gramoxone), and of ascorbic acid pretreatment followed by the LD_{50} of paraquat have been reported.[67] Ascorbic acid treatment increases the content of polyunsaturated fatty acids in the lung considerably (i.e., the pulmonary membrane fluidity decreases significantly in response to ascorbic acid). In the liver homogenate, the membrane fluidity is significantly increased by ascorbic acid pretreatment and significantly decreased by simultaneous ascorbic acid treatment. In renal tissue, the result of ascorbic acid pretreatment exhibits a similar, but more significant, result to that of the paraquat treatment. The administration of ascorbic acid together with paraquat does not cause a substantial change in the fluidity index compared to the control.[67]

BRAIN INJURY

Reactive oxygen species (ROS) have been shown to play a role in the pathophysiology of brain injury. Elangovan et al. reported that chronic oxidative stress exacerbates brain damage following closed head injury. They compared neurological recovery, edema, levels of low molecular weight antioxidants (LMWA), and markers of lipid peroxidation.[68] Diabetic rats under chronic oxidative stress showed greater neurological dysfunction associated with further lipid peroxidation following closed head injury. Vitamin C has also been demonstrated to attenuate amyotrophic lateral sclerosis and mitochondrial encephalomyopathy.[69,70]

ISCHEMIA-REPERFUSION INJURY

Ischemia-reperfusion injury (IRI) is a damaging process of tissues brought about by rapid oxidative activity after a prolonged period of ischemia due to inadequate blood flow. It is thought to be caused in large part by oxygen radicals. Rhee reported on the effects of antioxidants on hepatic IRI. They induced IRI by clamping the porta hepatis for 30 min. Vitamin C and vitamin E administration lowered the malondialdehyde levels and protected against catalase exhaustion. They concluded that antioxidants protected the liver tissue against IRI.[71] Similarly, vitamin C effects have been evaluated in myocardial infarction. The effect on infarction was estimated with Evans blue and triphenyl tetrazolium. The results demonstrated that vitamin E and ascorbic acid effectively reduced myocardial necrosis after ischemia.[72]

THERMAL INJURY AND OXYGEN RADICALS

After burn injury, a cascade of biochemical and physiologic events bring about not only further local damage but also a systemic response (Chapter 11). While some of this response is the result of local cytokines and other inflammatory mediators, current research suggests that oxygen radicals play an important role in increased vascular permeability, lipid peroxidation of the cell membrane, and initiation of local and systemic inflammation after burn injury.[73–76] In 1989, Friedl and associates proved that thermal injury in rats causes a release of histamine by mast cells, leading to an increase in xanthine oxidase activity for the first 15 min following thermal trauma.[77] They also demonstrated that increased vascular permeability is not entirely due to histamine effects. Instead, it results from damage to the microvascular endothelial cells caused by oxygen free radicals, produced by the breakdown of xanthine by xanthine oxidase to produce hypoxanthine.[78]

Increased xanthine oxidase (XO) was well described in an animal model of burn injury.[79] Hydroxyl radicals (OH^-), released from the hypoxanthine–xanthine oxidase system during the dermal ischemia of the early phase of burn injury (within 2 h after injury), may play a major role in lipid peroxidation at the burn injury site.

Tanaka et al. induced burn injuries on the backs of rats and measured the value of tissue malondialdehyde (MDA) concentration to determine the oxidative injury in this burn model.[80] Although a number of degradation products have been reported to measure lipid peroxidation, MDA by the thiobarbituric acid assay is the most commonly used technique.[79] The MDA is a final metabolite, which is the unsaturated fatty acid peroxidized by attacks from free radicals and is considered to be an index of the production of oxygen radicals within the burn tissue (Figure 8.10). In this study, they found that tissue MDA concentration increased rapidly 30 min after injury and then reached a peak value 1 or 2 h after infliction of the injury. This would suggest that not only are free radical moieties involved with the original free radical damage of burns, but that this process continues for some time period after the original injury.

Many drugs have been reported to significantly attenuate this phenomenon in several burn models by preburn administration of antioxidants such as catalase, Mn-SOD, GSH (glutathione), vitamin E, desferoxamine, allopurinol, and lodoxamine.[78,81,82] Unfortunately, burn injury is not anticipated; thus, prophylactic administration of these

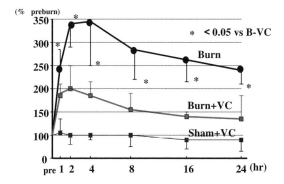

FIGURE 8.10 Changes lymphatic malondialdehyde (MDA) on burn hindpaw. The MDA (a lipid free radical end product) concentration of the lymph flow increased immediately after thermal injury and reached peak values 2 to 4 h after injury. The vitamin C administration group showed significantly lower values than that of control group. (*: $P < 0.05$ compared to the burn-vitamin-C administration group. (From Matsuda, T., *J. Burn Care. Rehabil.*, 14, 624, 1993. With permission.)

drugs is not feasible in a clinical setting. No clinically effective drug has been reported to date.

LABORATORY STUDIES OF VITAMIN C AND BURN INJURY

Applying the biochemical paradigm of vitamin C as a free radical scavenger, Tanaka evaluated the effectiveness of vitamin C on the early phase of burn injuries in several experimental models.

First, he studied 70% body surface area burn models in guinea pigs, which like humans, cannot synthesize vitamin C internally. In this guinea pig model, a dose of 170 mg/kg/24 h of vitamin C lessened increased vascular permeability in second-degree burns, and 340 mg/kg/24 h of vitamin C caused the same result in third-degree burns.[82,83] In the following study, the same animal model was used to examine the duration for continuous administration of vitamin C. This experiment revealed that a minimum of 8 h of continuous administration was needed to inhibit increased vascular permeability in third-degree burns (70%), with stable cardiac output and reduction in the water content of burn skin.[84]

More direct evidence of vitamin C efficacy on lipid peroxidation was found in lymph from burned canine hind paws.[85,86] Normally, extracellular fluid that leaks from blood vessels into the interstitial space immediately after burn injury is returned to the body fluids through the lymph vessels. By cannulation to these lymph vessels from the burn area, one may understand the direct changes within the cell that occur at a burn injury site. The degree of the increased protein leak was significantly less in the burned hind paws in the vitamin C administration group. In contrast, the control group demonstrated increased lymph flow accompanied by an increase in lymph-to-plasma-protein ratio, indicating that capillary permeability had increased in these burned hind paws. As seen in Figure 8.10, the MDA values of lymph flow were significantly reduced in the group administered vitamin C compared with the control group.

CLINICAL STUDIES OF VITAMIN C AND BURN INJURY

Based on this laboratory data, Tanaka et al. conducted clinical studies in humans. First, he examined the safety of continuous large-dose administration (66 mg/kg/h × 24 continuous hours; = 4.6 g/h in a 70 kg man) of vitamin C to 20 healthy adult volunteers.[87] This study revealed no abnormalities in liver function, kidney function, or blood clotting system for 7 d after administration of this dose, clearly indicating that high-dose vitamin C administration to humans appears to be safe.

The dose of vitamin C used in this study is fourfold higher than that used in guinea pigs. The optimum dose of vitamin C in humans has not been determined, but in a canine model of 50% total body surface area (TBSA) burn, similar benefits were observed using a dose of 66 mg/kg/h. It was speculated that large mammals may need larger doses of vitamin C, because they have more complex oxygen free radical generating systems.[88]

Finally, a clinical prospective randomized study was conducted in severe burn patients.[89] The study included consecutive patients with burns of more than 30% of their body surface area (BSA) who were admitted within 2 h postburn to the hospital. Inclusion criteria included those patients who were at least 15 yr but less than 70 yr of age. Patients having liver dysfunction or kidney dysfunction at the time of admission were excluded. Thirty-nine patients who met the criteria were used as subjects of this study during the 5-yr period. Nineteen patients were in the group administered vitamin C; 20 patients comprised the control group. The profiles of the two groups were similar regarding age, gender, body weight, and type of thermal injury, burn size (TBSA), percent of full thickness burn, and the presence of smoke inhalation. The experimental endpoints included the 24 h resuscitation fluid infusion volume, urinary output, changes in body weight, blood pressure, pulse, central venous pressure, hematocrit, total protein, albumin, MDA concentration in the blood, XOD (xanthine oxidase) activity in the blood, and changes in blood gases. These parameters were measured continuously over a period of 96 h. Furthermore, fluid infusion volume during the first 24 h was started immediately after admission using lactated Ringer's solution (L/R) according to the Parkland formula. The hourly infusion volume of the L/R was adjusted to maintain stable hemodynamic parameters (SBP > 90 mmHg) and urine output (0.5 to 1.0 ml/kg/h).

The results of this study are summarized in Figure 8.11. The 24-h resuscitation fluid volume requirement in the CTRL group was 5.5 ± 3.1 ml/kg/% burn, whereas the VC (vitamin C) group required only 3.0 ± 1.7 ml/kg/% burn, representing a 45.5% reduction in fluid requirements ($P < 0.004$), while adequate stable hemodynamic parameters and urine output were maintained. Burn wound edema at 24 h showed a significant reduction in the group administered vitamin C at 3.2 ± 1.3 ml/g per dry weight compared with 6.3 ± 1.6 ml/g per dry weight for the control group. Furthermore, by suppressing the increased vascular permeability, protein leakage

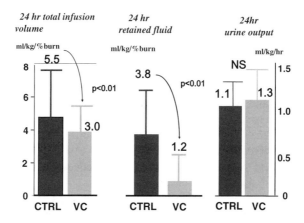

FIGURE 8.11 Patients treated with high-dose vitamin C (VC) vs. control (CTRL) burn patients required less fluid for resuscitation and retained less fluid while maintaining equivalent urine output to controls. (*: $P < 0.05$ compared to the VC.)

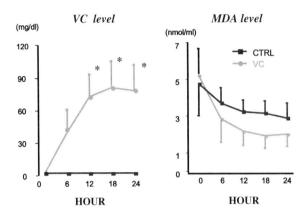

FIGURE 8.12 Burn patients receiving high-dose vitamin C (VC) had higher plasma concentration of vitamin C than controls (CTRL) and lower malondialdehyde (MDA) concentration than controls.

was inhibited, and total blood protein and albumin values were maintained at a significantly higher level for 12 to 72 h after the injury in the group administered vitamin C. However, no differences existed between the two groups in the hemodynamic (blood pressure, pulse, CVP pressure, and hematocrit value) parameters; thus, both groups had similar hemodynamics. Moreover, because the vitamin C solution was adjusted to the same sodium concentration and osmolality as lactated Ringer's solution, there were no significant differences between the two groups in the Na concentration in blood and in urine, or in osmolality in the blood and urine. A notable finding in the MDA concentration and XOD activity in the blood — both indicators of the lipid peroxidation and hydroxyl radical productivity of the burn tissue — was the decrease to a normal range after administration of vitamin C, in comparison to the control group (Figure 8.12).

Members of the group administered vitamin C had a higher PO_2/FiO_2 ratio from 18 to 72 h after injury. The length of mechanical ventilation in the group administered vitamin C was significantly shorter. It is clear from these results that the suppression of the edema generation and the effect of inhibiting the increased vascular permeability prevented respiratory dysfunction immediately after burn injury (Figure 8.13).

The goal of fluid resuscitation during the immediate postburn period is to maintain an adequate intravascular volume with minimum amount of fluid. The clinical benefits of the reduced fluid resuscitation volume with stable hemodynamic values that we observed using vitamin C led not only to a clear reduction in edema and body weight gain, but were also associated with reduced respiratory impairment and a reduced requirement for mechanical ventilation.

The present study involved a small number of patients showing the value of high-dose vitamin C therapy as an adjunct to resuscitation in severely burned patients. Oxygen radicals play an important role in increased vascular permeability, lipid peroxidation of the cell membrane, and initiation of local and systemic inflammation after burn injury. The authors conclude that even a small improvement of respiratory and hemodynamic parameters in the initial stage of burn injury may lead to a

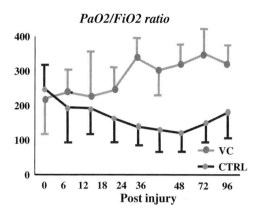

FIGURE 8.13 Burn patients receiving high-dose vitamin C (VC) vs. control (CTRL) demonstrated improved oxygenation (see text).

significant advance in the treatment of fluid resuscitation of thermal injury. One may conclude that vitamin C may prove extremely useful as an adjunctive therapy for the management of the burn shock period as well as for minimizing the progression of the severity of the burn wound in the early hours after injury.

In a similar fashion, Nathens et al. evaluated the efficacy of a combination of tocopherol (vitamin E) and vitamin C in a prospective randomized trial on critically ill surgical trauma patients.[28] In this study, 595 patients were enrolled. Those randomized to antioxidant supplementation received tocopherol (1000 IU) every 8 h per gastric tube and 1000 mg of ascorbic acid every 8 h intravenously for the period of time in the ICU or for 28 d. Measured outcomes included pulmonary morbidity, multiple organ system failure, duration of mechanical ventilation, length of intensive care stay, and mortality. Based on this treatment, pulmonary morbidity was significantly decreased, as was duration of mechanical ventilation and ICU stay.

While the above studies concerned patients with wounds, outcomes measured were primarily systemic endpoints rather than wound healing endpoints. However, as suggested elsewhere in this chapter and in this book (Chapter 1), one might anticipate improved wound healing either from the decrease in total metabolic stress or from a direct effect on the wound. Tanaka's studies clearly indicate decreased edema, which results in improved vascular density and decreased perfusion distances. Nathens' study would perhaps have an indirect influence on wound healing; pulmonary function was improved, allowing better tissue oxygenation and less total metabolic stress, leaving a metabolic reserve for improved wound healing.

TOXICITY OF VITAMIN C

Ascorbic acid appears to have very few toxic side effects. This is not surprising in view of the rate-limiting mechanisms of gastrointestinal absorption and the linearity in urinary excretion as described above. It would appear that it is impossible for the body to store significant quantities of vitamin C, thus minimizing adverse systemic effects.[1–4,10,27,31] These limitations in intestinal absorption are one of the arguments against high-dose oral vitamin C. It will result only in bathing the gastrointestinal tract with large quantities of ascorbate, but it will not increase plasma or tissue levels.[90]

Side effects of ascorbic acid have been reported in people taking ascorbic acid at 3 g/d. Complaints at this dose level include nausea, abdominal cramping, bloating, and diarrhea.[1,31] The upper limit of oral intake is, therefore, set at 2 g/d.[1,32] Nonetheless, some proponents of high-dose vitamin C intake for antioxidant value advocate 4 to 6 g/d of oral intake and anecdotally, these large doses seem to be tolerated.

One of the breakdown products of vitamin C is oxalate. In normal circumstances, oxalate accounts for 35 to 50% of the oxalate excretion by the body every day. However, this pathway of metabolic excretion is limited; therefore, large doses of vitamin C should not cause excessive oxaluria. In studies of normal people with no history of renal stones or kidney disease, increased vitamin C consumption did not increase kidney stone formation.[31] However, in patients with renal failure or known oxalate renal stone history, caution should be used, and vitamin C should be limited to 200 mg/d.[30,31]

In a similar fashion, because uric acid and ascorbic acid are both reabsorbed in the proximal tubule, there is concern that high-dose ascorbate intake could decrease renal absorption of uric acid, leading to gout. However, it appears that, because the tubular reabsorption of ascorbic acid is a saturable process, this concern is not valid. Studies have demonstrated in normal individuals that intakes of 4 to 12 g of ascorbic acid per day did not increase serum uric acid levels or urine uric acid or uric acid clearance.[31,91] Even in individuals with a history of gout, it is doubtful that large doses of ascorbate decrease uric acid excretion, although it would be prudent to be cautious in such individuals.

Because ascorbic acid facilitates absorption of nonheme iron by changing the redox state of the iron, there has been concern that elevated vitamin C intake could result in excessive iron storage. However, optimal promotion of iron absorption is induced with iron intakes of 25 to 50 mg per meal, suggesting that larger intakes would not result in excessive iron accumulation.[1,31,92] Cook et al. demonstrated that even 2 g/d of ascorbate taken in divided doses with meals did not induce increased iron stores over 18 months of observation in otherwise healthy individuals.[93] Nonetheless, caution should be used in patients with iron overload or in susceptible patients, such as those with sickle cell disease, sideroblastic anemia, thalassemia major, or those needing frequent blood transfusions.

Glucose-6-phosphate deficiency is a genetic disease that leads to hemolytic crises when the individual is exposed to oxidative stress. Hemolyis may be precipitated with intakes of oral doses of 6 g of vitamin C, with lower doses given by intravenous administration.[1,94]

As discussed above, Tanaka et al. examined the safety of continuous large-dose administration (66 mg/kg/h × 24 continuous hours; = 4.6 gm/h in a 70 kg man) of vitamin C to 20 healthy adult volunteers.[87] These studies revealed no abnormalities in liver function, kidney function, or the blood clotting system for 7 d after administration of this dose in healthy volunteers. This would suggest that even in extremely high doses given for short time periods, vitamin C has minimal adverse effects.

Vitamin C in doses of greater than 250 mg per day may cause false positive blood stool tests.[1,31] This must be considered in routine tests for occult blood. In a similar fashion, because ascorbate is excreted in the urine, it may interfere with urinary sugar tests.

Finally, certain adverse side effects that have been attributed to vitamin C must be mentioned only to indicate that they have not been proven to be true. It does not appear that vitamin C can cause hypoglycemia, rebound scurvy, infertility, mutagenesis, or destruction of vitamin B_{12}.[1,31]

RECOMMENDATIONS FOR VITAMIN C TO SUPPORT WOUND HEALING

The combined effect of ascorbic acid on collagen synthesis, antioxidant status, and immunomodulation make it an appropriate supplement for wound repair protocols. Research provides evidence for the use of low doses of vitamin C in vitamin C deficient individuals, but many practitioners believe larger doses of ascorbic acid in nondeficient individuals are indicated for optimal wound repair. In light of the discussion above, one must also decide if vitamin C is to be provided as an enzymatic cofactor or as an antioxidant.

While the literature is controversial, the authors suggest that to support collagen synthesis and immune function in otherwise healthy individuals with small wounds, such as pressure ulcers or elective small to moderate surgery, doses of 500 to 1000 mg should be given daily in two divided doses. Those with larger injury, such as large body surface area burns and multiple traumas, should be given doses of 1 to 2 g/d.

Proper doses to optimize antioxidant effect remain to be determined. The studies of Tanaka suggest 66 mg/kg/h intravenously for patients with large body surface area burns.[84–87,89] For multiple trauma patients Nathens et al. suggest an intake of only 1000 mg/d in three divided doses, as well as vitamin E.[28] Inadequate data exist to recommend doses to optimize the antioxidant effect in patients with smaller wounds and less metabolic stress. The low risk of toxicity suggests the liberal use of vitamin C.

FUTURE DIRECTIONS

Much of the controversy in the literature on vitamin C in wound healing revolves around the measured endpoints for optimal nutrition. Some studies measure plasma levels, some measure tissue levels, and others measure clinical parameters of vitamin C nutriture. In addition, some look at clinical parameters of collagen synthesis, immune competence, or free radical metabolism. Future studies should concentrate on functional assays of vitamin C deficiency. Serum and tissue levels are of uncertain value, even in healthy individuals, and will continue to be problematic when used to assess nutrition in the critically ill. Development of biochemical assays of collagen metabolism, immune function, and free radical metabolism that could be obtained as a clinical test rather than a laboratory research project would be invaluable to help in the healing of our wound patients.

Although the role of ascorbate in collagen metabolism has long been understood and extensively studied, further research on the other enzymatic cofactor functions and on its role in general protein synthesis must be better understood. The effect that these systems have on wound healing must also be elucidated.

Much of the future research in vitamin C will revolve around its use as a free radical scavenger. Its role in protecting against disease as well as in treating injury must be further understood, and proper safe intakes at these pharmacologic levels of ascorbate must be determined in a variety of clinical situations. The interaction of ascorbate and other antioxidants, such as glutathione and vitamin E, must be better understood to allow for the determination of proper clinical doses of vitamin C.

REFERENCES

1. Levine, M., Katz, A., Padayatty, S., Vitamin C, in *Modern Nutrition in Health and Disease,* Shils, M., Shike, M., Ross, A.C., Caballero, B., Cousins, R.J., Lippincott Williams & Wilkins, Philadelphia, 2006, chap. 31.
2. Hodges, R.E., Ascorbic acid, in *Modern Nutrition in Health and Disease,* Goodhart, R.S. and Shils, M.E., Lea & Febiger, Philadelphia, 1980, chap. 6K, p. 259.
3. Hirschmann, J.V. and Raugi, G.J., Adult scurvy, *J. Am. Acad. Dermatol.,* 41, 895, 1999.
4. Levensen, S.M. and Demetrious, A.A., Metabolic factors, in *Wound Healing: Biochemical and Clinical Aspects,* Cohen, I.K, Diegelman, R.F., and Lindblad, W.B., Eds., W.B. Saunders, Philadelphia, 1992, chap. 15, p. 248.
5. Food and Nutrition Board, National Academy of Sciences, *Recommended Daily Allowances,* 10th ed.,Washington, D.C., 1989, p. 115.
6. Blusztajn, J.K. and Wurtman, R.J., Choline and cholinergic neurons, *Science,* 221, 614, 1983.
7. Crandon, J.H. and Lund, C.C., Vitamin C deficiency in an otherwise normal adult, *N. Engl. J. Med.,* 222, 748, 1940.
8. Walter, R. and Robins, B., in *A Voyage Round the World in The Years MDCCXL, I, II, III, IV by George Anson,* Oxford University Press, London, 1974, p. 106.
9. Hemila, H., Vitamin C, respiratory infections and the immune system, *Trends in Immunol.,* 24, 579, 2003.
10. Padayatty, S. and Levine, M., New insights into the physiology and pharmacology of vitamin C, *CMAJ,* 164, 353, 2001.
11. Rumsey, S.C. and Levine, M., Absorption, transport, and disposition of ascorbic acid in humans, *J. Nutr. Biochem.,* 9, 116, 1998.
12. Gray, M. and Whitmey, J.D., Does vitamin C supplementation promote pressure ulcer healing, *JWOCN,* 30, 245, 2003.
13. Peterkofshy, B., Ascorbate requirements for hydroxylation and secretion of procollagen: relationship to inhibition of collagen synthesis in scurvy, *Am. J. Clin. Nutr.,* 54, 1135S, 1991.
14. ReGouche, C.J., Ascorbic acid and carnitine biosynthesis, *Am. J. Clin. Nutr.,* 54, 1147S, 1991.
15. Lindblad, B., Lindstedt, G., and Lindstedt, S., The mechanism of enzymic formation of homogentisate from *p*-hydroxyphenyl pyruvate, *J. Am. Chem. Soc.,* 92, 7446–7449, 1970.
16. Miller, E.J., Collagen types: structure, distribution and functions, in *Collagen Vol. II Biochemistry and Biomechanics,* Nimni, M.E., CRC Press, Boca Raton, FL, 1988, 139–156.
17. Ronchetti, I.P., Quaglino, D., and Bergaminni, G., Ascorbic acid and connective tissue, *Subcell. Biochem.,* 25, 249, 1996.

18. McCord, J.M., The superoxide free radical; its biochemistry and pathophysiology, *Surgery,* 94, 412, 1983.
19. Green, M.J. and Hao, H., Chemistry of dioxygen, *Meth. Enzymol.,* 105, 3–22.
20. Babior, B.M., Oxygen-dependent microbial killing by phagocytes, *N. Engl. J. Med.,* 298, 721, 1978.
21. Niki, E. et al., Inhibition of oxidation of methyl linoleate in solution by vitamin E and vitamin C, *J. Biol. Chem.,* 259, 4177, 1984.
22. Nishikimi, M., Oxidation of ascorbic acid with superoxide anion generated by the xanthine-xanthine oxidase system, *Biochem. Biophys. Res. Commun.,* 63, 463, 1975.
23. Bielski, B.H.J., Richter, H.W., and Chan, P.C., Some properties of the ascorbate free radical, *Ann. N.Y. Acad, Sci.,* 258, 231, 1975.
24. Bodannes, R.S. and Chan, P.C., Ascorbic acid as a scavenger of singlet oxygen, *FEBS Lett.,* 105, 195, 1979.
25. Shukla, A., Rasik, A.M., and Patnail, G.K., Depletion of reduced glutathione, ascorbic acid, vitamin E and antioxidant defence enzymes in a healing cutaneous wound, *Free Radic. Res.,* 26, 93, 1997.
26. Frei, B., Srocker, R., and Ames, B.N., Antioxidant defences and lipid peroxidation in human blood plasma, *Proc. Natl. Acad. Sci. U.S.A.,* 85, 9748, 1988.
27. Long, C.L. et al., Ascorbic acid dynamics in the seriously ill and injured, *J. Surg. Res.,* 109, 144, 2003.
28. Nathens, A.B. et al., Randomized, prospective trial of antioxidant supplementation in critically ill surgical patients, *Ann. Surg.,* 236, 814, 2002.
29. Dhariwal, K.R., Hartzwell, W.O., and Levine, M., Ascorbic acid and dehydroascorbic acid measurements in human plasma and serum, *Am. J. Clin. Nutr.,* 54, 712, 1991.
30. Dylewski, D.F. and Froman, D.M., Vitamin C supplementation in the patient with burns and renal failure, *J. Burn Care Rehabil.,* 13, 378, 1992.
31. Rivers, J.M., Safety of high level vitamin C ingestion, *Ann. N.Y. Acad. Science,* 498, 445, 1987.
32. Levine, M., Katz, A. et al., in *Modern Nutrition in Health and Disease*, Shils, M., Shike, M., Ross, A.C., Cabellero, B., and Cousins, R.J., Eds., Lippincott Williams & Wilkins, Philadelphia, 2005, p. 517, Figure 31.4.
33. Food and Nutrition Board, Vitamin C, in *Recommended Daily Allowances,* Commission on Life Sciences, National Research Council, The National Academies Press, Washington, D.C., 1989, pp. 115ñ124.
34. Scholl, D. and Langkamp-Henken, B., Nutrient recommendations for wound healing, *J. Intraven. Nurs.,* 24, 124, 2001.
35. Akikusa, J.D., Garrick, D., and Nash, M.C., Scurvy forgotten but not gone, *J. Paediatr. Child Health,* 39, 75, 2003.
36. Pugliese, P.T., The skinís antioxidant systems,*Dermatol. Nurs.,* 10, 401, 1998.
37. Rousseau, A.S. et al., Antioxidant vitamin status in high exposure to oxidative stress in competitive athletes, *Br. J. Nutr.,* 92, 461, 2004.
38. Tanzer, F. and Ozalp, I., Leukocyte ascorbic acid concentration and plasma ascorbic acid levels in children with various infections, *Mater. Med. Pol.,* 25, 5, 1993.
39. Hemila, H. and Douglas, R.M., Vitamin C and acute respiratory infections, *Int. J. Tuberc. Lung Dis.,* 3, 756, 1999.
40. Wolbach, S.B., Controlled formation of collagen and reticulum. A study of the source of intercellular substance in recovery from experimental scobutus, *Am. J. Path.,* 1X, 689, 1933.
41. Ronchetti, I.P., Quaglino, D., and Bergaminni, G., Ascorbic acid and connective tissue, *Subcell. Biochem.,* 25, 249, 1996.

42. Kaplan, B. et al., Relationship between tensile strength, ascorbic acid, hydroxy-proline, and zinc levels of rabbit full thickness incision wound healing, *Surg. Today,* 34, 747, 2004.

43. Crowley, L.V., Seifter, E., and Kriss, P., Effects of environmental temperature and femoral fracture on wound healing in rats, *J. Trauma,* 17, 436, 1977.

44. Schauble, J.F. et al., A study of the distribution of ascorbic acid in the wound healing of guinea pig tissue, *Surg. Gyn. Obstetrics,* 110, 314, 1960.

45. Levensen, S.M. et al., Effect of thermal burns on wound healing, *Ann. Surg.,* 146, 357, 1957.

46. Yung, S., Mayersohn, M., and Robinson, J., Ascorbic acid elimination in humans after intravenous administration, *J. Pharm. Sci.,* 67, 1491, 1978.

47. Taylor, T.V. et al., Ascorbic acid supplementation in the treatment of pressure sores, *Lancet,* 2, 544, 1974.

48. Reit, G.T., Kessel, A.G.H., and Knipschild, P.G., Randomized clinical trial of ascorbic acid in the treatment of pressure ulcers, *J. Clin. Epidemiol.,* 48, 1453, 1995.

49. Shukla, S.P., Plasma and urinary ascorbic acid levels in the postoperative period, *Experientia,* 25, 704, 1969.

50. Irvin, T.T., Chattopadhyay, D.K., and Smythe, A., Ascorbic acid requirements in postoperative patients, *Surg. Gyn. Obstetrics,* 147, 49, 1978.

51. Bartlett, M., Jones, C.M., and Ryan, A.E., Vitamin C and wound healing II: ascorbic acid content and tensile strength of healing wounds in human beings, *N. Engl. J. Med.,* 226, 474, 1942.

52. Ringsdorf, W.M. and Cheraskin, E., Vitamin C and human wound healing, *Oral Surg.,* 53, 231, 1982.

53. Afifi, A.M. et al., High dose ascorbic acid in the management of thalassalmia leg ulcers — a pilot study, *Br. J. Dermatol.,* 92, 339, 1975.

54. Shukla, A., Rasik, A.M., and Patnail, G.K., Depletion of reduced glutathione, ascorbic acid, vitamin E and antioxidant defence enzymes in a healing cutaneous wound, *Free Radic. Res.,* 26, 93, 1997.

55. Stadelmann, W.K., Digenis, A.G., and Tobtin, G.R., Physiology and healing dynamics of chronic cutaneous wounds, *Am. J. Surg.,* 176, 26S, 1998.

56. Barbul, A., Immune aspects of wound repair, *Clin. Plast. Surg.,* 17, 433, 1990.

57. Anderson, R. et al., The effect of ascorbate on cellular humoral immunity in asthmatic children, *S. Afr. Med. J.,* 58, 974, 1980.

58. Kennes, B. et al., Effect of vitamin C supplements on cell-mediated immunity in old people, *Gerontology,* 29, 305, 1983.

59. Anderson, R. et al., The effects of increasing weekly doses of ascorbate on certain cellular and humoral immune functions in normal volunteers, *Am. J. Clin. Nutr.,* 33, 71, 1980.

60. Rasik, A.M. and Shukla, A., Antioxidant status in delayed healing type of wounds, *Int. J. Exp. Pathol.,* 81, 257, 2000.

61. Long, C.L. et al., Ascorbic acid dynamics in the seriously ill and injured, *J. Surg. Res.,* 109, 144, 2003.

62. Nathens, A.B. et al., Randomized, prospective trial of antioxidant supplementation in critically ill surgical patients, *Ann. Surg.,* 236, 814, 2002.

63. Miyagantani, Y. et al., High dose vitamin C enhances hepatic glutathionine levels and increases survival of septic rats, *Surg. Forum XLIX,* 55, 1998.

64. Nathens, A.B. et al., Randomized, prospective trial of antioxidant supplementation in critically ill surgical patients, *Ann. Surg.,* 236, 814, 2002.

65. Nowak, D., Ruta, U., and Piasecka, G., Ascorbic acid inhibits polymorphonuclear leukocytes influx to the place of inflammation — possible protection of lung from phagocyte mediated injury, *Arch. Immunol. Ther. Exp.*, 37, 213, 1989.

66. Kovacikova, Z. and Ginter, E., Effect of ascorbic acid supplementation during the inhalation exposure of guinea pigs to industrial dust on bronchoalveolar lavage and pulmonary enzymes, *J. Appl. Toxicol.*, 15, 321, 1995.

67. Barabas, K. et al., Effects of ascorbic acid *in vivo* on the fatty acid composition of the tissues of mice treated with Gramoxone, *Gen. Pharmacol.*, 17, 363, 1986.

68. Elangovan, V., Kohen, R., and Shohami, E., Neurological recovery from closed head injury is impaired in diabetic rats, *J. Neurotrauma*, 17, 1013, 2000.

69. Nagano, S. et al., Benefit of a combined treatment with trientine and ascorbate in familial amyotrophic lateral sclerosis model mice, *Neurosci. Lett.*, 265, 159, 1999.

70. Ihara, Y. et al., Free radicals in the cerebrospinal fluid are associated with neurological disorders including mitochondrial encephalomyopathy, *Biochem. Mol. Biol. Int.*, 42, 937, 1997.

71. Rhee, J.E. et al., The effects of antioxidants and nitric oxide modulators on hepatic ischemic-reperfusion injury in rats, *J. Korean Med. Sci.*, 17, 502, 2002.

72. Mickle, D.A. et al., Myocardial salvage with trolox and ascorbic acid for an acute evolving infarction, *Ann. Thorac. Surg.*, 47, 553, 1989.

73. Demling, R.H. and Lalonde, C., Identification and modification of the pulmonary and systemic inflammatory and biochemical changes caused by a skin burn, *J. Trauma*, 30, 57, 1990.

74. Demling, R.H. et al., The immediate effect of burn wound excision on pulmonary function in sheep: the role of prostanoids, oxygen radicals, and chemoattractants, *Surgery*, 101, 44, 1987.

75. Demling, R.H. and Lalonde, C., Systemic lipid perioxidation and inflammation induced by thermal injury persists into the post resuscitation period, *J. Trauma*, 30, 69, 1990.

76. Friedle, H.P. et al., A mediator induced activation of xanthine oxidase in endothelial cells, *FASEB J.*, 3, 2512, 1989.

77. Friedle, H.P. et al., Role of histamine, complement and xanthine oxidase in thermal injury of skin, *Am. J. Pathol.*, 135, 203, 1989.

78. Till, G.O. et al., Role of xanthine oxidase in thermal injury of skin, *Am. J. Pathol.*, 135, 195, 1989.

79. Demling, R.H. and Lalonde, C., Relationship between lung injury and lung lipid perioxidation caused by recurrent endotoxemia, *Rev. Respir. Dis.*, 139, 1118, 1989.

80. Shimazaki, E. et al., Effects of the antiprotease Ulinastatin on mortality and oxidant injury in scalded rats, *Arch. Surg.*, 130, 99, 1995.

81. Ohkawa, H., Ohishi, N., and Yagi, K., Assay for lipid peroxides in animal tissues by thiobarbituric acid reaction, *Anal. Biochem.*, 95, 351, 1979.

82. Matsuda, T. et al., High dose vitamin C therapy for extensive deep dermal burns, *Burns*, 18, 127, 1992.

83. Matsuda, T. et al., Reduced fluid volume requirement for resuscitation of third degree burns with high dose vitamin C, *J. Burn Care Rehabil.*, 12, 525, 1991.

84. Tanaka, H. et al., How long do we need to give antioxidant therapy during resuscitation when its administration is delayed for two hours?, *J. Burn Care Rehabil.*, 13, 567, 1992.

85. Matsuda, T. et al., The effects of high dose vitamin C therapy on postburn lipid peroxidation, *J. Burn Care Rehabil.*, 14, 624, 1993.

86. Matsuda, T. et al., Effects of high dose vitamin C administration on postburn microvascular fluid and protein flux, *J. Burn Care Rehabil.,* 13, 560, 1992.

87. Matsuda, T. et al., Study of safety of continuous intravenous infusion of high dose vitamin C in healthy human volunteers, *J. Burn Care Rehabil.,* 17, 141, 1994.

88. Tolmasoff, J.M., Ono, T., and Culter, R.G., Superoxide dismutase: correlation with life span and specific metabolic rate in primate species, *Proc. Natl. Acad. Sci.,* 77, 2777, 1980.

89. Tanaka, H. et al., Vitamin C administration reduces resuscitation fluid volume in severely burned patients: a randomized, prospective study, *Arch. Surg.,* 135, 326, 2000.

90. Shane, B., Vitamin C pharmokinetics: it's déjà vu all over again, *Am. J. Clin. Nutr.,* 66, 1061, 1997.

91. Schmidt, K. et al., Urinary oxalate excretion after large intakes of ascorbic acid in man, *Am. J. Clin. Nutr.,* 34, 305, 1981.

92. Cacciola, E. et al., Ascorbic acid deficiency may be a cause of refractoriness to iron-therapy in the treatment of iron-deficiency anemia, *Haematologica,* 79, 96, 1994.

93. Cook, J.D. et al., The effect of high ascorbic acid supplementation on body iron stores, *Blood,* 64, 721, 1984.

94. Rees, D.C., Kelsey, H., and Richards, J.D., Acute haemolysis induced by high dose ascorbic acid in glucose-6-phosphate dehydrogenase deficiency, *BMJ,* 306, 841, 1993.

9 Fat-Soluble Vitamins and Wound Healing

Michele M. Gottschlich

CONTENTS

INTRODUCTION

The functions, uses, and salutary effects of fat-soluble vitamins in wound healing are described in this review. This encompasses supplementation options for a spectrum of conditions of repair from the treatment of dermatologic disorders to more serious wound conditions. Guidelines are presented for intake of vitamins A, D, E, and K in an effort to optimize wound healing. Adverse events (primarily associated with vitamin E) as well as the consequences of fat-soluble vitamin toxicity are discussed.

VITAMIN A

GENERAL METABOLISM

The term "vitamin A" is often employed generically for derivatives such as retinol, retinal, retinoic acid, and retinyl. It is acquired from the diet either as preformed vitamin A or as its provitamin A carotenoids. The term "provitamin A" is used to describe all carotenoids that show the biological activity of vitamin A. Of the ten forms of carotenoids, the most significant is beta-carotene. In mammals, β-carotene-15,15-dioxygenase catalyzes conversion of beta-carotene to retinal. This initial cleavage enzyme is rate limiting and noninducible. Beta-carotene's biologic activity is about one-sixth that of preformed vitamin A — making it less toxic. Dietary sources of vitamin A are summarized in Table 9.1.

After foods are ingested, preformed vitamin A of animal tissues and the provitamin carotenoids of vegetables and fruits are released from proteins by the action of proteolytic enzymes, first collecting in the stomach as fatty globules and then entering the duodenum. In the presence of bile salts, the globules are broken down into smaller lipid moieties that are further digested by pancreatic lipase and hydrolases. The resultant micelles are then readily absorbed into mucosal cells, mainly in the upper portion of the intestine. Under normal conditions, over 90% of vitamin A is stored in the liver.

The best elucidated role of vitamin A is in the visual process, where it is converted into the photopigments of rod and cone cells of the retina. Visual function is mediated by retinal, exclusively.

Although less well understood, the extra-retinal functions of vitamin A are of greater physiological impact than the visual function. Collectively referred to as "systemic" functions of the vitamin, this includes vital roles in differentiation, proliferation, and function of epithelial cells and on growth in general. That vitamin A plays a major role in epithelialization throughout the body (1), and that vitamin A deficiency has a detrimental effect on wound healing (2) has been known for many years.

Vitamin A also supports immunocompetence. Vitamin A deficient animals and humans are typically more susceptible to infection and have higher mortality rates than individuals with adequate vitamin A nutriture. Retinoids and carotenoids appear to affect immunity in different ways. Retinoids act on the differentiation of immune cells, increasing the number and nature of white blood cells and increasing phagocytosis of monocytes and macrophages involved in immune, inflammatory, and wound healing processes (3,4). Carotenoids seem to affect immunosurveilance of activated natural killer (NK) cells and T-helper cells by modifying the release of at least some cytokine-like products by activated lymphocytes and monocytes.

ROLE IN WOUND HEALING

Vitamin A has been effectively used pharmacologically in numerous inflammatory and dermatologic diseases, such as acne, atopic dermatitis, photodamage, striae, cellulite, and disorders of keratinization, including psoriasis and corneal healing (5–12). Pretreatment with retinoids before epidermal injury accelerates repair following cosmetic procedures such as chemical peels and dermabrasion (9,13–15).

Numerous studies have demonstrated the positive role of vitamin A in the treatment of open wounds. Known processes that influence healing that require vitamin A include epithelial growth, synthesis of glycoproteins and proteoglycans, cellular immunity, and the inflammatory reaction (3,4,7,16–20). Vitamin A can reverse the anti-inflammatory effect of steroids on wound healing. Reports by Hunt and colleagues (21–25) and others (26) have repeatedly shown that local or systemic administration of vitamin A to a steroid-retarded wound accelerates the formation of healthy granulation tissue and the healing rate. Vitamin A supplementation also increases collagen content and breaking strength in a variety of experimental models, including cutaneous wounds, flexor tendon repair, and intestinal anastomoses, to name a few (16,17,24,27–30). *In vitro*, vitamin A can accelerate fibroblast maturation and multiplication and increase the number of fibroblast receptors for epidermal growth factor (16,30). Additionally, both topical and enteral supplementation with this vitamin have been shown to facilitate wound healing in laboratory animals (3,17,18,26–28,31–36), as well as in the clinical repair (37,38) of wounds associated with fractures, burns, ulcerations, radiation, and antineoplastic therapies, or streptozotocin-induced diabetes.

CONSEQUENCES OF NUTRIENT DEFICIENCY

Table 9.1 highlights those at high risk of inadequate vitamin A status. Vitamin A deficient individuals experience replacement of normal mucous-secreting cells by cells that produce keratin (1), particularly in the conjunctiva and cornea, the trachea, the skin, and other ectodermal tissues. Deficiency symptoms include xerophthalmia (night blindness, conjunctival xerosis, Bitot's spots), respiratory ailments (pneumonia, bronchopulmonary dysplasia), increased susceptibility to infection, stunted growth, skin disorders, and delayed wound healing (21,39,40). Vitamin A deficiency impairs epithelialization, collagen synthesis, wound contraction, and cross-linking of newly formed collagen.

CONSEQUENCES OF NUTRIENT EXCESS

Short-term vitamin A supplementation with large amounts (150,000 IU) has not resulted in adverse side effects (3). However, prolonged high doses of vitamin A (over 50,000 IU/d) can be toxic (41). Clinical symptoms include nausea, vomiting, headache, dizziness, muscle weakness, gingivitis, alopecia, and peeling skin. An excessive inflammatory response, defects in cell-mediated immunity, visual and liver

TABLE 9.1
Fat-Soluble Vitamins in Wound Healing

Vitamin	Function in Wound Healing	Subjects at Risk of Deficiency [Reference]	Sources	Dietary Reference Intakes (DRI)	Recommendations to Optimize Wound Healing [Reference]
A	Major role in the differentiation and function of epithelial tissue; cofactor for collagen synthesis and cross-linkage; required for synthesis of glycoproteins and proteoglycans; stimulates fibroplasia and normalizes keritinization; inflammatory response is dependent on the presence of adequate vitamin A; counteracts the deleterious effects of glucocorticoids on cell membranes	Malnutrition, injury, burns [144–147], chronic wounds [148]	Vitamin A as retinol is found in animal products; good sources include liver, fish liver oils, enriched dairy products, and egg yolk; beta-carotene is found in plants, including yellow and orange fruits and vegetables such as carrots, sweet potato, squash, winter squash, dried apricots, peaches, and dark green leafy vegetables including spinach, broccoli, and lettuce	*Infants:* 0–6 months, 133* IU/d; 7–12 months, 1666* IU/d *Children:* 1–3 yr, **1000** IU/d; 4–8 yr, **1333** IU/d *Males:* 9–13 yr, **2000** IU/d; 14–18 yr, **3000** IU/d; 19–30 yr, **3000** IU/d; 31–50 yr, **3000** IU/d; 50–70 yr, **3000** IU/d; > 70 yr, **3000** IU/d *Females:* 9–13 yr, **2000** IU/d; 14–18 yr, **2333** IU/d; 19–30 yr, **2333** IU/d; 31–50 yr, **2333** IU/d; 50–70 yr, **2333** IU/d; > 70 yr, **2333** IU/d *Pregnancy:* ≤ 18 yr, **2500** IU/d; 19–30 yr, **2566** IU/d; 31–50 yr, **2566** IU/d *Lactation:* ≤ 18 yr, **4000** IU/d; 19–30 yr, **4333** IU/d; 31–50 yr, **4333** IU/d	Correct deficiency; daily enteric supplementation of 10,000–25,000 IU may enhance wound healing in patients with poor nutrient stores, malabsorption, severe injury or in those receiving steroids [16,37,39,46–48]

| D | Regulates the cutaneous immune system; downregulates epithelial proliferation and promotes differentiation | Elderly and house-bound people [52,81,88,89,149–152]; patients with burns; critically ill [89]; some breast-fed infants; long-term TPN [153,154]; anticonvulsant [155]; corticosteroid [156–158]; oxandrolone [50] or thyroxine [50] use protein deficiency [159]; liver disease [82,83,150]; renal disease [160,161]; malabsorptive disorders, such as tropical sprue; and regional enteritis [162–164]; systemic lupus erythematosis [158] | Exogenous and endogenous sources of vitamin D exist; vitamin D is produced in the skin; vitamin D_2 is found in food sources, such as saltwater fish (e.g., herring, mackerel, salmon, and sardines), liver and fat from seals and polar bears, eggs from hens that were fed vitamin D, fortified milk products, and other enriched food such as cereal | *Infants:*
0–6 months, 5* μg/d;
7–12 months, 5* μg/d
Children:
1–3 yr, 5* μg/d;
4–8 yr, 5* μg/d
Males:
9–13 yr, 5* μg/d;
14–18 yr, 5* μg/d;
19–30 yr, 5* μg/d;
31–50 yr, 5* μg/d;
50–70 yr, 10* μg/d;
> 70 yr, 15* μg/d
Females:
9–13 yr, 5* μg/d;
14–18 yr, 5* μg/d;
19–30 yr, 5* μg/d;
31–50 yr, 5* μg/d;
50–70 yr, 10* μg/d;
> 70 yr, 15* μg/d
Pregnancy:
≤ 18 yr, 5* μg/d;
19–30 yr, 5* μg/d;
31–50 yr, 5* μg/d
Lactation:
≤ 18 yr, 5* μg/d;
19–30 yr, 5* μg/d;
31–50 yr, 5* μg/d | Correct deficiency; vitamin D supplementation is recommended in patients with burns [50,51] |

(continued)

TABLE 9.1 (Continued)
Fat-Soluble Vitamins in Wound Healing

Vitamin	Function in Wound Healing	Subjects at Risk of Deficiency [Reference]	Sources	Dietary Reference Intakes (DRI)	Recommendations to Optimize Wound Healing [Reference]
E	Membrane antioxidant, influences wound healing by stabilizing cell walls and enhancing immune response	Long-term TPN [130,165]; premature infants [104,166]; those with burns and open wounds [108,111,112,146, 148,167,168]; malabsorption syndromes, such as celiac disease, biliary atresia, cystic fibrosis, pancreatitis [133]	Vegetable oils (primarily soybean, sunflower, and corn oils), unprocessed cereal grains, seeds, nuts, wheat germ, fruits, dark green leafy vegetables, legumes, meats	*Infants:* 0–6 months, 4* mg/d; 7–12 months, 5* mg/d *Children:* 1–3 yr, **6** mg/d; 4–8 yr, **7** mg/d *Males:* 9–13 yr, **11** mg/d; 14–18 yr, **15** mg/d; 19–30 yr, **15** mg/d; 31–50 yr, **15** mg/d; 50–70 yr, **15** mg/d; > 70 yr, **15** mg/d *Females:* 9–13 yr, **11** mg/d; 14–18 yr, **15** mg/d; 19–30 yr, **15** mg/d; 31–50 yr, **15** mg/d; 50–70 yr, **15** mg/d; > 70 yr, **15** mg/d *Pregnancy:* ≤ 18 yr, **15** mg/d; 19–30 yr, **15** mg/d; 31–50 yr, **15** mg/d *Lactation:* ≤ 18 yr, **19** mg/d; 19–30 yr, **19** mg/d; 31–50 yr, **19** mg/d	Until studies demonstrate optimal doses of vitamin E, high doses should be avoided; supplementation not to exceed 670 mg/d [132,139]

| K | Essential role in coagulation, which is required for healing | Malnutrition; use of broad-spectrum antibiotics [142,143,169–175]; critically ill, burn, and oncology patients [169,176]; renal or liver disease; elderly; long-term total parenteral nutrition; cystic fibrosis [177] | Vitamin K exists naturally in two forms: K_1 or K_2; K_1 is found in plants; K_2 is synthesized by certain bacteria in the GI tract; leafy green vegetables (collards, kale, cabbage, brussel sprouts, lettuce, spinach, broccoli) and some plant oils (soybean, canola, and olive oil) provide the best source in the diet; fruits and grains contain small amounts of K_1 | *Infants:*
0–6 months, 2.0* μg/d;
7–12 months, 2.5* μg/d
Children:
1–3 yr, 30* μg/d;
4–8 yr, 55* μg/d
Males:
9–13 yr, 60* μg/d;
14–18 yr, 75* μg/d;
19–30 yr, 120* μg/d;
31–50 yr, 120* μg/d;
50–70 yr, 120* μg/d;
> 70 yr, 120* μg/d
Females:
9–13 yr, 60* μg/d;
14–18 yr, 75* μg/d;
19–30 yr, 90* μg/d;
31–50 yr, 90* μg/d;
50–70 yr, 90* μg/d;
> 70 yr, 90* μg/d
Pregnancy:
≤ 18 yr, 75* μg/d;
19–30 yr, 90* μg/d;
31–50 yr, 90* μg/d
Lactation:
≤ 18 yr, 75* μg/d;
19–30 yr, 90* μg/d;
31–50 yr, 90* μg/d | 5–10 mg (orally or intramuscularly 1–3 times weekly in high-risk patients) [142,143] |

Note: The table (adapted from the DRI reports, www.nap.edu) presents recommended dietary allowances (RDAs) in bold type and adequate intakes (AIs) in ordinary type followed by an asterisk (*).

disturbances, coma, and connective tissue disorders can also result from excessive vitamin A (21,41–44). Signs of vitamin A intoxication are usually reversed upon cessation of exposure.

RECOMMENDATIONS TO OPTIMIZE WOUND HEALING

Proper wound healing depends upon adequate, and in some situations, augmented vitamin A status of the host. Any deficiency of existing vitamin A deficiency should be corrected as soon as possible so that wound healing may progress at an appropriate rate.

Although vitamin A has thus far yielded promising results for the treatment of wounds, research-based guidelines for the pharmacologic modulation of wound healing cannot be made at present. There are surprisingly few clinical outcome studies that examine optimal dosage. Nevertheless, it has been recommended that 1000 IU/d be administered to malnourished individuals before and after elective surgery (45). In addition, experts suggested supplementation from 10,000 to 25,000 IU of vitamin A per day in patients with severe injuries, burns, and gastrointestinal dysfunction, and those with fractures or tendon repairs and those being treated with high-dose radiation therapy or steroids (16,37,39,46–48). The strength of these recommendations is unclear, and further investigation is required.

VITAMIN D

GENERAL METABOLISM

Two principal forms exist: cholecalciferol (vitamin D_3) and ergocalciferol (vitamin D_2). Vitamin D_2 is obtained from the diet (Table 9.1), in which case it is absorbed, with the help of bile salts, in the small intestine. Vitamin D_3 is produced endogenously by keratinocytes in the skin via biosynthesis from 7-dehydrocholesterol upon exposure to ultraviolet light. The epidermis is where the greatest amount of vitamin D production occurs (49). It is conceivable that large cutaneous wounds and scarring impair the process of epidermal vitamin D synthesis (50,51). Burn scar and normal skin adjacent to the wound show a fivefold decrease in the ability to transform 7-dehydrocholesterol to vitamin D_3 (51).

As vitamin D enters the circulation, both vitamin D_2 and vitamin D_3 are biologically inert and must undergo hydroxylation to produce their biological responses. Vitamin D is hydroxylated sequentially in the liver and kidney, first to 25-hydroxyvitamin D (the major circulating form), and then to its most physiologically active form, 1,25-dihydroxyvitamin D. This conversion is regulated through concentrations of serum calcium, phosphorus, and parathyroid hormone. Vitamin D functions in a manner analogous to the steroid hormones. Important actions include its role in calcium and phosphorus absorption, calcium and phosphorus homeostasis, and endochondral bone formation (52).

ROLE IN WOUND HEALING

Apart from the calciotropic tissues (e.g., bone, intestine, and kidney), recent research suggests a biological role for vitamin D in wound repair (53,54). It has been shown that vitamin D has the ability to regulate growth and differentiation of other cell types, including cancer cells, B and T lymphocytes, melanocytes, fibroblasts, endothelial cells, and monocyte/macrophages (55–61). Furthermore, 1,25-dihydroxyvitamin D_3 reverses corticosteroid-induced epidermal atrophy (62) and promotes the differentiation and proliferation of normal epidermal keratinocytes (59,63–69). In contrast, inhibitory effects of 1,25-dihydroxyvitamin D_3 on proliferation of hyperplastic epidermis occurs (52,70–72), possibly mediated through growth factors and cytokines (73). Pharmacologic amounts of 1,25-dihydroxyvitamin D_3 has been used as an effective agent for inhibiting hyperproliferative diseases, such as psoriasis (52,71,72) and cancer (52,59,74–76).

Time course and specificity studies demonstrated that daily topical application of 1,25-dihydroxyvitamin D_3 significantly accelerated healing of full thickness cutaneous wounds in rats at 1 to 5 d after wounding (54). Another study in rats demonstrated intraperitonial D_3 to produce a significant increase in wound breaking strength and improved epithelialization (53).

1,25-Dihydroxyvitamin D_3 has been shown to stimulate the synthesis of fibronectin, a prominent component of wound healing (77,78). Macrophages may also play an important role in the 1,25-dihydroxyvitamin D_3 mediated wound healing process. It has been reported by Abe et al. (57) that 1,25-dihydroxyvitamin D_3 activates the maturation of macrophages (cells actively involved in wound healing). Thus, vitamin D has numerous activities that affect the process of wound healing.

CONSEQUENCES OF NUTRIENT DEFICIENCY

A deficiency of vitamin D results in inadequate intestinal absorption and renal reabsorption of calcium and phosphorus. As a consequence, serum calcium and phosphate concentrations drop, and serum alkaline phosphatase activity increases. In response to low serum calcium levels, hyperparathyroidism may occur. Vitamin D deficiency has been associated with adverse effects on the skeletal (50,79–87), neuromuscular (88,89), endocrine (47,90,91), and immune (58–61,92–94) systems. Clinical symptoms include growth arrest in children, low bone mineral density, increased fracture incidence, and impaired healing.

CONSEQUENCES OF NUTRIENT EXCESS

Vitamin D toxicity does not occur from prolonged exposure of the skin to ultraviolet (UV) light. Pharmacologic doses are also usually well tolerated (95,96). Few data from which to establish vitamin D safety and toxicity limits exist. Vieth and colleagues (97) and Heaney et al. (98) demonstrated that doses of 75–125 µg/kg daily are well tolerated in healthy adults. Gottschlich et al. (50) have shown this to also be the case while administering up to 100 µg/d in pediatric burn patients. However, toxicity may be of concern in those patients receiving prolonged treatment with supplemental vitamin D. For example, a few reports of overdosage and toxicity exist from extreme amounts (in the range of 250 µg/d for 4 months to 5000 µg of vitamin D daily for 2 weeks) (99–101). Intoxication is associated with elevated plasma 25-hydroxyvitamin D concentration (rather than high 1,25-dihydroxy vitamin D), causing hypercalcemia with attendant decreases in serum parathyroid hormone (PTH). Other symptoms include hypercalciuria, anorexia, nausea, vomiting, headache, diarrhea, thirst, polyuria, muscle weakness, fatigue, joint pain, demineralization of bones, pruritus, nervousness, disorientation, psychosis, and tremor. Hypervitaminosis D is a serious problem, because it can result in irreversible deposition of calcium and phosphorus in the heart, lungs, kidneys, and other soft tissues. Therefore, it is important to detect early signs of vitamin D toxicity. It is fortunate that serum 25-hydroxyvitamin D is the best screen for both hypervitaminosis and hypovitaminosis D (102).

RECOMMENDATIONS TO OPTIMIZE WOUND HEALING

Those presenting with a heightened risk of hypovitaminosis D (Table 9.1) merit assessment of vitamin D status with therapeutic correction of low serum levels in an effort to minimize the adverse effects of classic deficiency symptoms (delayed growth and osteoporosis) as well as to address more recent findings demonstrating benefits of vitamin D as it pertains to the immune system and epithelial proliferation. In the future, 1,25-dihydroxyvitamin D_3 may represent a new avenue in wound medication; however, more research is needed to define its clinical application in wound healing.

VITAMIN E

GENERAL METABOLISM

The term "vitamin E" refers to a group of at least eight compounds — α-, β-, γ-, and δ-tocopherols and α-, β-, γ-, and δ-tocotrienols. All eight isomers are widely distributed in nature. α-Tocopherol has the highest biological activity.

Table 9.1 lists food sources of vitamin E. Only 20 to 40% of orally ingested tocopherol or its esters are absorbed. Efficiency of absorption is enhanced by the presence of dietary lipids. Medium-chain triglycerides in particular enhance absorption, whereas polyunsaturated fatty acids are inhibitory. Both bile and pancreatic juice are necessary for maximal absorption of vitamin E.

Vitamin E is an antioxidant and free radical scavenger that helps prevent the oxidation of cell membranes, which is very important for their stability and structure (103–107). In this role, vitamin E is considered a significant line of defense against lipid peroxidation, offsetting oxidative damage that occurs with disease, injury, inflammation, and environmental insult (105,108–113).

Several other functions of vitamin E have been identified, which are likely not related to its antioxidant capacity (113,114). Vitamin E has a role in the immune response, inflammation, platelet aggregation, platelet adhesion, protein kinase C activation, lipoprotein transport, nucleic acid and protein metabolism, mitochondrial function, and hormonal production (104,114–118). Vitamin E spares selenium (a component of the enzyme glutathione peroxidase) and protects vitamin A from destruction in the body.

ROLE IN WOUND HEALING

The role of vitamin E in the healing of wounds is controversial. In chronic wounds, necrotic tissue, bacteria, and ischemia trigger inflammatory cascades that enhance liberation of free radicals (119). Vitamin E may decrease damage to the wound induced by excessive free radical release. Vitamin E is also thought to facilitate wound healing by enhancing the immune response (115,116).

Lee (120) conducted the first controlled study of the effect of vitamin E on wound healing in humans. He described 57 patients who had been under care for stasis ulcers for at least 3 months. Lee found that 28 patients receiving vitamin E supplementation had improved frequency of healing and healing time as compared to 29 patients on placebo.

Researchers likewise reported some animal studies in which rats receiving oral vitamin E experienced accelerated wound healing. For example, Taren et al. (121) demonstrated increased breaking strength of wounds in rats pretreated with systemic vitamin E and then irradiated. In addition, oral and topical vitamin E has been shown to enhance wound closure and breaking strength in rats following burns and surgery (122,123).

Vitamin E has achieved an unusually prominent role in the mind of the lay public as being beneficial for healing and for the prevention of scar formation (124,125). However, it is prudent to note that many claims are anecdotal, and existing in the literature as well are scientific reports implicating vitamin E as a negative effector of the wound healing process. For example, Greenwald (29) found that vitamin E interfered with collagen synthesis and decreased tensile strength of wounds and impaired tendon healing in chickens. Ehrlich et al. (32) reported that microscopic sections from rats treated with a massive amount of vitamin E had the appearance of less collagen and cells, and demonstrated decreased breaking strength of the wounds, along with an inhibited inflammatory response and a reduction in the number of fibroblasts.

Antiproliferative effects of vitamin E (114) suggest that it might be beneficial in the clinical setting in preventing the development of keloids or hypertrophic scarring. Unfortunately, efforts to date using either topical or systemic vitamin E have not consistently demonstrated benefit, although only three controlled studies have been reported. One clinical trial found that vitamin E improved the effect of silicon bandages on the treatment of large, well-established keloid scars (126). Favorable results were not apparent when vitamin E was evaluated as a means of scar prevention. For example, Jenkins et al. (127) evaluated the topical use of vitamin E on acute scar formation, change in graft size, cosmetic appearance, and range of motion. In that study, 159 procedures involving reconstructive surgery were random-ized to postoperative treatment for 4 months with topical steroid, topical vitamin E, or placebo. Neither topical steroid nor vitamin E was effective in reducing scar formation. Furthermore, 19.9% showed adverse reactions in the form of rash or itching, requiring discontinuation of the vitamin E. Likewise, Baumann and Spencer (124) showed that topically applied vitamin E did not improve scar appearance, and it led to a 33% incidence of contact dermatitis in patients who had undergone skin cancer removal surgery. Adverse follicular and papular dermatitis has also been associated with the use of vitamin E in cosmetics (128,129).

CONSEQUENCES OF NUTRIENT DEFICIENCY

It is generally accepted that the prevalence of vitamin E deficiency in humans is rare. During conditions of vitamin E inadequacy, there is damage to many cells, particularly the red blood cells, T and B cells, and muscle and nerve cells (111,115,116,130,131). The various clinical signs of vitamin E deficiency are believed to be manifestations of membrane dysfunction resulting from the oxidative degradation of polyunsaturated membrane phospholipids or the disruption of other critical cellular processes. Deficiency symptoms include increased platelet aggregation, decreased red blood cell survival, hemolytic anemia, neurologic abnormalities (e.g., altered reflexes, gait disturbances, limb weakness, sensory loss in the arms or legs), and excessive creatinuria (132–134).

CONSEQUENCES OF NUTRIENT EXCESS

The toxicity of vitamin E is very low (95,135–137). There is no evidence of adverse effects from the consumption of vitamin E naturally occurring in foods. Side effects of a minor nature can occur from very high doses of vitamin E supplements (> 670 mg/d). Symptoms include headache, nausea, double vision, fatigue, dermatitis, and retarded wound repair. Intake of high levels can also exacerbate the blood coagulation defect of vitamin K deficiency (138) and antagonize the wound healing effects of vitamin A (32).

RECOMMENDATIONS TO OPTIMIZE WOUND HEALING

Purported beneficial effects have been widely variable. Certainly, correction of vitamin E deficiency is always warranted. The benefits of pharmacologic vitamin E, with the intent of modulating surgical wound healing and acute scar formation, have not been reliably demonstrated.

Conservative use of vitamin E supplements is recommended in lieu of the dubious effects of this vitamin on the healing process. Goodson and Hunt (139) report patients whose healing was retarded by doses of vitamin E over 1000 IU/d. Horwitt (132) recommends < 1000 mg as an upper limit for vitamin E. Certainly, high doses should be avoided until studies demonstrate the optimal route and level of vitamin E supplementation for wound repair.

VITAMIN K

GENERAL METABOLISM

Vitamin K exists naturally in two forms: as K_1 or phylloquinone, and as K_2 or menaquinone. Phylloquinone is found in plants. Green leafy vegetables constitute the major source of vitamin K in the diet. The second source of vitamin K is the menaquinones, which are synthesized by certain bacteria including intestinal microflora.

Under normal conditions, vitamin K is moderately well absorbed from the jejunum and ileum. As with other fat-soluble vitamins, absorption depends on a normal flow of bile and pancreatic secretions and is enhanced by dietary fat.

The metabolic role of vitamin K is to act as a cofactor for a microsomal enzyme (vitamin K dependent carboxylase) which promotes the modification of specific glutamic acid residues to carboxyglutamic acid (gla) in certain proteins referred to as being "vitamin K dependent." These gla-containing proteins are known to occur in a variety of tissues, such as kidney, placenta, pancreas, spleen, and lungs. Specific gla-proteins are required for thenormal function of blood clotting. As such, vitamin K is involved in the hepatic biosynthesis of factors II (prothrombin), VII (proconvertin), IX (antihemophilic factor B), and X (Stuart–Prower factor). In addition, a major protein of the bone matrix, osteocalcin, has also been found to be vitamin K dependent.

Role in Wound Healing

Vitamin K has no known direct role in the wound. The relevance of vitamin K to wound healing involves its function in coagulation, which is a prerequisite of healing. Optimal wound healing requires the prevention of hemorrhage and hematoma formation, which impair wound healing.

Consequences of Nutrient Deficiency

Vitamin K deficiency presents with clinical features ranging from mild bruising to life-threatening hemorrhage. Impaired coagulation can have a detrimental effect on wound healing, as bleeding disorders and wound hematomas predispose to infection and poor tissue repair.

Consequences of Nutrient Excess

The administration of supplements containing natural vitamin K is assumed to be safe and have neglible adverse effects. One case report suggestive of anaphylactoid toxicity exists in the literature (140). The actual prevalence of anaphylactoid reactions to vitamin K is believed to be rare, given the prevalence of use of intravenous vitamin K (141).

Recommendations to Optimize Wound Healing

People at risk of vitamin K deficiency, particularly those expected to have prolonged periods of restricted food intake while requiring antibiotics, should be monitored and treated, because normal coagulation is required for optimal wound healing. The precise dose of supplemental vitamin K that high-risk patients should receive is unknown; however, amounts administered in the range of 5 to 10 mg (orally or intramuscularly) one to three times weekly are common (142,143).

FUTURE DIRECTIONS

Nutrition plays a significant role in the wound healing process. This chapter focused on the importance of the fat-soluble vitamins for tissue regeneration. Clinical experience and research have shown that deficiency of vitamins A, D, E, or K may be associated with impaired wound healing. Likewise, there exists suggestive evidence that pharmacologic therapy with each of the fat-soluble vitamins may be associated with enhanced wound repair, although the specific benefit and amount of supplementation in patients who are not clinically deficient remains controversial. Before pharmacologic use of these vitamins for wound therapy becomes routine, further research is clearly justified, as no vitamin reviewed here has been the subject of a large, double-blind clinical study.

REFERENCES

1. Wolbach, S.B. and Howe, P.R., Tissue changes following deprivation of fat soluble A vitamin, *J. Exp. Med.*, 1925; 42: 753–777.
2. Brandaleone, H. and Papper, E., The effect of the local and oral administration of cod liver oil on the rate of wound healing in vitamin A deficient and normal animals, *Ann. Surg.*, 1941; 114: 791–798.
3. Barbul, A., Thysen, B., Rettura, G., Levenson, S.M., and Seifter, E., White cell involvement in the inflammatory, wound healing and immune actions of vitamin A, *JPEN*, 1978; 2: 129–138.
4. Fusi, S., Kupper, T.S., Green, D.R., and Ariyan, S., Reversal of postburn immunosuppression by the administration of vitamin A, *Surgery*, 1984; 95: 330–334.
5. Shapiro, S.S. and Saliou, C., Role of vitamins in skin care, *Nutrition*, 2001; 17: 839–844.
6. Gollnick, H.P. and Krautheim, A., Topical treatment in acne: current status and future aspects, *Dermatology*, 2003; 206: 29–36.
7. Wolf, J.E., Potential anti-inflammatory effects of topical retinoids and retinoid analogues, *Adv. Ther.*, 2002; 19: 109–118.
8. Kenney, M.C., Shih, L.M., Labermeir, V., and Satterfield, D., Modulation of rabbit keratocyte production of collagen, sulfated glycosaminoglycans and fibronectin by retinol and retinoic acid, *Biochim. Biophys. Acta*, 1986; 889: 156–162.
9. Elson, M.L., The role of retinoids in wound healing, *J. Am. Acad. Dermatol.*, 1998; 39: S79–S81.
10. Weiss, J.S., Ellis, C.N., Headington, J.T., Tincoff, T., Hamilton, T.A., and Voorhees, J.J., Topical tretinoin improves photoaged skin, *JAMA*, 1988; 259: 527–532.
11. Smolin, G., Okumoto, M., and Friedlaender, M., Tretinoin and corneal epithelial wound healing, *Arch. Ophthalmol.*, 1979; 97: 545–546.
12. Smolin, G. and Okumoto, M., Vitamin A acid and corneal epithelial wound healing, *Ann. Ophthalmol.*, 1981; 13: 563–566.
13. Mandy, S., Tretinoin in the preoperative and postoperative management of dermabrasion, *J. Am. Acad. Dermatol.*, 1986; 15(Suppl.): 878–879.
14. Vagotis, F.L. and Brundage, S.R., Histologic study of dermabrasion and chemical peel in an animal model after pre-treatment with Retin-A, *Aesthet. Plast. Surg.*, 1995; 19: 243–246.

15. Hevia, O., Nemeth, A.J., and Taylor, J.R., Tretinoin accelerates healing after trichloroacetic acid chemical peel, *Arch. Dermatol.*, 1991; 127: 678–682.

16. Levenson, S.M. and Demetriou, A.A., Metabolic factors, in *Wound Healing: Biochemical and Clinical Aspects*, Cohen, I.K., Diegelmann, R.F., and Lindblad, W.J., Eds., W.B. Saunders, Philadelphia, 1992: 248–273.

17. Seifter, E., Crowley, L.V., Rettura, G., Nakao, K., Gruber, C.A., Kan, D., and Levenson, S.M., Influence of vitamin A on wound healing in rats with femoral fracture, *Ann. Surg.*, 1975; 181: 836–841.

18. Seifter, E., Rettura, G., Padawer, J., Impaired wound healing in streptozotocin diabetes: prevention by supplemental vitamin A, *Ann. Surg.*, 1981; 194: 42–50.

19. Sporn, M.B., Dunlop, N.M., Newton, D.L., and Henderson, W.R., Relationship between structure and activity of retinoids, *Nature*, 1976; 262: 110–113.

20. DeLuca, L.M., Bhat, P.V., Sasak, W., and Adamo, S., Biosynthesis of phosphoryl and glycosyl phosphoryl derivatives of vitamin A in biological membranes, *Fed. Proc.* 1979; 38: 2535–2539.

21. Hunt, T.K., Vitamin A and wound healing, *J. Am. Acad. Dermatol.*, 1986; 15: 817–821.

22. Ehrlich, H.P. and Hunt, T.K., Effects of cortisone and vitamin A on wound healing, *Ann. Surg.*, 1968; 167: 324–328.

23. Hunt, T.K., Ehrlich, H.P., Garcia, J.A., and Dunphy, J.E., Effect of vitamin A on reversing the inhibitory effect of cortisone on healing of open wounds in animals and man, *Ann. Surg.*, 1969; 170: 633–640.

24. Wicke, C., Halliday, B., Allen, D., Roche, N.S., Scheuenstuhl, H., Spencer, M., Roberts, A.B., and Hunt, T.K., Effects of steroids and retinoids on wound healing, *Arch. Surg.*, 2000; 135: 1265–1270.

25. Ehrlich, H.P., Tarver, H., and Hunt, T.K., Effects of vitamin A and glucocorticoids upon inflammation and collagen synthesis, *Ann. Surg.*, 1973; 177: 222–227.

26. Phillips, J.D., Kim, C.S., Fonkalsrud, E.W., Zeng, H., and Dindar, H., Effects of chronic corticosteroids and vitamin A on the healing of experimental intestinal anastomoses, *Am. J. Surg.*, 1992; 163: 71–77.

27. Winsey, K., Simon, R.J., Levenson, S.M., Seifter, E., and Demetriou, A.A., Effect of supplemental vitamin A on colon anastomotic healing in rats given preoperative irradiation, *Am. J. Surg.*, 1987; 153: 153–156.

28. de Waard, J.W.D., Wobbes, T., van der Linden, C.J., and Hendriks, T., Retinol may promote fluorouracil-suppressed healing of experimental intestinal anastomoses, *Arch. Surg.*, 1995; 130: 959–965.

29. Greenwald, D.P., Scharzer, L.A., Padawer, J., Levenson, S.M., and Seifter, E., Zone II flexor tendon repair: effects of vitamin A, E and beta-carotene, *J. Surg. Res.*, 1990; 49: 98–102.

30. Demetriou, A.A., Levenson, S.M., Rettura, G., and Seifter, E., Vitamin A and retinoic acid:Induced fibroblast differentiation *in vitro*, *Surgery*, 1985; 98: 931–934.

31. Levenson, S.M., Gruber, C.A., Rettura, G., Gruber, D.K., Demetriou, A.A., and Seifter, E., Supplemental vitamin A prevents the acute radiation-induced defect in wound healing, *Ann. Surg.*, 1984; 200: 494–512.

32. Ehrlich, H.P., Tarver, H., and Hunt, T.K., Inhibitory effects of vitamin E on collagen synthesis and wound repair, *Ann. Surg.*, 1972; 175: 235–240.

33. Raju, S.S. and Kulkarni, D.R., Vitamin A reverses the wound healing suppressant effect of cyclophosphamide, *Indian J. Pharmacol.*, 1986; 18: 154–157.

34. Maymood, T., Tenenbaum, S., Niu, X.T., Levenson, S.M., Seifter, E., and Demetriou, A.A., Prevention of duodenal ulcer formation in the rat by dietary vitamin A supplementation, *JPEN*, 1986; 10: 74–77.

35. Terkelsen, L.H., Eskild-Jensen, A., Kjeldsen, H., Barker, J.H., and Hjortdal, V.E., Topical application of cod liver oil ointment accelerates wound healing: an experimental study in wounds in the ears of hairless mice, *Scand. J. Plast. Reconstr. Hand Surg.*, 2000; 34: 15–20.

36. Weinzweig, J., Levenson, S.M., and Returra, G., Supplemental vitamin A prevents the tumor-induced defect in wound healing, *Ann. Surg.*, 1990; 211: 269–276.

37. Levitsky, J., Hong, J.J., Jani, A.B., and Ehrenpreis, E.D., Oral vitamin A therapy for a patient with severely symptomatic postradiation anal ulceration: report of a case, *Dis. Colon Rectum*, 2003; 46: 679–682.

38. Paquette, D., Badiavas, E., and Falang, V., Short-contact topical trentinoin therapy to stimulate granulation tissue in chronic wounds, *J. Am. Acad. Dermatol.*, 2001; 45: 382–386.

39. Levenson, S.M. and Seifter, E., Dysnutrition, wound healing, and resistance to infection, *Clin. Plast. Surg.*, 1977; 4: 375–388.

40. Freiman, M., Seifter, E., Connerton, C., and Levenson, S.M., Vitamin A deficiency and surgical stress, *Surg. Forum*, 1970; 21: 81–82.

41. Kuroiwa, K., Trocki, O., Alexander, J.W., Tchervenkov, J., Inoue, S., and Nelson, J.L., Effect of vitamin A in enteral formulae for burned guinea, *Burns*, 1990; 16: 265–272.

42. Jarrett, A. and Spearman, R.I.C., Vitamin A and the skin, *Br. J. Dermatol.*, 1970; 82: 197–199.

43. Gamble, J.G. and Ip, S.C., Hypervitaminosis A in a child from megadosing, *J. Pediatr. Orthop.*, 1985; 5: 219–221.

44. Smith, F.R. and Goodman, D.S., Vitamin A transport in human vitamin A toxicity, *N. Engl. J. Med.*, 1976; 294: 805–808.

45. Scholl, D. and Langkamp-Henken, B., Nutrient recommendations for wound healing, *J. Intraven. Nurs.*, 2001; 24: 124–132.

46. Marian, M.J. and Winkler, M.F., Wound healing, in *Nutrition Support: Dietetics Core Curriculum*, Gottschlich, M.M., Matarese, L.E., and Shronts, E.P., Eds., American Society for Parenteral and Enteral Nutrition, 1993: 397–407.

47. Pollack, S., Wound healing: a review. III. Nutritional factors affecting wound healing, *J. Dermatol. Surg. Oncol.*, 1979; 5: 615–619.

48. Gottschlich, M.M. and Warden, G.D., Vitamin supplementation in the patient with burns, *J. Burn Care Rehab.*, 1990; 11: 275–279.

49. Holick, M.F., MacLaughlin, J.A., and Doppelt, S.H., Factors that influence the cutaneous photosynthesis of previtamin D_3, *Science*, 1981; 211: 590–593.

50. Gottschlich, M.M., Mayes, T., Khoury, J., and Warden, G.D., Hypovitaminosis D in pediatric burn patients, *J. Am. Diet. Assoc.*, 2004; 104: 931–941.

51. Klein, G.L., Chen, T.C., Holick, M.F., Langman, C.B., Price, H., Celis, M.M., and Herndon, D.N., Synthesis of vitamin D in skin after burns, *Lancet*, 2004; 363: 291–292.

52. Holick, M.F., Vitamin D — new horizons for the 21st century, *Am. J. Clin. Nutr.*, 1994; 60: 619–630.

53. Ramesh, K.V., Mahindrakar, M.B., and Bhat, E.P., A new role for vitamin D: cholecalciferol promotes dermal wound strength and re-epithelization, *Indian J. Exp. Biol.*, 1993; 31: 778–779.

54. Tian, X.Q., Chen, T.C., and Holick, M.F., 1,25-dihydroxyvitamin D_3: a novel agent for enhancing wound healing, *J. Cell. Biochem.*, 1995; 59: 53–56.

55. Stumpf, W.E., Sar, M., and Reid, F.A., Target cells for 1,25-dihydroxyvitamin D_3 in intestinal tract, stomach, kidney, skin, pituitary, and parathyroid, *Science*, 1979; 206: 1188–1190.

56. Tanaka, H., Abe, E., Miyaura, C., Kuribayashi, T., Konno, K., Nishii, Y., and Suda, T., 1 α,25-dihydroxycholecalciferol and a human myeloid leukaemia cell line, *Biochem. J.*, 1982; 204: 713–719.

57. Abe, E., Shiina, Y., Miyaura, C., Tanaka, H., Hayashi, T., Kanegasaki, S., Saito, M., Nishii, Y., DeLuca, H.F., and Suda, T., Activation and fusion induced by 1,25-dihydroxyvitamin D_3 and their relation in alveolar macrophages, *Proc. Natl. Acad. Sci. U.S.A.*, 1984; 81: 7112–7116.

58. Bhalla, A.K., Amento, E.P., and Krane, S.M., Differential effects of 1,25-dihydroxyvitamin D_3 on human lymphocytes and monocyte/macrophages: inhibition of interleukin-2 and augmentation of interleukin-2 and augmentation of interleukin-1 production, *Cell. Immunol.*, 1986; 98: 311–322.

59. Kragballe, K., The future of vitamin D in dermatology, *J. Am. Acad. Dermatol.*, 1997; 37: S72–S76.

60. Bhalla, A.K., Amento, E.P., and Clemens, T.L., Specific high affinity receptors for 1,25 dihydroxy vitamin D_3 in human peripheral blood mononuclear cells: presence in monocytes and induction in T-lymphocytes following activation, *J. Clin. Endocrinol. Metab.*, 1983; 57: 1308–1310.

61. Rigby, W.F.C. and Waugh, M.G., Decreased accessory cell function and costimulatory activity by 1,25 dihydroxyvitamin D_3 treated monocytes, *Arthritis Rheum.*, 1992; 35: 110–119.

62. Gniadecki, R., Gniadecki, M., and Serup, J., Inhibition of glucocorticoid-induced epidermaland dermal atrophy with KH 1060 — a potent 20-epi analogue of 1,25 dihydroxyvitamin D_3, *Br. Med. Pharmacol.*, 1994; 113: 439–444.

63. Bikle, D.D. and Pillai, S., Vitamin D, calcium and epidermal differentiation, *Endocr. Rev.*, 1993; 14: 3–19.

64. Chen, T.C., Persons, K., Uskokovic, M.R., Horst, R.L., and Holick, M.F., An evaluation of 1,25-dihydroxyvitamin D_3 analogues on the proliferation and differentiation of cultured human keratinocytes, calcium metabolism and the differentiation of human HL-60 cells, *J. Nutr. Biochem.*, 1993; 4: 49–57.

65. Bikle, D.D., Pillai, S., Gee, E., and Hincenbergs, M., Regulation of 1,25-dihydroxyvitamin D production in human keratinocytes by interferon-gamma, *Endocrinology*, 1989; 124: 655–660.

66. Smith, E.L., Walworth, N.C., and Holick, M.F., Effect of 1 α,25-dihydroxyvitamin D_3 on the morphologic and biochemical differentiation of cultured human epidermal keratinocytes grown in serum-free conditions, *J. Invest. Dermatol.*, 1986; 86: 709–714.

67. Lutzow-Holm, C., DeAngelis, P., Grosvik, H., and Clausen, O.P., 1,25 dihydroxyvitamin D_3 analogue KH 1060 induces hyperproliferation in normal mouse epidermis, *Exp. Dermatol.*, 1993; 2: 113–120.

68. Gniadecki, R. and Serup, J., Stimulation of epidermal proliferation in mice with 1,25 dihydroxyvitamin D_3 and receptor-active 20-epi analogues of 1,25 dihydroxyvitamin D_3, *Biochem. Pharmacol.*, 1995; 49: 621–624.

69. Hosomi, J., Hosoi, J., Abe, E., Suda, T., and Kuroki, T., Regulation of terminal differentiation of mouse cultured epidermal cells by 1,25 dihydroxyvitamin D_3, *Endocrinology*, 1983; 113: 1950–1957.

70. Kato, T., Terui, T., and Tagami, H., Topically active vitamin D_3 analogue, 1,24 dihydroxycholecalciferol, has an antiproliferative effect on the epidermis of guinea pig skin, *Br. J. Dermatol.*, 1987; 117: 528–530.

71. Kragballe, K., Steijlen, B., Ibsen, H.H., van de Kerkhof, P.C., Esmann, J., Sorensen, L.H., and Axelsen, M.B., Efficacy, tolerability, and safety of calcipotriol ointment in disorders of keratinization, *Arch. Dermatol.*, 1995; 131: 556–560.

72. van der Kerhof, P.C., Biological activity of vitamin D analogues in the skin, with special reference to antipsoriatic mechanisms, *Br. J. Dermatol.*, 1995; 132: 675–682.

73. Gurlek, A., Pittelkow, M.R., and Kumar, R., Modulation of growth factor/cytokine synthesis and signaling by 1,25 dihydroxyvitamin D₃: implications in cell growth and differentiation, *Endocrine Rev.*, 2002; 23: 763–786.

74. Bao, B.Y., Hu, Y.C., Ting, H.J., and Lee, Y.F., Androgen signaling is required for the vitamin D-mediated growth inhibition in human prostate cancer cells, *Oncogene*, 2004; 23: 3350–3360.

75. Eisman, J.A., Barkla, D.H., and Tutto, J.M., Suppression of *in vivo* growth of human cancer solid tumor xenografts by 1,25 dihydroxyvitamin D₃, *Cancer Res.*, 1987; 47: 21–25.

76. Bower, M., Colston, K.W., Stein, R.C., Hedley, A., Gazet, J.C., Ford, H.T., and Combes, R.C., Topical calcipotriol treatment in advanced breast cancer, *Lancet*, 1991; 337: 701–702.

77. Brown, L.F., Dubin, D., Lavigne, L., Logan, B., Dvorak, H.F., and Van de Water, L., Macrophages and fibroblasts express embryonic fibronectins during cutaneous wound healing, *Am. J. Pathol.*, 1993; 142: 793–801.

78. Fransson, J. and Hammar, H., Epidermal growth in the skin equivalent, *Arch. Dermatol. Res.*, 1992; 284: 343–348.

79. Klein, G.L., Langman, C.B., and Herndon, D.N., Vitamin D depletion following burn injury in children: a possible factor in post-burn osteopenia, *J. Trauma*, 2002; 52: 346–350.

80. Wray, C.J., Mayes, T., Khoury, J., Warden, G.D., and Gottschlich, M., Metabolic effects of vitamin D on serum calcium, magnesium and phosphorus in pediatric burn patients, *J. Burn Care Rehab.*, 2002; 23: 416–423.

81. Dawson-Hughes, B., Harris, S.S., Krall, E.A., and Dallal, G.E., Effect of calcium and vitamin D supplementation on bone density in men and women 65 years of age or older, *N. Engl. J. Med.*, 1997; 337: 670–676.

82. Heubi, J.E., Hollis, B.W., Specker, B., and Tsang, R.C., Bone disease in chronic childhood cholestasis. I. Vitamin D absorption and metabolism, *Hepatology*, 1989; 9: 258–264.

83. Heubi, J.E., Hollis, B.W., and Tsang, R.C., Bone disease in chronic childhood cholestasis. II. Better absorption of 25-OH vitamin D than vitamin D in extrahepatic biliary atresia, *Pediatr. Res.*, 1990; 27: 26–31.

84. Davies, M., Heys, S.E., Selby, P.L., Berr, J.L., and Mawer, E.B., Increased catabolism of 25-hydroxyvitamin D levels. Implications for metabolic bone disease, *J. Clin. Endocrinol. Metab.*, 1997; 82: 209–212.

85. Gartner, L.M., Greer, F.R., and the Section on Breast Feeding and Committee on Nutrition, Prevention of rickets and vitamin D deficiency. New guidelines for vitamin D intake, *Pediatrics*, 2003; 111: 908–910.

86. Bordier, P., Rasmussen, H., Marie, P., Miravet, L., Gueris, J., and Ryckwaert, A., Vitamin D metabolites and bone mineralization in man, *J. Clin. Endocrinol. Metab.*, 1978; 46: 284–294.

87. Valimaki, V., Alfthan, H., Lehmuskallio, E., Loyttyniemi, E., Sahi, T., Stenman, U., Suominen, H., and Valimaki, M.J., Vitamin D status as a determinant of peak bone mass in young Finnish men, *J. Clin. Endocrinol. Metab.*, 2004; 89: 76–80.

88. Janssen, H.C.J.P., Samson, M.M., and Verbaar, H.J., Vitamin D deficiency, muscle function, and falls in elderly people, *Am. J. Clin. Nutr.*, 2002; 75: 611–615.

89. Rimaniol, J.M., Authier, F.J., and Chariot, P., Muscle weakness in intensive care patients. Initial manifestation of vitamin D deficiency, *Intensive Care Med.*, 1994; 20: 591–592.

90. Vu, D., Ong, J.M., Clemens, T.L., and Kern, P.A., 1,25-dihydroxyvitamin D induces lipoprotein lipase expression in 3T3-L1 cells in association with adipocyte differentiation, *Endocrinology*, 1996; 1137: 1540–1544.

91. Hypponen, E., Laara, E., Reunanen, A., Jarvelin, M.R., and Virtanen, S.M., Intake of vitamin D and risk of type I diabetes: a cohort study, *Lancet*, 2001; 358: 1500–1503.

92. Tsoukas, C.D., Provvedini, D.M., and Manolagas, S.C., 1,25 Dihydroxyvitamin D_3: a novel immunoregulatory hormone, *Science*, 1984; 224: 1438–1439.

93. Manolagas, S.C., Provvedini, D.M., and Tsoukas, C.D., Interaction of 1,25-dihydroxyvitamin D_3 and the immune system, *Mol. Cell. Endocrinol.*, 1985; 43: 113–122.

94. Binderup, L., Latini, S., Binderup, E., Bretting, C., Calverley, M., and Hansen, K., 20-epi-vitamin D_3 analogues: a novel class of potent regulators of cell growth and immune responses, *Biochem. Pharmacol.*, 1991; 42: 1569–1575.

95. Tsai, A.C., Kelley, J.J., Peng, B., and Cook, N., Study on the effect of megavitamin supplementation in man, *Am. J. Clin. Nutr.*, 1978; 31: 831–837.

96. Kitagawa, M. and Mino, M., Effects of elevated D-(RRR)-tocopherol dosage in man, *J. Nutr. Sci. Vitaminol.*, 1989; 35: 133–142.

97. Vieth, R., Chan, P.C.R., and MacFarlane, G.D., Efficacy and safety of vitamin D_3 intake exceeding the lowest observed adverse effect level, *Am. J. Clin. Nutr.*, 2001; 73: 288–294.

98. Heaney, R.P., Davies, K.M., Chen, T.C., Holick, M.F., Barger-Lux, M.J., Human serum 25-hydroxycholecalciferol response to extended oral dosing with cholecalciferol, *Am. J. Clin. Nutr.*, 2003; 77: 204–210.

99. Vieth, R., Vitamin D supplementation, 25-hydroxyvitamin D concentrations, and safety, *Am. J. Clin. Nutr.*, 1999; 69: 842–856.

100. Hayes, K.C. and Hegsted, D.M., Toxicity of the vitamins, in *Committee on Food Protection Toxicants Occurring Naturally in Foods*, 2nd ed., National Academy of Sciences, Washington, D.C., 1973; 239–242.

101. American Academy of Pediatrics, The prophylactic requirement and the toxicity of vitamin D, *Pediatrics*, 1963; 31: 512–523.

102. Adams, J.S., Bone density and vitamin D intoxication, *Ann. Intern. Med.*, 1998; 128: 508.

103. Hinder, R.A. and Stein, H.J., Oxygen-derived free radicals, *Arch. Surg.*, 1991; 124: 104–105.

104. Bieri, J.G., Corash, L., and Hubbard, V.S., Medical uses of vitamin E, *N. Engl. J. Med.*, 1983; 308: 1063–1071.

105. Lopez-Torres, M., Thiele, J.J., Shindo, Y., Han, D., and Packer, L., Topical application of -tocopherol modulates the antioxidant network and diminishes ultraviolet-induced oxidative damage in murine skin, *Br. J. Dermatol.*, 1998; 138: 207–213.

106. Tappel, A.L., Free-radical lipid peroxidation damage and its inhibition by vitamin E and selenium, *Fed. Proc.*, 1965; 24: 73–78.

107. Sata, K., Niki, E., and Shimasaki, H., Free radical-mediated chain oxidation of low density lipoprotein and its synergistic inhibition by vitamin E and vitamin C, *Arch. Biochem. Biophys.*, 1990; 279: 402–405.

108. Nguyen, T.T., Cox, C.S., Traber, D.L., Gasser, H., Ridl, H., Schlag, G., and Herndon, D.N., Free radical activity and loss of plasma antioxidants, vitamin E and sulfhydryl groups in patients with burns, *J. Burn Care Rehabil.*, 1993; 14: 602–609.

109. Williams, R.J., Motteram, J.M., Sharp, C.H., and Gallagher, P.J., Dietary vitamin E and the attenuation of early lesion development in modified Watanabe rabbits, *Atherosclerosis*, 1992; 94: 153–159.

110. Jurkiewicz, B.A., Bissett, D.L., and Buettner, G.R., Effect of topically applied toco-pherol on ultraviolet radiation-mediated free radical damage in skin, *J. Invest. Dermatol.*, 1995; 104: 484–488.

111. Sasaki, J., Cottam, G.L., and Baxter, C.R., Lipid peroxidation following thermal injury, *J. Burn Care Rehabil.*, 1983; 4: 251–254.

112. Mingjian, Z., Qifang, W., Lanxing, G., Hong, J., and Zongyin, W., Comparative observation of the changes in serum lipid peroxides influenced by the supplementation of vitamin E in burn patients and healthy controls, *Burns*, 1992; 18: 19–21.

113. Brigelius-Flohe, R., Kelly, F.J., Salonen, J.T., Neuzil, J., Zingg, J.M., and Azzi, A., The European perspective on vitamin E: current knowledge and future research, *Am. J. Clin. Nutr.*, 2002; 76: 703–716.

114. Traber, M.G. and Packer, L., Vitamin E: beyond antioxidant function, *Am. J. Clin. Nutr.*, 1995; 62: 1501S–1509.

115. Rundus, C., Peterson, V.M., Zapata-Sirvent, R., Hansbrough, J., and Robinson, W.A., Vitamin E improves cell-mediated immunity in the burned mouse: a preliminary study, *Burns*, 1984; 11: 11–15.

116. Tanaka, J., Fujiwara, H., and Torisu, M., Vitamin E and immune response: I. Enhancement of helper T-cell activity by dietary supplementation of vitamin E in mice, *Immunology*, 1979; 38: 727–734.

117. Violi, F., Pratico, D., Ghiselli, A., Alessandri, C., Iuliano, L., Cordova, C., Balsano, F., Inhibition of cyclooxygenase-independent platelet aggregation by low dose vitamin E concentration, *Atherosclerosis*, 1990; 82: 247–252.

118. Steiner, M., Influence of vitamin E on platelet function in humans, *J. Am. Coll. Nutr.*, 1991; 10: 466–473.

119. Baxter, C.R., Immunologic reactions in chronic wounds, *Am. J. Surg.*, 1994; 167(S): 12–14.

120. Lee, M., An investigation into the value of *d*-1-tocopherol acetate (vitamin E) in the treatment of gravitational ulcers, *Br. J. Dermatol.*, 1953; 65: 131–138.

121. Taren, D.L., Chvapil, M., and Weber, C.W., Increasing the breaking strength of wounds exposed to preoperative irradiation using vitamin E supplementation, *Int. J. Vit. Nutr. Res.*, 1987; 57: 133–137.

122. Melkumian, A.S., Tumanian, E.L., and Agadzhanov, M.I., Histological evaluation of the regenerative capacity of the skin in the treatment of burn wounds with a vitamin E based ointment, *Zh. Eksp. Klin. Med.*, 1978; 18: 52–54.

123. Vandenboer, H., Schmidt, E., Fajardo, C., Buttler, I., Assis, G., and Vianna, L.M., Effect of α-tocopherol on wound healing, *Clin. Nutr.*, 1999; 18: 59.

124. Baumann, L.S. and Spencer, J., The effects of topical vitamin E on the cosmetic appearance of scars, *Dermatol. Surg.*, 1999; 25: 311–315.

125. Havlik, R.J., Vitamin E and wound healing, *Plast. Reconstr. Surg.*, 1997; 100: 1901–1902.

126. Palmieri, G., Vitamin E added silicone gel sheets for treatment of hypertrophic scars and keloids, *Int. J. Dermatol.*, 1995; 34: 506–509.

127. Jenkins, M., Alexander, J.W., MacMillan, B.G., Waymack, J.P., and Kopcha, R., Failure of topical steroids and vitamin E to reduce postoperative scar formation following reconstructive surgery, *J. Burn Care Med.*, 1986; 7: 309–312.

128. Fisher, A.A., Three faces of vitamin E topical allergy, *Cutis*, 1991; 48: 272–274.

129. Perrenoud, D., Homberger, H.P., Auderset, P.C., Emmenegger, R., Frenk, E., Saurat, J.H., and Hauser, C., An epidemic outbreak of papular and follicular dermatitis to tocopheryl linoleate in cosmetics, *Dermatology*, 1994; 189: 225–233.

130. Kelly, F.J. and Sutton, G.L.J., Plasma and red blood cell vitamin E status in patients on total parenteral nutrition, *JPEN*, 1989; 13: 510–515.

131. Kuroiwa, K., Nelson, J.L., Boyce, S.T., Alexander, J.W., Ogle, C.K., and Inoue, S., Metabolic and immune effect of vitamin E supplementation after burn, *JPEN*, 1991; 15: 22–26.

132. Horwitt, M.K., Critique of the requirement for vitamin E, *Am. J. Clin. Nutr.*, 2001; 73: 1003–1005.

133. Carpenter, D., Vitamin E deficiency, *Sem. Neurol.*, 1985; 5: 283–287.

134. Sokol, R.J., Vitamin E deficiency and neurologic disease, *Ann. Rev. Nutr.*, 1988; 8: 351–373.

135. Farrell, P.M. and Bieri, J.G., Megavitamin E supplementation in man, *Am. J. Clin. Nutr.*, 1975; 28: 1381–1386.

136. Weber, P., Bendich, A., and Machlin, L., Vitamin E and human health: rationale for determining recommended intake levels, *Nutrition*, 1997; 13: 450–460.

137. Bendich, A. and Machlin, L.J., Safety of oral intake of vitamin E, *Am. J. Clin. Nutr.*, 1988; 48: 612–619.

138. Kappus, H. and Diplock, A.T., Tolerance and safety of vitamin E: a toxicological position report, *Free Rad. Biol. Med.*, 1992; 13: 55–74.

139. Goodson, W.H. and Hunt, T.K., Wound healing, in *Nutrition and Metabolism in Patient Care*, Kinney, J.M., Jeejeebhoy, K.N., and Hill, G.L., Eds., W.B. Saunders, Philadelphia, 1988: 635–642.

140. de la Rubia, J., Grau, E., Montserrat, I., Zuazu, I., and Paya, A., Anaphylactic shock and vitamin K_1 [letter], *Ann. Intern. Med.*, 1989; 110: 943.

141. Bossee, G.M., Mallory, M.N., and Malone, G.J., The safety of intravenously administered vitamin K, *Vet. Hum. Toxicol.*, 2002; 44: 174–176.

142. Shevchuk, Y.M. and Conly, J.M., Antibiotic-associated hypoprothrombinemia: a review of prospective studies 1966–1988, *Rev. Infect. Dis.*, 1990; 12: 1109–1126.

143. Shearer, M.J., Bechtold, H., Andrassy, K., Koderisch, J., McCarthy, P.T., Trenk, K., Jahnchen, E., and Ritz, E., Mechanism of cephalosporin-induced hypoprothrombinemia: relation to cephalosporin side chain, vitamin K metabolism, and vitamin K status, *J. Clin. Pharmacol.*, 1988; 28: 88–95.

144. Rai, K. and Courtemanche, A.D., Vitamin A assay in burned patients, *J. Trauma*, 1975; 15: 419–424.

145. Cynober, L., Desmoulins, D., Lioret, N., Aussel, C., Hirsch-Marie, H., and Saizy, R., Significance of vitamin A and retinol binding protein serum levels after burn injury, *Clin. Chim. Acta*, 1985; 148: 247–253.

146. Rock, C.L., Dechert, R.E., Khilnani, R., Parker, R.S., and Rodriguez, J.L., Carotenoids and antioxidant vitamins in patients after burn injury, *J. Burn Care Rehabil.*, 1997; 18: 269–278.

147. Szebeni, A., Negyesi, G., and Feuer, L., Vitamin A levels in the serum of burned patients, *Burns*, 1980; 7: 313–318.

148. Rojas, A.I. and Phillips, T.J., Patients with chronic leg ulcers show diminished levels of vitamins A and E, carotenes, and zinc, *Dermatol. Surg.*, 1999; 25: 601–604.

149. Thomas, M.K., Lloyd Jones, D.M., Thadhani, R.I., Shaw, A.C., Deraska, D.J., Kitch, B.T., Vamvakas, E.C., Dick, I.M., Prince, R.L., and Finkelstein, J.S., Hypovitaminosis D in medical inpatients, *N. Engl. J. Med.*, 1998; 338: 777–783.

150. Freaney, R., McBrinn, Y., and McKenna, M.J., Secondary hyperparathyroidism in elderly people: combined effect of renal insufficiency and vitamin D deficiency, *Am. J. Clin. Nutr.*, 1993; 58: 187–191.

151. Jacques, P.F., Felson, D.T., Tucker, K.L., Mahnken, B., Wilson, P.W., Rosenberg, I.H., and Rush, D., Plasma 25-hydroxyvitamin D and its determinants in an elderly population, *Am. J. Clin. Nutr.*, 1997; 66: 929–936.
152. MacLaughlin, J. and Holick, M.F., Aging decreases capacity of human skin to produce vitamin D₃, *J. Clin. Invest.*, 1985; 76: 1536–1538.
153. Klein, G.L., Horst, R.L., and Norman, A.W., Reduced serum levels of 1,25-dihydroxyvitamin D during long term total parenteral nutrition, *Ann. Intern. Med.*, 1981; 94: 638–643.
154. Shike, M., Harrison, J.E., Sturtridge, W.C., Tam, C.S., Bobechko, P.E., Jones, G., Murray, T.M., and Jeejeebhoy, K.N., Metabolic bone disease in patients receiving long term total parenteral nutrition, *Ann. Intern. Med.*, 1980; 92: 343–350.
155. Baer, M.T., Kozlowski, B.W., Blyler, E.M., Trahms, C.M., Taylor, M.L., and Hogan, M.P., Vitamin D, calcium and bone status in children with developmental delay in relation to anticonvulsant use and ambulatory status, *Am. J. Clin. Nutr.*, 1997; 65: 1042–1051.
156. Buckley, L.M., Leib, E.S., Cartularo, K.S., Vacek, P.M., and Cooper, S.M., Calcium and vitamin D₃ supplementation prevents bone loss in the spine secondary to low dose corticosteroids in patients with rheumatoid arthritis, *Ann. Intern. Med.*, 1996; 125: 961–968.
157. Sambrook, P., Birmingham, J., Kelly, P., Kempler, S., Nguyen, T., Pocock, N., and Eisman, J., Prevention of corticosteroid osteoporosis: a comparison of calcium, calcitriol, and calcitonin, *N. Engl. J. Med.*, 1993; 328: 1747–1752.
158. Barnes, T.C. and Bucknall, R.C., Vitamin D deficiency in a patient with systemic lupus every thematosus, *Rheumatology*, 2004; 43: 393–394.
159. Mayes, T., Gottschlich, M.M., James, L., and Warden, G.D., An evaluation of the relationship between protein status and vitamin D nutriture in burned infants, *J. Burn Care Rehabil.*, 2004; 25: S147.
160. Cannata-Andia, J.B. and Alonso, C.G., Vitamin D deficiency: a neglected aspect of disturbed calcium metabolism in renal failure, *Nephrol. Dial. Transplant*, 2002; 17: 1875–1878.
161. Wilson, L., Felsenfeld, A., Drezner, M.K., and Llach, F., Altered divalent ion metabolism inearly renal failure: role of 1,25(OH)₂D, *Kidney Int.*, 1985; 27: 565–573.
162. Rosen, J.F. and Chesney, R.W., Circulating calcitriol concentrations in health and disease, *J. Pediatr.*, 1983; 103: 1–17.
163. Compston, J.E., Ayers, A.B., Horton, L.W., Tighe, J.R., and Creamer, B., Osteomalacia after small intestinal resection, *Lancet*, 1978; 1: 9–12.
164. Lo, C.W., Paris, P.W., Clemens, T.L., Nolan, J., and Holick, M.F., Vitamin D absorption in healthy subjects and in in-patients with intestinal malabsorption syndromes, *Am. J. Clin. Nutr.*, 1985; 42: 644–649.
165. Vandewoude, M.G., Vandewoude, M.F.J., and DeLeeuw, I.H., Vitamin E status in patients on parenteral nutrition receiving Intralipid, *JPEN*, 1986; 10: 303–305.
166. Lloyd, J.K., The importance of vitamin E in human nutrition, *Acta Pediatr. Scand.*, 1990; 79: 6–11.
167. Shukla, A., Rasik, A.M., and Patnaik, G.K., Depletion of reduced glutathione, ascorbic acid, vitamin E and antioxidant defence enzymes in a healing cutaneous wound, *Free Radic. Res.*, 1997; 26: 93–101.
168. Gupta, A., Singh, R.L., and Raghubir, R., Antioxidant status during cutaneous wound healing in immunocompromised rats, *Mol. Cell. Biochem.*, 2002; 241: 1–7.

169. Jenkins, M.E., Gottschlich, M.M., Kopcha, R., Khoury, J., and Warden, G.D., A prospective analysis of serum vitamin K in severely burned pediatric patients, *J. Burn Care Rehabil.*, 1998; 19: 75–81.

170. Alperin, J.B., Coagulopathy caused by vitamin K deficiency in critically ill, hospitalized patients, *JAMA*, 1987; 258: 1916–1919.

171. Shevchuk, Y.M. and Conly, J.M., Antibiotic-associated hypoprothrombinemia: a review of prospective studies 1966–1988, *Rev. Infect. Dis.*, 1990; 12: 1109–1126.

172. Conly, J.M., Ramotar, K., Chubb, H., Bow, E.J., and Louie, T.J., Hyproprothrombinemia in febrile, neutropenic patients with cancer: association with antimicrobial suppression of intestinal microflora, *J. Infect. Dis.*, 1984; 150: 202–212.

173. Carlin, A. and Walker, W.A., Rapid development of vitamin K deficiency in an adolescent boy receiving total parenteral nutrition following bone marrow transplantation, *Nutr. Rev.*, 1991; 49: 179–183.

174. Allison, P.M., Mummah-Schendel, L.L., Kindberg, C.G., Harms, C.S., Bang, N.U., and Suttie, J.W., Effects of a vitamin K-deficient diet and antibiotics in normal human volunteers, *J. Lab. Clin. Med.*, 1987; 110: 180–188.

175. Bhat, R.V. and Deshmukh, C.T., A study of vitamin K status in children on prolonged antibiotic therapy, *Indian Pediatr.*, 2003; 40: 36–40.

176. Ansell, J.E., Kumar, R., and Deykin, D., The spectrum of vitamin K deficiency, *JAMA*, 1977; 238: 40–42.

177. Verghese, T. and Beverley, D., Vitamin K deficient bleeding in cystic fibrosis, *Arch. Dis. Child*, 2003; 88: 553–555.

10 Trace Elements and Wound Healing

Thomas G. Baumgartner

CONTENTS

Wound healing is a complex, tightly regulated process, consisting of three distinct phases. In each phase of wound healing, macronutrients and micronutrients are required. In other chapters of this book, the other macronutrients and micronutrients are discussed, but the complex interaction of trace elements with all other nutrients merits some additional review here. Chronic wounds (such as pressure ulcers) have been extensively investigated as to the risk of development, prevention, and cure. The combination of chronic wounds and malnutrition in the aged is particularly unfortunate. Malnutrition is frequently associated with skin anergy and immobility because of mental apathy and muscle wasting. Further, impaired nutritional intake and the risk of pressure ulcer formation are interrelated.

When considering nutritional support, oral supplementation should be weighed against tube feeding, as the associated morbidity of tube feeding (i.e., insufficient intake because of procedures, aspiration risk, diarrhea, constipation, translocation liability, and restricted mobility) might obscure the favorable effects of adequate nutrition. Total parenteral nutrition (TPN) should be used when the gastrointestinal tract cannot be used or cannot be used enough.

Attention should be focused on early recognition of a depleted nutritional status and an adequate and supervised intake of the following:

- Energy (as tolerated and up to 35 kcal/kg)
- Protein (up to 1 g of oral or enteral amino acids [AAs]/kg/d or up to 2 g parenteral AA/kg/d) with provision of the recommended daily allowances of micronutrients that will usually will require 1 to 1.5 l of any selected enteral feeding formula[1]

Parenteral nutrition should be reserved for the patient who cannot enterally ingest or cannot enterally eat enough.

Pressure ulcers affect one out of ten patients in hospitals, and older people are at highest risk for decubitus. The correlation between the lack of nutritional intake and the development of pressure ulcers is supported by several studies, but the results are inconsonant. Although it is difficult to draw any firm conclusions on the effect of enteral and parenteral nutrition on the prevention and treatment of pressure ulcers,[2] nutrition support intuitively provides precursors for every messenger mediator involved in the healing process and consequently plays a key role in the process of healing.

Primary wound healing mechanisms are contraction, epithelialization, and connective tissue deposition. In turn, micronutrients (electrolytes, trace elements, and vitamins) are intimately related to all of these physiologic responses in wound healing.

CONTRACTION

Although wound contraction begins almost concurrently with collagen synthesis, contraction does not appear to depend on collagen synthesis. Contraction, defined as the centripetal movement of wound edges that facilitates closure of a wound defect, is maximal at 5 to 15 days after injury. Contraction results in a decrease in wound size. The maximal rate of contraction is 0.75 mm/d and depends on the degree of tissue laxity and shape of the wound. Wound contraction depends on the myofibroblast located at the periphery of the wound, its connection to components of the extracellular matrix, and myofibroblast proliferation. Cell division inhibition (i.e., radiation, medications) will delay wound contraction. Topical zinc, for example, has been shown to decrease contraction.

EPITHELIALIZATION

Epithelialization is the formation of epithelium over a denuded surface within hours of injury. Epithelialization of an incisional wound involves the migration of cells at the wound edges over a distance of less than 1 mm from one side of the incision to the other. Incisional wounds are epithelialized within 24 to 48 h after injury. This epithelial layer provides a seal between the underlying wound and the environment. Epidermal cells at the wound edges undergo structural changes, allowing them to detach from their connections to other epidermal cells and to their basement membrane.

Intracellular actin microfilaments are formed, allowing the epidermal cells to creep across the wound surface. As the cells migrate, they dissect the wound and separate the overlying eschar from the underlying viable tissue. Epidermal cells secrete collagenases that break down collagen and plasminogen activator, which stimulates the production of plasmin. Plasmin promotes clot dissolution along the path of epithelial cell migration. The extracellular wound matrix over which epithelial cells migrate has received increased emphasis in wound healing research. Migrating epithelial cells interact with a provisional matrix of fibrin cross-linked to fibronectin and collagen. The matrix components may be a source of cell signals to facilitate epithelial cell proliferation and migration. In particular, fibronectin seems to promote keratinocyte adhesion to guide these cells across the wound base. Epithelial cell migration also may be facilitated in wound beds containing critical water content. Wounds with adequate tissue humidity demonstrate a faster and more direct course of epithelialization. Occlusive and semiocclusive dressings applied in the first 48 h after injury may maintain tissue humidity and optimize epithelialization. When epithelialization is complete, the epidermal cell assumes its original form and new desmosomal linkages to other epidermal cells and hemidesmosomal linkages to the basement membrane are restored. Zinc and saline wet dressings, for example, have been shown to promote epithelialization followed by faster healing.

CONNECTIVE TISSUE

Connective tissue deposition or collagen remodeling during the maturation phase depends on continued collagen synthesis in the presence of collagen destruction. Collagenases and matrix metalloproteinases in the wound assist in the removal of excess collagen, although synthesis of new collagen persists. Tissue inhibitors of metalloproteinases limit these collagenolytic enzymes so that a balance exists between formation of new collagen and removal of old collagen.

During remodeling, collagen becomes more organized. Fibronectin gradually disappears, and hyaluronic acid and glycosaminoglycans are replaced by proteoglycans. Type III collagen is replaced by type I collagen. Water is resorbed from the scar. These events allow collagen fibers to lie closer together, facilitating collagen cross-linking and ultimately decreasing scar thickness. Intramolecular and intermolecular collagen cross-links result in increased wound bursting strength. Remodeling begins approximately 21 d after injury, when the net collagen content of the wound is stable and may continue indefinitely.

The tensile strength of a wound is a measurement of its load capacity per unit area. The bursting strength of a wound is the force required to break a wound regardless of its dimension. Bursting strength varies with skin thickness. Peak tensile strength of a wound occurs approximately 60 d after injury. A healed wound reaches only approximately 80% of the tensile strength of unwounded skin. The roles of topical manganese, calcium, zinc, and ascorbic acid dressings in the treatment of chronic wounds and positive steps in tensile strength remain to be elucidated.

The zinc- and calcium-dependent family of proteins called the matrix metalloproteinases is collectively responsible for the degradation of the extracellular matrix. Members of this family, such as the collagenases, stromelysins, and the gelatinases, are involved in the routine tissue remodeling processes, such as wound healing, embryonic growth, and angiogenesis. Imbalance between the active enzymes and their natural inhibitors leads to the accelerated destruction of connective tissue associated with the pathology of diseases such as rheumatoid arthritis and osteoarthritis (Figure 10.1). Micronutrients, and particularly trace elements, again, are constituents of complex physiologic processes dealing with all of these stages.

Angiogenesis (via platelet inhibition) launches the collagen/extracellular matrix interaction that initiates the release of clotting factors, growth factors, and cytokines.

In short, following this period of hemostasis, neutrophils, and the business of phagocytosis to remove foreign materials, bacteria and damaged tissue move to the forefront. Macrophages help with the engulfment of foreign materials and release additional growth

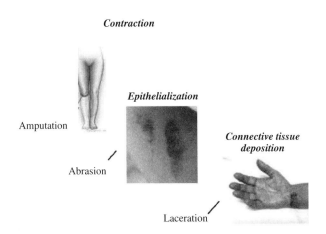

FIGURE 10.1 Wound healing mechanisms. So-called wound healing stages associated with these wound healing mechanisms include hemostasis, inflammation, proliferation, and remodeling.

TABLE 10.1
Wound Healing Stages

Stage	Cellular Components	Cellular Mediators and Activity
Hemostasis	Endothelial cells, platelets	Fibronectin, platelet-derived growth factor
Inflammation	Neutrophils, macrophages, lymphocytes	Cytokines, interleukins, proteases
Proliferation	Endothelial cells, fibroblasts, cytokines, epithelial cells	Collagen synthesis
Remodeling	Fibroblasts, epithelial cells	Collagenases, gelatinases, degradation, metalloproteinases, stromelysins

factors to clean up the wounded area. If this inflammation with associated reactive oxygen species (ROS) and catabolic enzymes is not halted, healing will not occur.

Once inflammation is controlled, new extracellular matrix is then formed with fibroblasts that begin the so-called proliferative phase. Fibrotic lesions (often in association with increased densities of mast cells) are characterized by excessive matrix deposition and reduced remodeling.

The cellular components and associated mediators of these stages can be found in Table 10.1.

Interleukins (about 20 have been identified) are cytokines produced by lymphocytes, monocytes, and macrophages. They regulate the cell-mediated response of the immune system. For example, interleukin-1 (IL-1) is involved in the triggering of the immune response, starting acute inflammation and maintaining chronic inflammation. Interleukin-2 (IL-2) is produced by helper T cells and induces proliferation of immune cells, both T and B. Interleukin-3 (IL-3) promotes the differentiation and proliferation of stem cells of the leukocyte family. Interleukin-6 (IL-6) is produced by various cells, including tumor cells, and acts as a stimulant of plasma proteins and B and T cells. Interleukin-12 (IL-12), produced by a range of cells, activates T cells and natural killer cells and promotes the response to a range of pathogens, including the human immunodeficiency viruses (HIV) of IL-2. It appears to be one of the most promising interleukins for the control of viral, bacterial, and protozoal infections.

Zinc, for example, is a trace element that is essential for immune functions. It directly induces monokine secretion by monocytes. There is also a specific inhibition of IL-1 receptor-associated protein kinase (IRAK) by zinc ions. Therefore, in contrast to an indirect stimulation of T cells due to zinc-induced monokines, higher concentrations of zinc directly inhibit T cell functions by means of specific inhibition of IRAK and subsequent signaling events, such as NFκB activation. The complex natures of these tiny nutrients are further illustrated by these divergent effects of zinc on different cell populations that depend on zinc concentration.[3,4]

Interferons are also cytokines belonging to a family of antiviral proteins that occur naturally in the body. α-Interferon and β-interferon probably exert an overall suppressive effect on the immune system. γ-Interferon is produced by immune system cells and enhances T cell recognition of antigens.

TABLE 10.2
Growth Factors and Cytokines

Colony-stimulating factor (CSF)
Epidermal growth factor (EGF)
Fibroblast growth factor (FGF)
Insulin-like growth factor (IGF)
Interleukins (ILs)
Interferon-α (INF-α) and INF-α 2b
Platelet-derived growth factor (PDGF)
Transforming growth factor-β (TGF-β)

Growth factors (GFs), unlike steroids that penetrate the cell, attach to the cell membrane, and their actions are primarily autocrine (action is on the cell that produced the GF), juxtacrine (action is on the adjacent cell), paracrine (action is on the local environment), and, of least importance, endocrine (action is on a distant cell).

Fibroblast GF and GF-α and GF-β have shown to be of little benefit in wound healing; however, platelet-derived GF (AA, AB, and B) and particularly recombinant platelet-derived GF (becaptermin) have been shown to be of value in diabetic foot ulcer healing.

Platelet-rich plasmas (PRPs) are used in a variety of clinical applications, based on the premise that higher growth factor content should promote better healing. PRP supernatants promote strong osteoblast and endothelial cell divisions, supporting the concept that PRPs may be beneficial in wound healing.[5–7] There are approximately 6 kg of protein in a 70-kg human. Losing one third of this compartment almost always leads to death. Weight loss and impaired nutritional status are associated with increased complications following injury or surgery. There is a significant reduction in the plasma C-reactive protein response in malnourished patients but no difference from controls in the responses of α-1-antitrypsin, α-1-acid glycoprotein, or in the trace elements iron or zinc, which reflect induction of ferritin and metallothionein, respectively.

There is an early increase in IL-6, soluble receptors of tumor necrosis factor (TNF), and in IL-1 receptor antagonist in both groups, but there is no detectable increase in plasma TNF or IL-1. There is no difference between the well-nourished and malnourished group for any of these markers of cytokine network activation. Weight loss is therefore associated with a reduction in aspects of the acute phase response, but this is due to impaired effectiveness rather than to reduced magnitude of the cytokine response.[8]

To sum up, in addition to this complex array of wound mediators, appropriate nutrition support, meticulous debridement, and vigilant infection control play important roles in the arena of wound healing. The extent of nutritional repletion and its impact on wound healing continues to deserve aggressive study.

Savvy clinicians would intuitively agree that good nutritional status is key for patient wellbeing and in turn must play an essential role in the wound healing process. Ignoring nutritional status may compromise the patient's ability to heal and subsequently prolong the stages of wound healing.

PROTEIN

Protein deficiency contributes to poor healing rates through reduced collagen formation and wound dehiscence. High exudate loss can result in a deficit of as much as 100 g of protein in 1 d. There is a correlation between low serum albumin and body mass index (BMI) and the development of pressure ulcers. Also, low serum albumin and high Waterlow score have a positive association. The body automatically renews tissue while we are asleep, but this does not mean that protein synthesis does not take place during our wakeful hours. Glucose provides the body with its power source for wound healing, and this gives energy for angiogenesis and the deposition of new tissue. Therefore, it is vital that the body receives adequate amounts of glucose to provide additional energy for wound healing. Fatty acids are essential for cell structure and play an important role in the inflammatory process. Vitamins, particularly those associated with skin integrity (vitamins A, D, and C), are also important in wound healing.[9]

Protein synthesis at the wound site must be increased for collagen deposition and healing to occur. Patients with protein–calorie malnutrition have diminished hydoxyproline accumulation (an index of collagen deposition) in subcutaneously implanted polytetrafluoroethylene catheters compared with normally nourished controls.[10]

AMINO ACIDS

The administration of individual sulfur-containing amino acids has been shown to abrogate the impaired healing in protein-deficient rats, as evidenced by increased fibroblastic proliferation and collagen accumulation.[11,12]

Recently, acetylcysteine is being investigated with respect to its ability to squelch oxygen radicals and provide antioxidant action for wound healing.[13]

The branched-chain amino acids (valine, leucine, and isoleucine) have been used to treat liver disease and have an additional role in retaining nitrogen in sepsis, trauma, and burns. Branched-chain amino acids support protein synthesis after injury and decrease muscle proteolysis. Serving as caloric substrates, branched-chain amino acids can be metabolized as an energy source independent of liver function.[14–21]

Glutamine is the most abundant amino acid in the body, and it accounts for approximately 20% of the total circulating free amino acid pool and 60% of the free intracellular amino acid pool. The process of gluconeogenesis involves the shuttling of alanine and glutamine to the liver for conversion to glucose, which is used peripherally as fuel to power certain aspects of wound healing. Glutamine is also an important precursor for the synthesis of nucleotides in cells, including fibroblasts and macrophages. Glutamine is an energy source for lymphocytes and is essential for lymphocyte proliferation. Finally, glutamine has a crucial role in stimulating the inflammatory immune response occurring early in wound healing.

Given the abundant roles of glutamine in the numerous cells involved in wound healing, it is not surprising that after injury there is a rapid fall in plasma and muscle glutamine levels, which is greater than that of any other amino acid. Although efficacy of supplemental glutamine administration has been shown in some clinical situations, it has not been proved to have any dramatic effect on wound healing.[24–34]

Arginine is absorbed from the intestine by a transport system shared with lysine, ornithine, and cysteine in an energy-dependent and sodium-dependent fashion with substrate specificity. Arginine also shares a common uptake and transport system into fibroblasts and leukocytes with these amino acids.[35]

Arginine is synthesized in adequate quantities to sustain muscle and connective tissue mass but in insufficient quantities for optimal protein biosynthesis and healing. In situations of stress or injury, in which synthesis of arginine is insufficient to meet the demands of increased protein turnover, arginine becomes an indispensable amino acid in the process of wound healing and maintenance of a positive nitrogen balance.

Arginine supplementation has no effect on the rate of epithelialization of the skin defect; the predominant effect of arginine is on wound collagen deposition. The beneficial effects of supplemental arginine on wound healing are similar to the effects of growth hormone; specifically, enhanced wound breaking strength and collagen deposition.[36–38]

Arginine has been identified as the unique substrate for the generation of the highly reactive radical nitric oxide (NO). Several studies suggest that NO plays a crucial role in wound healing. Inhibitors of NO have been shown to significantly impair healing of cutaneous incisional wounds and colonic anastomosis in rodents.[39,40] The inducible NO synthase (iNOS) pathway is at least partially responsible for the enhancement of wound healing observed with the administration of arginine.[41]

Nitric oxide is synthesized by the enzyme nitric oxide synthase, which converts the amino acid L-arginine to citrulline and NO. NO functions in biological systems in two very important ways. First, it has been found to be a messenger by which cells communicate with one another (signal transduction); second, it plays a critical role in the host response to infection. In this second function, it appears that the toxic properties of NO have been harnessed by the immune system to kill or at least slow the growth of invading organisms. The nonspecific chemical reactivity with key cellular targets is responsible for this action. In signaling, NO directly activates the enzyme soluble guanylate cyclase (sGC). Once activated, sGC converts cyclic guanosine triphosphate (GTP) to cyclic guanosine monophosphate (cGMP) and pyrophosphate. The cGMP formed is responsible for the well-documented actions of NO, such as blood vessel dilation. With the initial discovery of NO signaling, several important questions emerged that centered largely on the issue of how a signaling system functions when the signaling agent is chemically reactive (short lived), highly diffusible, and toxic. Critical, especially in signaling, are the control of NO biosynthesis and interaction with the biological receptors in due time at a concentration that will not harm the host.[42]

DEXTROSE AND LIPID

Protein is composed of approximately 20 amino acids and although protein can be gluconeogenically converted to carbohydrate (that in turn can promote hypertriglyceridemia), the desired energy substrates (to drive α-nitrogen into muscle) are dextrose and essential fatty acids and not protein.

Careful repletion of carbohydrate and lipid macronutrients will avoid adverse outcome. For example, overfeeding with carbohydrate is associated with hypercapnia, osmotic dehydration, and nonenzymatic glycosylation leading to immune compromise. The delivery of more than 5 mg/kg/d of dextrose will result in steatosis and the need for exogenous insulin. In addition, deleterious effects of hyperinsulinemia include antinaturetic effects and microalbuminuria.

The omission of long-chain fatty acids in nutrition regimens will lead to essential fatty acid deficiency in as little as 1 d (5 d are cited in the package inserts for intravenous lipid). As much as one third of hepatic phase I (oxidation/reduction) action will fall off if there is no fat in the diet.[43]

Macronutrients (protein, carbohydrate, and lipids) in turn must always be accompanied by micronutrients (electrolytes, trace elements, and vitamins) and water to promote anabolism. The remainder of this chapter will touch on electrolyte and vitamin micronutrients and will then specifically focus on the faces of trace elements and their relationship to wound healing processes.

MICRONUTRIENTS

Although micronutrients comprise only a small portion of the body's overall nutritional needs, their importance is highlighted by the cellular machinery that carries out wound healing.

ELECTROLYTES AND WOUND HEALING

Acid/base status must be ascertained to provide the correct salts for needed electrolytes based on serial trends of abnormal blood concentrations and excrements. Chloride, sulfate, and phosphate will provide passive acidification, and acetate, citrate, lactate, and gluconate are the anions of choice for passive alkalinization.

Sodium, potassium, calcium, magnesium, and phosphate will be the most important electrolytes to follow in the wound healing process.

An electrocardiogram is the most sensitive method to measure potassium and calcium status, but whole blood (as well as plasma and serum) concentration complemented by excrement assessment are used clinically. The most difficult electrolyte to measure is likely magnesium, because it is decreased stalwartly by stress or catecholamine shower.

Magnesium (Mg) is a macromineral that is essential for wound repair and is a cofactor for many enzymes that are involved in the process of protein synthesis. The primary role of magnesium is to provide structural stability to ATP, which powers many of the processes used in collagen synthesis, making it a factor essential to wound repair.[44,45]

Magnesium modulates cellular events involved in inflammation. Severe experimental Mg deficiency in the rat induces after a few days a clinical inflammatory syndrome characterized by polymorphonuclear (PMN) leukocyte and macrophage activation, release of inflammatory cytokines and acute phase proteins, and excessive production of free radicals. An increase in Mg concentration decreases the inflammatory response, and reduction in the extracellular Mg results in cell activation. Because Mg acts as a natural calcium antagonist, the molecular basis for inflammatory response is probably the result of modulation of intracellular calcium concentration. Mg deficiency contributes to an exaggerated response to immune stress, hyperlipemia, atherosclerosis, endothelial dysfunction, thrombosis, hypertension, and free radical damage.[46]

As with other electrolytes, whole blood (plasma or serum), intracellular stores (i.e., mononuclear leukocyte content), or excretory load will be useful indicators of status integrated with clinical appreciation. In the case of magnesium, urine is the most precise assessment of magnesium status. When sufficient excretion is evident (i.e., greater than 50% of intake), intracellular magnesium concentration is said to be sufficient. Magnesium and zinc are essential elements in all biological systems. They are both essential for enzymatic activity, maintaining three-dimensional structures of proteins, for the synthesis of nucleic acids and proteins, and so forth.

Low phosphate indicators are likely the most important parameters to respect in wound healing, because low 2,3-diphosphoglycerate content in the erythrocyte is very much a part of hemoglobin: oxygen tightening (so-called shift to the left in the hemoglobin:oxygen curve). This is amplified with concurrent clinical happenings, such as hypothermia, alkalemia, and hypocapnia, resulting in poor wound healing.

Overall, electrolyte concentrations must be normalized for favorable wound healing to occur. Serial measurement must guide the clinician to provide adequate but not excessive supplementation via an administration route that will not result in additional morbidity yet will guarantee appropriate needs.

Vitamins and Wound Healing

Vitamin A increases the inflammatory response in wounds that is thought to occur by an enhanced lysosomal membrane lability, increased macrophage influx and activation, and stimulation of collagen synthesis. *In vitro* studies have shown an increased presence of epidermal growth factor receptors and increased collagen synthesis of fibroblast cell cultures in the presence of vitamin A.[47,48]

Serious injury or stress leads to increased vitamin A requirements. Large doses of corticosteroids also deplete hepatic stores of vitamin A. Decreased serum levels of vitamin A, retinol binding protein, retinyl esters, and β-carotene have been noted after burns, fractures, and elective surgery. The clinician must be ever mindful, however, of the disease states (i.e., acute or chronic renal failure) associated with hypervitaminosis A to avoid the toxicities of vitamin A overload (i.e., osteolytic effects).[49–51] In the severely injured, doses of vitamin A of 25,000 IU/d (five times the recommended daily dose) have been advocated and used without any significant side effects. Larger doses of vitamin A do not improve further wound healing, and prolonged excessive intake can be toxic.[52] It is generally appreciated that zinc and other nutrients, such as a vitamin A derivative, are needed to avoid age-related macular degeneration. Several chronic diseases also associated with alterations in zinc status are bronchial asthma, rheumatoid arthritis, and Alzheimer's disease.

Vitamin E, or tocopherol, maintains and stabilizes cellular membrane integrity, primarily by protection against destruction by oxidation.[53] Vitamin E also possesses anti-inflammatory properties similar to those of steroids, as shown by the reversal of wound healing impairment imposed by vitamin E after administration of vitamin A in the first days after wounding.[54] Vitamin E also has been shown to affect various host immune functions. As an antioxidant, it has been proposed that vitamin E could reduce injury to the wound by squelching excessive free radicals. The liberation of free radicals from inflamed tissue cascades in necrotic tissue, tissue colonized with microbial flora, ischemic tissue, and chronic wounds can result in the depletion of free radical scavengers such as vitamin E.[55,56]

Vitamin K is known as the antihemorrhage vitamin and is required for the carboxylation of glutamate in clotting factors II, VII, IX, and X. Vitamin K contributes little to wound healing, but its absence or deficiency leads to decreased coagulation, which consequently affects the initial phases of healing. Vitamins A and E antagonize the homeostatic properties of vitamin K.

Formation of hematomas within the wound can impair healing and predispose to wound infection. The enteral absorption of fat-soluble vitamins (vitamins A, D, E, and K) requires the action of lipid and bile acids. These are absorbed via the jejunal/ileal parenchyma.

Cyanocobalamin (B_{12}) and folic acid (B_9), as well as copper and calcium, are inherently associated with hematological homeostasis. Pyridoxine (B_6) is intimately aligned with protein supplementation. Vitamins B_1 (important for the treatment of lactic acidemia), B_2, and B_3 (thiamine, riboflavin, and niacin, respectively) are similarly dosed as per caloric supplementation. Vitamin C or ascorbic acid decreases capillary fragility and provides antioxidant action to promote collagen synthesis.

Vitamins provide the coenzymatic machinery in the work of healing wounds. In addition to the superior free radical squelching of the sulfurated amino acids (i.e., acetylcysteine, cysteine, serine, threonine), much has been written about the antioxidant actions of vitamins A, C, and E. Daily supplementation of fat- and water-soluble vitamins will be required for optimum wound healing to occur.

TRACE ELEMENTS

Trace element and vitamin (and other indirect reflections of) status can be measured in plasma, serum or whole blood, and excrements. Again, pragmatic supplementation designed to avoid deficiencies or excesses will be a mandate. The clinician must be ever vigilant for signs and symptoms of deficiency or excess. It will be particularly difficult to associate deficits in trace elements (Table 10.3) to impairment in wound healing, because deficiencies of micronutrients are almost always accompanied by coexisting metabolic or other nutritional disturbances. Most of the trace elements do not influence wound healing directly; rather, they serve as cofactors or part of an enzyme that is essential to healing and homeostasis. Clinicians became more aware of deficiencies of these elements after the introduction of long-term parenteral nutrition solutions that did not include supplemental trace elements. It is often easier to prevent these deficiencies than to diagnose them clinically.

Copper, zinc, and iron have the closest relationship to wound healing. Copper is a required cofactor for cytochrome oxidase and the cytosolic antioxidant superoxide dismutase. Lysyl oxidase is a key copper enzyme used in the development of connective tissue, where it catalyzes the cross-linking of collagen and strengthens the collagen framework.[57]

Zinc is a cofactor for RNA and DNA polymerase and, consequently, is involved in DNA synthesis, protein synthesis, and cellular proliferation. Zinc deficiency

TABLE 10.3
Essential Trace Elements in Humans

Arsenic	Manganese
Cadmium	Molybdenum
Chromium	Nickel
Cobalt	Selenium
Copper	Silicon
Fluorine	Tin
Iron	Vanadium
Lead	Zinc
Lithium	

impairs the crucial roles each of these processes play in wound healing. Zinc levels less than 100 mg/100 ml have been associated with impairments in wound healing.

In zinc deficiency, fibroblast proliferation and collagen synthesis are decreased, leading to decreased wound strength and delayed epithelialization. These defects are readily reversed with repletion of zinc to normal levels. Cellular and humoral immunity are impaired with zinc deficiency, resulting in an increased susceptibility to wound infection and resultant increased possibility of delayed healing. Zinc levels can be severely depleted in settings of major stress,[58] and in patients receiving long-term steroids. In these settings, it is recommended that patients receive vitamin A and zinc supplements to improve wound healing.

The current recommended daily allowance for elemental zinc is 15 mg, remembering that approximately 25% of zinc sulfate is elemental and only 20% is absorbed. No studies have shown improvement in wound healing after the administration of zinc to patients who are not zinc deficient.

Zinc should be avoided during the acute phase response, because it has been associated with an increase in the febrile response.[59]

Iron is required for the hydroxylation of proline and lysine, and as a result, severe iron deficiency can result in impaired collagen production. As a part of the oxygen transport system, iron can affect wound healing, but this occurs only in settings of severe iron-deficiency anemia. In the clinical setting, iron deficiency is common and can result from blood loss, infectious causes, malnutrition, or an underlying hematopoietic disorder.

Determination of the presence or absence of a deficiency of one or more of the micronutrient minerals can be a complex problem, frequently requiring the integration of clinical, nutritional, and biochemical data. Using a combination of techniques, it is usually possible to determine with confidence whether an individual subject or small groups of subjects have a deficiency of specific trace elements, but simple reliable tests that can be used in population studies are still lacking an emphasis on the importance of sign and symptom recognition.[60]

In addition, disease states add to the complexity of trace element status assessment. For example, micronutrient deficiencies may occur in patients with malignancy due to a variety of possible causes, including unbalanced or insufficient dietary intake and adverse effects of treatment. Further, many cancer patients show signs of a chronic inflammatory response that can affect circulating concentrations of certain vitamins and trace elements. Blood concentrations of zinc and selenium are frequently lower than their respective reference ranges, although copper and manganese concentrations rise above their respective reference ranges. However, interestingly, none of these micronutrients show significant correlation with C-reactive protein.[61]

More recently, the ratio of neutrophils to lymphocytes has received considerable attention and is said to be of more value in terms of understanding the relationship of inflammation to mortality and heart disease.[62]

The surface of learning has barely been scratched with regard to the physiologic roles of trace elements. Table 10.4 summarizes the most common roles for the most important trace elements.

The assessment of trace element status is fraught with problems. Unreliable histories, contamination concentrations in medications and nutrients, analytical techniques, bioavailability, and excretion are all problematic. Because pragmatic serum levels leave much to be desired, assumption of a period without adequate nutrition should be presumed, and supplementation from day 1 of any so-called artificial feeding may be in the best interests of the patient.

Concentrations of trace elements in human tissues characteristically vary widely. Examination of some of the factors that contribute to the marked variability and skewness of the concentrations revealed that distributions of concentrations are satisfactorily normal (Gaussian) after logarithmic transformation, ash weight is the best frame of reference in which to report results, the distributions of metal concentrations are not further normalized by adjustments that assume that tissue lipid or collagen contains a fixed fraction of the metal found in the parenchyma, and the choice of sample site (i.e., hepatic) is often of minimal significance.[64]

To illustrate the frustration of trace element assessment, aluminum, copper, zinc, and selenium levels were determined in serum, urine, and tissue samples of burned patients. Relationships between wound healing and trace elements were evaluated. Trace element levels were determined using atomic absorption spectrophotometry. During 20 d of treatment, a significant rise in aluminum levels was determined in serum, urine, and tissue samples of patients. After day 5 of treatment, copper levels increased significantly only in urine samples. Zinc levels decreased in serum and tissue samples. However, high values of zinc in urine were measured within the first week, and then the levels returned to the initial value. There was a significant decrease in zinc in serum and tissue samples taken from patients with burns during treatment. Urine selenium levels showed a significant rise within the first 15 d.[65]

A variety of sources (Table 10.5) were proposed to assess functional, regulatory, sequestrated, and transport/storage sites.

Finally, the kinetics of trace elements (Table 10.6) must be appreciated. Meticulous review of biological systems must take place. Needs, toxicities, nutritional state, and disease all play a role in determining dosing.

Oral or enteral feeding requirements, respectively, can only be presumed sufficient, with corroborating calorie counts by a competent registered dietitian, and with the tolerability evidence of at least 1 to 2 L of most commercially available enteral

TABLE 10.4
Trace Element Primary and Secondary Roles in Wound Healing

Trace Elements of Primary Importance in Wound Healing

Copper
- Maintains iron utilization, because it is a cofactor for ceruloplasmin (94% serum binding)
- Oxidase necessary for the formation of transferrin (carrier of iron)
- Associated with the maintainance of normal synthetic rates for red blood cells and white blood cells

Iron
- Oxygen transport — component of heme that is the nonprotein portion of hemoglobin (Hgb); combines with Hgb in lungs and distributes to the tissue; also found in myoglobin
- Cytochrome content — normal cellular respiration; ATP storage through iron coupling reactions
- T-cell immunity and cognitive function roles

Zinc
- Functions with hundreds of enzymes (e.g., carbonic anhydrase, alkaline phosphatase, lactic acid dehydrogenase, alcohol dehydrogenase, RNA and DNA polymerases, and superoxide dismutase), wound healing, taste, increases oxygen affinity in normal and sickle cell patients, component of bone, synthesis of nucleic acid, glutathione, connective tissue, and collagen precursors

Trace Elements of Secondary Importance in Wound Healing

Chromium
- Maintains protein, carbohydrate, and lipid metabolism
- Glucose tolerance factor (GTF) — cofactor with insulin
- Important in peripheral nerve function

Iodine
- Sole function in man, incorporation into thyroid hormones (T3 and T4) — regulates cellular metabolism, temperature, and normal growth

Manganese
- Activator for several enzymes — glycotransferase activation (mucopolysaccharides formation)
- Found in association with vitamin K deficiencies — glycotransferase activation in prothrombin synthesis
- Found in association with squalene — precursor of cholesterol and sex hormones
- Found in association with protein synthesis, carbohydrate and lipid (activates lipoproteinlipase) metabolism

Molybdenum
- Constituent of three enzymes — aldehyde oxidase, sulfite oxidase, and xanthine oxidase
- Causes increased mobilization of copper from tissue and increases urinary excretion

Selenium
- Glutathione peroxidase (antioxidant) component — protects the cell from lipid oxidation; functions with and can substitute for vitamin E

Source: From Baumgartner, T.G., *Nutr. Clin. Pract.*, 8, 251, 1993. With permission.

TABLE 10.5
Tissues and Trace Element Analysis

Essential Function Sites
Hemoglobin (iron)
Liver (zinc)

Regulatory Sites
Intestinal mucosa (iron)
Thyroid (iodine)
Liver (manganese or chromium)

Sequestrian Tissues
Lung
Kidney
Reticuloendothelial
Nails
Hair
Stratum corneum of the skin

Transport and Storage Sites
Serum concentration
Urine concentration
Bone marrow

---

formulas. Baseline and serial assessment of both signs and symptoms should continue throughout the course of parenteral therapy and during the transitional period to enteral use, because bioavailability may not yet be in place. Recommended daily dietary allowances, estimated safe and adequate daily dietary intakes, and intravenous dosage recommendations can be found in Table 10.7 through Table 10.9.

Boron

Many anecdotal alternative treatments with clandestine sources of trace elements abound in the literature. For example, matrix metalloproteinase (MMP)-2 and MMP-9 are involved in keratinocyte migration and granulation tissue remodeling during wound healing. Thermal water cures are sometimes proposed as complementary treatment for accelerating healing of wounds resulting from burns or surgery, but their mechanisms of action remain unknown. Some thermal waters are rich in trace elements, such as boron and manganese. Clinical studies have also shown beneficial effects of trace elements, such as boron and manganese, for human wound healing.[67]

Chromium

Assessment of chromium status includes blood (plasma, serum, whole), red blood cell, hair, and urinary concentrations.

Conditions that increase circulating glucose and insulin concentrations increase urinary chromium output. Chromium is probably excreted in the form of the

TABLE 10.6
Trace Element Kinetics

Chromium

Absorption is minimal (i.e., 0.5 to 2%). Chromium, not unlike iron, uses a transferrin vehicle for transport to target sites. Mean serum concentrations are 0.16 ng/ml. The excretion of chromium is 0.2 to 0.6 mcg/l urine, and diets high in simple carbohydrates may increase urinary excretion up to threefold.

Copper

Absorption is about 30 to 60%. Copper absorption is impaired by Zn supplements providing 22.5 mg/d, even when the supplement is taken independently of meals. Distribution is principally (94%) via binding to ceruloplasmin; however, there also is binding to transcuprein, albumin, and amino acids. Plasma concentrations are approximately 1 mcg/ml with principal excretion in bile (80%). Intestinal and urine excretion account for 16 and 4% excretion, respectively.

Iodine

Absorption is greater than 50% and up to 100% is from gut. Iodine is also absorbed from skin. Dietary iodized salt is a major source of this trace element. The distribution of iodine is mainly via triiodothyronine (T3) and thyroxine (T4). Plasma concentrations are about 60 ng/ml, and excretion is principally in urine with rapid turnover (i.e., two thirds of absorbed iodide is excreted within 2 to 3 d).

Iron

Absorption is approximately 5 to 15% as the ferrous ion. Once absorbed, it is converted to the ferric ion in the mucosal cells of the intestine and binds to apoferritin that forms ferritin (regulates absorption of iron); transferrin binds iron in the plasma and transports iron to the liver, spleen, and bone marrow (where it is stored again as ferritin). Nascent distribution is bound to transferrin and is influenced by interleukin I (leukocyte endogenous mediator). The plasma concentration is approximately 1 mcg/ml and is excreted principally in bile, but also via skin and urine.

Manganese

Absorption is about 3 to 4%; however, absorption may be decreased with iron, cobalt, calcium, and phosphate. The distribution of manganese is bound extensively to transferrin or transmanganin. There is a small amount bound to $_1$globulin. Plasma concentrations are about 0.6 to 2 ng/ml. Excretion is extensive in bile (greater than 99%), and excretion (not absorption) regulates homeostasis.

Molybdenum

Absorption is about 40 to 100% in duodenum. The plasma concentration is about 2 to 6 ng/ml, and although excretion is principally in the urine, great gastrointestinal losses can occur.

Selenium

Absorption is 35 to 85% in duodenum; however, absorption is dependent on selenium solubility and the ratio of selenium to sulfur. Plasma concentrations are approximately 100 to 130 ng/ml, and excretion is principally in the urine; however, as with molybdenum, great intestinal losses can occur. Patients with burns (greater than 20% of body surface area) will need 200 mcg selenium for at least 2 weeks.

Zinc

Absorption is about 10 to 40% with 2.5 to 4 mg absorbed per day in duodenum and proximal jejunem. Absorption will be diminished if given with copper; iron:zinc ratio of 2 to 3:1 and vitamin D may increase zinc bioavailability. Zinc metallothionein regulates zinc metabolism and absorption.

Distribution is via binding to albumin, transferrin, ceruloplasmin, and -globulin. Plasma concentrations are approximately 1 mcg/ml, and excretion in biliary and pancreatic losses may account for up to 25% of daily losses (12 mg/l fistula, 17 mg/kg stool). Sweat losses can be as high as 1 mcg/ml.

TABLE 10.7
Trace Elements That Have Recommended Daily Dietary Allowances

Trace Element	Daily Dose Range[a]
Iodine	40 to 200 mcg
Iron	6 to 15 mg
Selenium	10 to 75 mcg
Zinc	5 to 16 mg

[a] Dosing is dependent on age, sex, pregnancy, and the duration of female lactation.

oligopeptide chromodulin. Chromodulin may be the key to understanding the role of chromium at a molecular level, as the molecule has been found to bind to activated insulin receptor, stimulating its kinase activity.[68]

The clinical consequences of chromium deficiency include glucose intolerance (and increased insulin requirements), hyperlipidemia, metabolic encephalopathy, and neuropathy.

Chromium plays a pivotal role in all macronutrient (protein, carbohydrate, and lipid) metabolism. It is, however, crucial in the synthesis of glucose tolerance factor (GTF), a cofactor in insulin action. Trivalent chromium is an essential nutrient and has a key role in lipid and glucose metabolism. Supplementation with chromium does not appear to reduce glucose levels in euglycemia. It may, however, have some efficacy in reducing glucose levels in hyperglycemia. The effects of chromium on lipid levels are variable. Chromium in doses less than 1000 mcg or 1 mg/d appear to be safe for short-term administration to type 2 diabetic patients.[69]

No specific manifestations of chromium toxicity are anticipated from parenteral administration. Chromium as an element, however, has a recognized potential for toxicity, with the chromate form being much more injurious than the chromic form and organic compounds much more toxic than elemental forms. Orally, chromium

TABLE 10.8
Trace Elements That Have Estimated Safe and Adequate Daily Dietary Intakes

Trace Element	Daily Dose Range[a]
Chromium	10 to 200 mcg
Copper	0.4 to 3 mg
Fluoride	0.1 to 4 mg
Manganese	0.3 to 5 mg
Molybdenum	15 to 250 mcg

[a] Dosing is dependent solely on age.

TABLE 10.9
Suggested Daily Intravenous Intake of Essential Trace Elements 66

	Pediatric (μg/kg)[a]	Adult		
		Stable	Acute Catabolic[b]	GI Losses[b]
Zinc	300[c]	2.5 to 4 mg	Additional 2 mg	Add 12.2 mg/l small bowel fluid lost; 17.1 mg/kg of stool or ileostomy output[e]
	100[d]			
Copper	20	0.5 to 1.5 mg	—	—
Chromium	0.14 to 0.2	10 to 15 μg	—	20 μg
Manganese	2	0.15 to 0.8 mg	—	—

[a] Limited data are available for infants weighing less than 1500 g. Their requirements may be more than the recommendations because of their low body reserves and increased requirements for growth.
[b] Frequent monitoring of blood concentrations in these patients is essential to provide proper dosage.
[c] Premature infants (weight less than 1500 g) up to 3 kg of body weight. Thereafter, the recommendation for full-term infants applies.
[d] Values derived by mathematical fitting of balance data from a 71-patient-week study in 24 patients.
[e] Mean from balance study.

Source: From Nutrition Advisory Group, American Medical Association, *J. Parenter. Enteral. Nutr.,* 3, 263, 1979. With permission.

can lead to cognitive, perceptual, and motor dysfunction at doses of 200 to 400 mcg/d. It can also cause anemia, thrombocytopenia, hemolysis, hepatic dysfunction, and renal failure when given in dosages of 1200 to 2400 mcg/d.[70] Chromium picolinate might affect dopamine, serotonin, and norepinephrine metabolism in the brain, due to the picolinic acid component.[71]

Studies show that people with type 2 diabetes have lower blood levels of chromium than those without the disease. Insulin resistance is the common denominator in a cluster of cardiovascular disease risk factors. One out of every five Americans has metabolic syndrome. It affects 40% of people in their 60s and 70s. Insulin resistance, with or without the presence of metabolic syndrome, significantly increases the risk of cardiovascular disease. Insulin resistance is present in two serious health problems in women — polycystic ovarian syndrome (PCOS) and gestational diabetes. Several studies have demonstrated that chromium supplements enhance the metabolic action of insulin and lower some of the risk factors for cardiovascular disease, particularly in overweight individuals. Chromium picolinate, specifically, has been shown to reduce insulin resistance and to help reduce the risk of cardiovascular disease and type 2 diabetes. It must be remembered that dietary chromium is poorly absorbed, and chromium levels decrease with age. Supplements containing 200 to 1000 mcg chromium as chromium picolinate taken each day have been found to improve blood glucose control. Chromium picolinate appears to be the most efficacious form of chromium supplementation.[72]

Chromium is of particular importance in wound healing. Chromium can alter the immune response by immunostimulatory or immunosuppressive processes, as shown by its effects on T and B lymphocytes, macrophages, cytokine production, and the immune response that may induce hypersensitivity reactions.[73]

More recently, researchers conducting a randomized, placebo-controlled, double-blind study of supplementation in patients with impaired glucose tolerance suggested that chromium supplementation does not improve glucose tolerance, insulin sensitivity, or lipid profile.[74]

Further, a meta-analysis from 15 randomized, controlled trials showed no effect of chromium on glucose or insulin concentrations in nondiabetic subjects.[75]

Therefore, the role of chromium (as part of glucose tolerance factor in insulin, the chief anabolic hormone in humans) in wound healing remains somewhat unclear. Yet, particularly in type 2 diabetics, there are suggestions that chromium supplementation may serve to avoid hyperglycemia and associated glycation that leads to complement fixation compromise and infection.

Copper

Copper is an indispensable trace element for life. Several points are key, in that copper is combined with essential enzymatic systems (see Table 10.10), is necessary for inclusion of iron in hemoglobin, has a primordial role in the metabolism of hemoglobin, and has a pristine role in the metabolism of collagen and elastin, and some vascular diseases (aneurysms) are closely related to a lack of it. Finally, an increase in plasma copper can be found in patients with cancerous diseases, which is significant early on and its increase is usually proportional to the malignancy evolution.[76]

More specifically, the physiological role of copper in the human organism is to reduce the excesses of free radicals, biogenic amines, and cholesterol, to aid in the proper synthesis of hemoglobin, elastin, collagen, and probably thyroid hormones, and to assist in energy formation in the respiratory chain needed for biochemical syntheses and proper physical activity (Table 10.11 and Table 10.12).

TABLE 10.10
Selected Functions of Cuproenzymes with Oxidation and Reduction Activity in Human Enzyme Function

Amine oxidases	Deamination of primary amines
Catechol oxidase	Synthesis of melanin
Ceruloplasmin	Ferroxidase
Cytochrome-c oxidase	Electron transport, terminal oxidase
Dopamine-b-monooxygenase	Dopamine/norepinephrine
Peptidylglycine monooxygenase	α-Amidation of neuropeptides
Protein-lysine 6-oxidase	Collagen and elastin cross-linking
Superoxide dismutase	Superoxide dismutation

TABLE 10.11
Selected Functions of Copper-Binding Proteins in Humans

Physiologic Role	Copper-Binding Proteins
Blood coagulation	Factors V and VIII
Ferroxidase activity	Ferroxidase I
	Ferroxidase II
Metal transport	Albumin
	Ferroxidase I
	Metallothionein
	Transcuprein
Radical scavenging	Ferroxidase I
	Metallothionein
	Superoxide dismutase
Synthesis of adenosine	Adenosylhomocysteinase homocysteine

The common feature of reactions catalyzed by cuproenzymes is the involvement of molecular oxygen or a derivative; thus, unlike the metalloenzymes of zinc, cuproenzymes almost universally govern the rate-limiting steps in the respective biochemical pathways. Therefore, unlike zinc, most of the clinical expression of copper deficiency in humans (except for the hematological manifestations) can be explained on a molecular basis in terms of the deficiency of one or another metalloenzyme of copper.[77]

Dietary copper bioavailability (40 to 60%) can be affected by other nutrients and the status of its primary binding protein, ceruloplasmin. Copper stores (approximately 120 mg) are mainly in the liver and are secreted in saliva, gastric and pancreatic juice, and bile. A copper–metallothionein complex present in intestinal mucosal cells is shed into the intestinal lumen.

Medications such as estrogen stimulate ceruloplasmin and therefore increase mean serum copper concentrations in females. Even higher serum coppers are found in women who are pregnant (during the third trimester), in patients with hyperthyroidism, and in those using oral contraceptives.[78] Copper and ceruloplasmin concentrations are also higher in those who smoke and in those with conditions involving chronic inflammation (e.g., rheumatoid arthritis), chronic infection, and some neoplasms. Serum copper concentrations in patients with burns over 15% of their bodies remain within normal limits, and hypozincemia was found in patients irrespective of burn surface area. Long-term monitoring of patients with burns over 70% of their bodies shows initial hypocupremia and hypozincemia.[79]

Although typically bound to proteins, copper may be released and become free to catalyze the formation of highly reactive hydroxyl radicals. Data obtained from *in vitro* and cell culture studies are largely supportive of copper's capacity to initiate oxidative damage and interfere with important cellular events. Oxidative damage has been linked to chronic copper overload and exposure to excess copper caused by accidents, occupational hazards, and environmental contamination. Additionally,

TABLE 10.12
Selected Physiologic Roles of Copper

Antioxidant action
Bone mineralization
Catecholamine metabolism
Collagen cross-linking
Elastin
Erythropoiesis
Iron turnover
Leukopoiesis
Melanin formation

copper-induced oxidative damage has been implicated in disorders associated with abnormal copper metabolism and neurodegenerative changes. Interestingly, a deficiency in dietary copper also increases cellular susceptibility to oxidative damage. A number of nutrients have been shown to interact with copper and alter its cellular effects. Vitamin E is generally protective against copper-induced oxidative damage. Although most *in vitro* or cell culture studies show that ascorbic acid aggravates copper-induced oxidative damage, results obtained from available animal studies suggest that the compound is protective. High intakes of ascorbic acid and zinc may provide protection against copper toxicity by preventing excess copper uptake. Zinc also removes copper from its binding site, where it may cause free radical formation.

β-Carotene, α-lipoic acid, and polyphenols have also been shown to attenuate copper-induced oxidative damage.[80]

Copper status is assessed using serum, plasma, erythrocyte, leukocyte, serum ceruloplasmin, serum amine oxidase, hemoglobin, and urinary concentrations.

Microcytic hypochromic anemia (similar to iron deficiency) and neutropenia are the most common hematological manifestations of copper deficiency. Hair depigmentation, demineralization of skeleton, and central nervous system anomalies may also be found with deficiency.

Kinky hair disease, first described in 1962, is a sex-linked disorder, with its gene located on the long arm of the X chromosome close to the centromere. The condition is marked by intellectual deterioration, seizures, and poorly pigmented, friable hair. Bony changes resembling scurvy, tortuosities of the cerebral and systemic vasculature, and diverticuli of the bladder are also seen. Biochemically, the most diagnostic alteration is a marked reduction in blood copper and ceruloplasmin levels. Even though parenteral copper administration will correct the biochemical abnormalities, such treatment will not arrest cerebral deterioration.[81] In central nervous system demyelination, hematologic recovery followed copper supplementation, both initially and after relapse off copper therapy, while serum zinc levels remained high, and the neurologic abnormalities only stabilized.[82]

Copper toxicity includes nausea, vomiting, bloody diarrhea, hypotension, hemolytic anemia, uremia, and cardiovascular collapse. Chronic exposure symptoms include sporadic fever, vomiting, epigastric pain, diarrhea, and jaundice. Renal failure and death can occur with ingestion of as little as 1 g of copper sulfate.[83]

Angiogenesis plays a central role in wound healing. Among many known growth factors, vascular endothelial growth factor (VEGF) is believed to be the most prevalent, efficacious, and long-term signal that is known to stimulate angiogenesis in wounds. Whereas a direct role of copper in facilitating angiogenesis was evident two decades ago, the specific targets of copper action remained unclear. This report presents the first evidence showing that inducible VEGF expression is sensitive to copper and that the angiogenic potential of copper may be harnessed to accelerate dermal wound contraction and closure. At physiologically relevant concentrations, copper sulfate induced VEGF expression in primary as well as transformed human keratinocytes. Copper shared some of the pathways utilized by hypoxia to regulate VEGF expression. Topical copper sulfate accelerated the closure of an excisional murine dermal wound allowed to heal by secondary intention. Copper-sensitive pathways regulate key mediators of wound healing, such as angiogenesis and extracellular matrix remodeling. The use of copper-based therapeutics represents a feasible approach to promote dermal wound healing.[84]

Copper is a required cofactor for cytochrome oxidase and the cytosolic antioxidant superoxide dismutase. Lysyl oxidase is a key copper enzyme used in the development of connective tissue, where it catalyzes the cross-linking of collagen and strengthens the collagen framework. Experimentally, impaired healing has been noted secondary to decreased copper stores in patients with Wilson's disease and in animal models after the administration of penicillamine.[85]

Copper ions can adopt distinct redox states, oxidized Cu(II) or reduced (I), allowing the metal to play a pivotal role in cell physiology as a catalytic cofactor in the redox chemistry of enzymes, mitochondrial respiration, iron absorption, free radical scavenging, and elastin cross-linking. If present in excess, free copper ions can cause damage to cellular components, and a delicate balance between the uptake and efflux of copper ions determines the amount of cellular copper. In biological systems, copper homeostasis has been characterized at the molecular level. It is coordinated by several proteins, such as glutathione, metallothionein, Cu-transporting P-type ATPases, Menkes and Wilson proteins, and cytoplasmic transport proteins called copper chaperones to ensure that it is delivered to specific subcellular compartments and thereby to copper-requiring proteins.

Iodine

Iodine is important in the cellular oxidative processes associated with thyroid functions. Brain development in humans is remarkably resistant to permanent damage from protein-energy malnutrition. Iodine deficiency is the most important and widespread nutrient deficiency; it causes endemic cretinism, associated with deaf mutism and cerebral palsy. The minimum requirement of adults has been estimated at 50 to 75 µg/d; children and pregnant women have a higher requirement. The principal role of iodine in man is its incorporation into thyroid hormones (T3 and T4) that regulate cellular metabolism, temperature, and normal growth. About two thirds of total body iodine is found in the thyroid. More than one half of oral iodine is absorbed; two thirds of that amount is excreted in the next 48 to 72 h. Goitrogens (e.g., cabbage, phthlates, resorcinol, rutabaga, thiocyanate, turnips) may inhibit thyroid uptake of iodine. Pulmonary insufficiency and dysphagia should trigger an examination of the thyroid gland and could possibly lead to a goiter. A goiter can occur, however, without hypothyroidism. Weakness, cold intolerance, weight gain, puffiness of face/eyelids, thinning of the hair, and brittle nails combined with pallor, hoarseness, decreased sweating, constipation, and anginal pain may be part of the signs and symptoms of hypothyroidism. Topical administration of iodine complexes has also been associated with thyrotoxicosis.[86]

Iron

The principal role of iron is to deliver oxygen to tissues. It binds with heme, the nonprotein portion of hemoglobin (Hgb), in the lungs and is distributed to tissues where it is also found as myoglobin. Cellular respiration, adenosine triphosphate storage using iron-coupling reactions, and possibly T-cell immunity and cognitive function actions are other roles that may require iron.

Absorption of iron usually takes place in the duodenum and occurs as the ferrous ion. Acidification with vitamin C is said to increase the bioavailability, whereas alkalinizers (e.g., antacid or basic ash foods, such as fruits and vegetables) may hinder absorption. Once absorbed, iron is then converted to ferric ion in the intestinal mucosal cells and binds to apoferritin, which forms ferritin (a storage protein said to regulate iron absorption). Transferrin binds iron and chromium in the plasma and transports iron to the liver, spleen, and bone marrow, where iron is again stored as ferritin. Iron is excreted principally in the feces.

Iron deficiency is associated with insufficient intake, excessive blood loss, achlorhydria, and malabsorption. Symptoms may include fatigue, dyspnea, palpitations, angina, tachycardia, and presentation of a hypochromic, microcytic anemia. Toxicity, namely hemosiderosis (mainly in males as a result of saturation of hemosiderin stores), can result from multiple blood transfusions, because blood contains about 0.5 mg iron/ml. In order to remain in iron balance, the daily iron intake of men, as well as of postmenopausal women, must be 0.5 to 1 mg. Because only 10% of iron will be absorbed, 10 times this requirement must be given orally as elemental iron. Although parenteral iron is 100% bioavailable, target site delivery, incorporation into the erythrocyte, takes at least 3 weeks. Menstruating women may require an additional 0.3 to 1 mg/d. The iron requirement is increased during pregnancy, due in particular to the increase in the total erythrocyte volume. This need is met partly by mobilization of iron reserves, which are restored postpartum when the total erythrocyte volume falls again. Parenteral iron may not need to be repleted during short periods of parenteral feeding if iron stores are adequate prior to the initiation of parenteral therapy. A test dose of 25 mg (0.5 ml of iron dextran) over 5 min will be needed, because there are reports of anaphylaxis. Sympathomimetics and antihistaminics should be available if there is an adverse reaction. If the infusion is delivered peripherally, there will be less phlebitis if the vehicle is sodium chloride. A maximum daily dose of 100 mg is recommended, but total dose repletion is frequently infused over several hours. Patients with Crohn's disease may trap parenteral iron in the reticular endothelium with resultant adverse reactions, suggesting the possible undesirability of this dosage form in inflammatory states. Patients who are infected should not receive parenteral iron, because iron is typically sequestered to the liver during infective processes. When given intramuscularly, the product must be given via a Z-track technique; that is, the depression and lateral movement of the gluteal areas, upper, and outer quadrant, should ensure prevention of retrograde leak and staining of the subcutaneous fatty areas with iron.

Manganese

Mn-superoxide dismutase and pyruvate carboxylase are the two most important metalloenzymes of manganese. Evidence for the occurrence of overt manganese deficiency in human subjects has not been adequately described. Nonetheless, homeostasis of the metabolic synthesis of proteins, such as mucopolysaccharides and prothrombin, as well as carbohydrate and lipid (e.g., activates lipoprotein lipase activation, cholesterol, and sex hormone precursors) are important roles of manganese. Stores are found in the mitochondria of hepatic, renal, pancreatitic, bone, and skeletal muscle parenchyma. Deficiencies have been manifested as tardive dyskinesia, epilepsy, diabetes mellitus, pancreatic insufficiency, and malnutrition. Deficiency has also been related to hair color changes, hypercholesterolemia, and prolonged prothrombin times. Manganese may accumulate in hepatically compromised patients.

Several experiences of manganese toxicity in individuals with cholestasis, including some confirmed by basal ganglia deposition as revealed by magnetic resonance imaging (MRI), were reported.[87]

Selenium

Glutathione peroxidase, an enzyme that protects the cell from lipid oxidation and functions with (and can substitute for) *in vivo* vitamin E, contains selenium. Selenium is associated with the degradation of intracellular peroxides and the oxidation of glutathione. Selenium is absorbed principally in the duodenum (80%) and is dependent on a number of variables. In particular, sulfurated amino acids can increase absorption significantly. Selenium is principally excreted in the urine, with extraordinary fecal losses occurring in the setting of bowel compromise. Total body content of selenium varies according to the relative amount present in the soil. The highest concentrations are found in the kidney, followed by the liver, muscle, and skin. Muscle contains almost half the total body selenium content. Myositis with concurrent complaints of muscle pain coupled with cardiomyopathy and abnormal elevations of creatine phosphokinase serum concentrations provide evidence for empiric selenium supplementation.

Selenium prevents the occurrence of Keshan disease, a juvenile cardiomyopathy precipitated by very low dietary selenium intake. The disease is characterized by congestive heart failure with moderate to severe enlargement of the heart and facial edema, which may involve a predisposing condition not yet clarified.

Inadequate selenium nutriture has additionally been linked to Kashin–Beck disease, an endemic osteoarthritis.[88]

Selenium appears to be capable of selectively regulating the generation of functional lymphocyte subsets *in vitro*. Such selective regulation could explain the published effects of selenium on immunity and would be consistent with a role for immunity in the observed reduction of cancer incidence associated with elevated selenium intake.[89]

Silicon

Silicon performs an important role in connective tissue, especially in bone and cartilage. Silicon's primary effect in bone and cartilage appears to be on the formation of the organic matrix. Bone and cartilage abnormalities are associated with a reduction in matrix components, resulting in the establishment of a requirement for silicon in collagen and glycosaminoglycan formation. Additional support for silicon's metabolic role in connective tissue is provided by the finding that silicon is a major ion of osteogenic cells, especially high in the metabolically active state of the cell. Further studies also indicate that silicon participates in the biochemistry of subcellular enzyme-containing structures. Silicon also forms important relationships with other elements. Although it is clear from the body of recent work that silicon performs a specific metabolic function, a structural role has been proposed for silicon in connective tissue. A relationship established between silicon and aging is likely associated with glycosaminoglycan changes.[90]

Silver

Pure silver, through the release of silver ions, has been reported to be effective in preventing infections as well as in improving wound healing. Silver appears to kill microbes by blocking the respiratory enzymes required for energy production. Although silver's potent antimicrobial properties are well studied, scientific data on the healing effects of silver are lacking.

Over the past 40 years, silver has been combined with more stable complexes, such as nitrate and sulfadiazine, for topical use on wounds. This approach that maintains silver's antimicrobial properties, however, may actually impede the reepithelialization process.[91]

Zinc

The physiological functions of zinc in humans include cell growth/proliferation, sexual maturation/reproduction, dark adaptation/night vision, gustatory acuity, wound healing, and host immune defenses. The actions of zinc with metalloenzymes, as a component of cysteine residues, in organelle membranes and polyribosomes are particularly important.

Wound healing response to zinc supplementation may begin as early as 24 h.

As a result of zinc deficiency, growth is affected adversely in many animal species and in man. Inasmuch as zinc is needed for protein and DNA synthesis and cell division, it is believed that the growth effect of zinc is related to its effect on protein synthesis.[92]

TABLE 10.13
Trace Element Dosing

Chromium	0.01 to 0.2 mg
Copper	0.4 to 3 mg
Fluoride	0.1 to 4 mg
Iodine	0.04 to 0.2 mg
Iron	6 to 15 mg
Manganese	0.3 to 0.5 mg
Molybdenum	0.015 to 0.25 mg
Selenium	0.01 to 0.075 mg
Zinc	5 to 16 mg

There are approximately 2 to 3 g zinc stores, of which about one fifth is in bone and one half is in the liver. Much of the remaining zinc is in the skeletal muscle. Serum binding is about 55% albumin and 40% to an α-macroglobulin (a zinc metalloprotein). Zinc is lost in fistula output and diarrhea (12 and 17 mg/l, respectively).

Treatment of zinc deficiency may require up to tenfold increments of the parenteral zinc dosages. If infused steadily over the course of 24 h, dosages of 50 to 100 mg/d elemental zinc can be tolerated. Zinc deficiency signs and symptoms include alopecia, diarrhea, glucose intolerance, hypospermia, impaired chemotaxis, night blindness, depression, apathy, and delayed wound healing.

Zinc, like chromium, also works in concert with insulin. About one fourth of oral zinc is absorbed daily in the duodenum and proximal jejunum. Other divalent trace elements, such as copper and iron, may suppress zinc absorption. Vitamin D may increase zinc bioavailability. Human peripheral blood lymphocytes have the capacity to produce metallothioneins (MTs) as a protective response to heavy metal exposure. Zinc, like iron, is redistributed to the liver under the direction of leukocytic endogenous mediator (LEM, IL-1) during infection. Sweat (up to 1 mg zinc per liter) and skin losses become important with dermatologic patients or those with burns, because muscle, bone, and liver account for greater than 2 g of total body stores. A marked decrease in skin zinc concentration may contribute to skin lesions and to impaired wound healing in skin.

Adverse reactions to zinc include nausea, vomiting, anorexia, and hyperamylasemia. The reciprocal relationship of zinc and molybdenum to copper must also be respected, particularly because copper can be depressed with zinc loading over long periods of time. The sideroblastic anemia that results is manifested by an iron-like microcytic, hypochromic anemia, and neutropenia. Other zinc deficiency signs and symptoms include skin lesions, dermatological anergy, growth retardation, impaired taste, immunological impairment, glucose intolerance (similar to chromium deficiency), alopecia, hypogonadism, hypospermia, mental depression, and diarrhea. Serum testosterone concentrations, seminal volume, and total seminal zinc loss per ejaculate are sensitive to short-term zinc depletion in young men. Diseases (sickle cell anemia, malignancies, diabetes, inflammatory or infectious conditions) and medications (e.g., estrogens, caffeine, theophylline, and corticosteroids) can result in greater zinc losses.

Zinc protects against ultraviolet (UV) radiation, enhances wound healing, contributes to immune and neuropsychiatric functions, and decreases the relative risk of cancer and cardiovascular disease. All body tissues contain zinc; in skin, it is five to six times more concentrated in the epidermis than the dermis. Zinc is required for the normal growth, development, and function of mammals. It is an essential element of hundreds of metalloenzymes, including superoxide dismutase. Zinc is also important for the proper functioning of the immune system and for glandular, reproductive, and cell health. Abundant evidence demonstrates the antioxidant role of zinc. Topical zinc, in the form of divalent zinc ions, has been reported to provide antioxidant photoprotection for skin. Two antioxidant mechanisms have been proposed for zinc: zinc ions may replace redox active molecules, such as iron and copper, at critical sites in cell membranes and proteins; alternatively, zinc ions may induce the synthesis of MT, sulfhydryl-rich proteins that protect against free radicals. Topical zinc ions may provide an important and helpful antioxidant defense for skin.[93]

Metallothionein

No treatise of trace elements would be complete without a discussion of binding proteins. The binding proteins for trace elements are of paramount importance for distribution to target sites of metabolism and excretion. These include a variety of proteins to include albumin, ceruloplasmin, α-glycoprotein, transferrin, and MT.

MTs, a family of low molecular weight-binding proteins (containing approximately 30% cysteine) for cadmium, copper, and zinc, are increased in several organs during the early phase of infection and are associated with redistribution of both essential and nonessential trace elements. This may be a normal response in common infections that could adversely influence the pathogenesis when the host is concomitantly exposed to potentially toxic trace elements, even at levels in the physiological range.[94]

Metalloenzymes have an important role in repair and regenerative processes in skin wounds. Demands for different enzymes vary according to the phase in the healing cascade and constituent events. Sequential changes in the concentrations of calcium, copper, magnesium, and zinc were studied in the incisional wound model in the rat over a 10 d period. Copper levels remained low (< 10 μ/g dry weight) throughout, but calcium, magnesium, and zinc increased from wounding, and peaked at about 5 d at a time of high inflammation, granulation tissue formation, and epidermal cell proliferation. Metal concentrations declined to normal by 7 d when inflammation had regressed, reepithelialization of the wound site was complete, and the "normalization" phase had commenced. Although the wound was overtly healed by day 10, the epidermis was still moderately hyperplastic. In view of competitive binding of trace metals at membrane receptors and carrier proteins, the ratio or balance between these trace metals was studied. Using immunocytochemistry, increases in MT immunoreactivity as an indication of zinc and copper activity were shown in the papillary dermis and in basal epidermal cells (near the wound margin 1 to 5 d after wounding). This is consistent with metalloenzyme requirements in inflammation and fibrogenesis. Calmodulin, a major cytosolic calcium-binding protein, was highest in maturing keratinocytes and in sebaceous gland cells of normal skin; it was notably more abundant in the epidermis near the wound margin and in reepithelializing areas at a time when local calcium levels were highest.[95]

Expression of the MT gene is upregulated in the skin following topical application of zinc and copper, and in wound margins, particularly in regions of high mitotic activity. This induction of MT in the wound margin may reflect its role in promoting cell proliferation and reepithelialization. The action of MTs in these processes may result from the large number of zinc-dependent and copper-dependent enzymes required for cell proliferation and matrix remodeling. In addition, selected growth factors may modulate MT gene expression and hence the ability of cells to proliferate.

MTs play a pivotal role in zinc-related cell homeostasis because of their high affinity for this trace element which is, in turn, relevant against oxidative stress and for the efficiency of the entire immune system, including natural killer (NK) cell activity. In order to accomplish this role, MTs sequester or dispense zinc during stress and inflammation to protect cells against reactive oxygen species. The gene expression of MT is affected by IL-6 for a prompt immune response. Concomitantly, MTs release zinc for the activity of antioxidant zinc-dependent enzymes, including poly(ADP-ribose)polymerase-1(PARP-1), which is involved in base excision DNA repair. This role of MTs is peculiar in young adult age during transient stress and inflammation, but not in aging, because stress-like and inflammatory conditions are persistent. This may lead MTs to turn off from a role of protection in young age to a deleterious one in aging, with subsequent appearance of age-related diseases (severe infections). The aim is to study the role played by MTs/IL-6/PARP-1 in the interplay on NK cell activity in the elderly population, in infected older patients (acute and remission phases by bronchopneumonia infection), and in healthy nonagenarian/centenarian subjects. MTmRNA (metallothionein messenger RNA) is high in lymphocytes from older people coupled with high IL-6, low zinc ion bioavailability, decreased NK cell activity, and impaired capacity of PARP-1 in base excision DNA repair. The same trend in this altered physiological cascade during aging also occurs in infected older patients (both acute and remission phases) with more marked immune damage, inflammatory condition, and very impaired PARP-1 in base excision DNA repair. By contrast, centenarian subjects display low MTmRNA, good zinc ion bioavailability, satisfactory NK cell activity, and higher capacity of PARP-1 in base excision DNA repair. These findings clearly demonstrate that the sequestering of zinc by MTs in aging is deleterious, because it leads to low zinc ion bioavailability with subsequent impairment of PARP-1 and NK cell activity and eventual appearance of severe infections. Physiological zinc supply (12 mg Zn(++)/d) for 1 month in the elderly and in infected older patients (remission phase) restores the activity of NK cells to values observed in healthy centenarians. Therefore, the zinc ion bioavailability by zinc-bound MT homeostasis is pivotal to reach healthy longevity and successfully age.[96]

Wound repair is initiated with the aggregation of platelets, formation of a fibrin clot, and release of growth factors from the activated coagulation pathways, injured cells, platelets, and extracellular matrix (ECM), followed by migration of inflammatory cells to the wound site. Thereafter, keratinocytes migrate over the wound, angiogenesis is initiated, and fibroblasts deposit and remodel the granulation tissue.

Cell migration, angiogenesis, degradation of provisional matrix, and remodeling of newly formed granulation tissue all require controlled degradation of the ECM. Disturbance in the balance between ECM production and degradation leads to formation of chronic ulcers with excessive ECM degradation, or to fibrosis, for example, hypertrophic scars or keloids characterized by excessive accumulation of ECM components. Matrix metalloproteinases (MMPs) are a family of zinc-dependent endopeptidases, which as a group can degrade essentially all ECM components. To date, 20 members of the human MMP family have been identified. Based on their structure and substrate specificity, they can be divided into subgroups of collagenases, stromelysins, stromelysin-like MMPs, gelatinases, membrane-type MMPs (MT-MMPs), and other MMPs.[97]

TRACE ELEMENT IMPLICATIONS IN WOUND REPAIR

To reiterate, the normal wound repair process consists of three phases — inflammation, proliferation, and remodeling — that occur in a predictable series of cellular and biochemical events.

Growth factors play a role in cell division, migration, differentiation, protein expression, and enzyme production, and they have the potential to heal wounds by stimulating angiogenesis and cellular proliferation, affecting the production and the degradation of the extracellular matrix, and by being chemotactic for inflammatory cells and fibroblasts. There are seven major families of growth factors: epidermal growth factor (EGF), transforming growth factor-α (TGF-β), insulin-like growth factor (IGF), platelet-derived growth factor (PDGF), fibroblast growth factor (FGF), interleukins (ILs), and colony-stimulating factor (CSF).

Cytokines, especially interferon-α (IFN-α) and IFN-α-2b, may also reduce scar formation. These cytokines decrease the proliferation rate of fibroblasts and reduce the rate of collagen and fibronectin synthesis by reducing the production of mRNA. Nitric oxide synthase (NOS) and heat shock proteins (HSP) have an important role in wound healing, as do trace elements.

The normal healing response begins the moment the tissue is injured. As the blood components spill into the site of injury, the platelets come into contact with exposed collagen and other elements of the extracellular matrix. This contact triggers the platelets to release clotting factors as well as essential growth factors and cytokines, such as PDGF and TGF-β. Following hemostasis, the neutrophils enter the wound site and begin the critical task of phagocytosis to remove foreign materials, bacteria, and damaged tissue. As part of this inflammatory phase, the macrophages appear and continue the process of phagocytosis as well as release more PDGF and TGF-β. Once the wound site is cleaned out, fibroblasts migrate in to begin the proliferative phase and deposit new extracellular matrix. The new collagen matrix then becomes cross-linked and organized during the final remodeling phase. In order for this efficient and highly controlled repair process to take place, numerous cell-signaling events are required. In pathologic conditions, such as nonhealing pressure ulcers, this efficient and orderly process is lost, and the ulcers are locked into a state of chronic inflammation characterized by abundant neutrophil infiltration with associated ROS and destructive enzymes.

Healing proceeds only after the inflammation is controlled. On the opposite end of the spectrum, fibrosis is characterized by excessive matrix deposition and reduced remodeling. Often, fibrotic lesions are associated with increased densities of mast cells.[98] Trace elements are intimately involved with all aspects of the healing spectrum.

TRACE ELEMENT AND INFLAMMATORY PHASE IMPLICATIONS

Highly potent substances are produced by the immune system. These substances include both cytokines and oxidant molecules, such as hydrogen peroxide, free radicals, and hypochlorous acid. The purpose of immune cell products is to destroy invading organisms and damaged tissue, bringing about recovery. However, oxidants and cytokines can damage healthy tissue. Excessive or inappropriate production of these substances is associated with mortality and morbidity after inflammation, infection, and trauma. Oxidants enhance IL-1, IL-8, and tumor necrosis factor (TNF) production in response to inflammatory stimuli by activating the nuclear transcription factor, NFκB. Sophisticated antioxidant defenses directly and indirectly protect the host against the damaging influence of cytokines and oxidants. Indirect protection is afforded by antioxidants, which reduce activation of NFκB, thereby preventing upregulation of cytokine production by oxidants. Cytokines increase both oxidant production and antioxidant defenses, thus minimizing damage to the host. Although antioxidant defenses interact when a component is compromised, the nature and extent of the defenses are influenced by dietary intake of sulfur amino acids, for glutathione synthesis, and vitamins E and C. In animal studies, *in vivo* and *in vitro* responses to inflammatory stimuli are influenced by dietary intake of copper, zinc, selenium, *N*-acetylcysteine, cysteine, methionine, taurine, and vitamin E. Information from animal studies has yet to be fully translated into a clinical context. However, *N*acetylcysteine, vitamin E, and a cocktail of antioxidant nutrients have reduced inflammatory symptoms in inflammatory joint disease, acute and chronic pancreatitis, and adult respiratory distress syndrome.[99]

It is widely appreciated that copper, iron, selenium, and zinc modulate immune function and influence the susceptibility of the host to infection. Nevertheless, the effect of individual trace elements or other micronutrients on components of innate immunity is difficult to design and interpret.

Zinc and iron concentrations in pus exceed normal serum. Calcium and magnesium levels in pus were two- to threefold lower and higher, respectively, than normal serum values. Lactoferrin concentrations were 880 ± 48 µg/ml, and ferritin levels were $20,726 \pm 2667$ ng/ml. Growth of an *Escherichia coli* strain was inhibited in pus at pH 5.5 but not at pH 7.4, and growth was enhanced by the addition of iron or zinc to *E. coli* suspended in pus at pH 6.7. Therefore, host defense mechanisms are enhanced by the restriction of the bioavailability of zinc and iron in suppurative infection.[100]

Zinc undernutrition results in lymphoid atrophy and reduced capacity to respond to many T-cell-dependent antigens. The plaque-forming cell response to heterologous erythrocytes is decreased, as is the function of B cells. In zinc-deficient rodents, the generation of cytotoxic lymphocytes in the spleen is reduced. Antibody-dependent cell-mediated cytotoxicity is largely unchanged. In acrodermatitis enteropathica, the lymphocyte proliferation response to mitogens is decreased, and there are significant changes in delayed hypersensitivity responses and in the proportion of various T-cell subsets. Neutrophil function is not changed by zinc deficiency. Iron deficiency results in a slight decrease in the number of rosette-forming T cells and a significant impairment of lymphocyte response to mitogens and antigens. Polymorphonuclear leukocytes are unable to kill ingested bacteria and fungi in an efficient manner. Copper deficiency impairs cell-mediated immunity, as does selenium deficiency, when it is associated with vitamin E deficiency.[101]

As a constituent of selenoproteins, selenium is needed for the proper functioning of neutrophils, macrophages, NK cells, T lymphocytes, and some other immune mechanisms. Elevated selenium intake may be associated with reduced cancer risk and may alleviate other pathological conditions, including oxidative stress and inflammation. Selenium appears to be a key nutrient in counteracting the development of virulence and inhibiting HIV progression to AIDS. It is required for sperm motility and may reduce the risk of miscarriage. Selenium deficiency has been linked to adverse mood states. Some findings suggest that selenium deficiency may be a risk factor in cardiovascular diseases.[102]

Lipopolysaccharide (LPS) produces ROS and NO in macrophages. These molecules are involved in inflammation associated with endotoxic shock. Selenium (Se), a biologically essential trace element, modulates the functions of many regulatory proteins involved in signal transduction and affects a variety of cellular activities, including cell growth and survival. Se attenuated LPS-induced ROS and NO production in murine macrophage cultures *in vitro*. This Se-decreased production of NO was demonstrated by decreases in both mRNA and protein expression for inducible NO synthase (iNOS). The preventive effects of Se on iNOS were p38 mitogen-activated protein kinase and NF-B dependent. Se specifically blocked the LPS-induced activation of p38 but not that of c-jun-*N*-terminal kinase and extracellular signal-regulated kinase; the p38-specific pathway was confirmed using p38 inhibitor SB 203580.

These results suggest the mechanism by which Se may act as an anti-inflammatory agent and that Se may be considered as a possible preventive intervention for endotoxemia, particularly in Se-deficient geographical locations.[103] Long-term intake greater than 0.4 mg/d Se in adults can produce adverse effects. In burn patients, balance studies have shown the need for 200 mcg Se per day for 2 weeks and then 60 mcg/d.[104]

Again, selenium represents a trace element foundin antioxidant enzyme glutathion-peroxidase. Its anti-inflammatory activity is based on the elimination of hydroperoxides produced in the site of inflammation.[105]

Patients with systemic inflammatory response syndrome (SIRS) and sepsis exhibit decreased plasma selenium and glutathione peroxidase activity. Moreover, the degree of selenium deficiency correlates with the severity of the disease and the incidence of mortality. Patients with SIRS and sepsis are exposed to severe oxidative stress. Selenoenzymes play a major role in protecting cells against peroxidation, especially lipid peroxidation, and are involved in the regulation of inflammatory processes.[106]

In bacterial infections, septicemia, pneumonia, erysipelas, and meningitis, the plasma concentrations of selenium, iron, and zinc are decreased. Plasma copper was unchanged in patients with erysipelas but increased in other types of bacterial infections. Although the patients with viral infections showed similar shifts of the trace elements as were observed in patients with bacterial infections, the changes were not as pronounced. A low plasma selenium level less than 0.8 mumol/l was found in only 6% of the patients with viral infections in contrast to 63% of the patients with septicemia or 57% of the patients with pneumonia. Furthermore, in viral infections 60% of the zinc values were below the mean level of 12.8 mumol/l observed in healthy controls as compared with 90% of the values in patients with sepsis or 92% of the values in patients with pneumonia. The onset of change in trace elements occurred within a few days and persisted for several weeks. These changes seem to be nonspecific and are independent of the agent causing infection. The different types of infections were followed by changes in most of the plasma proteins, which are known to be associated with an inflammatory reaction. The changes in plasma proteins were most pronounced in patients with sepsis and pneumonia. Therefore, patients with sepsis having a high degree of inflammation did not show a positive correlation between the severity of the disease — as judged by plasma proteins — and the alterations of trace elements.[107]

The addition of copper and zinc salts to human peripheral blood leukocytes cultured in complete medium containing endotoxin and fetal calf serum stimulated tumor necrosis factor (TNF) secretion in a concentration-dependent manner. The secretion of interleukin-1β (IL-1β) and interleukin-6 (IL-6) was inhibited by copper under the same culture conditions, although zinc stimulated IL-1β secretion in a concentration-dependent manner and had no effect on leukocyte IL-6 release. Both copper and zinc induced increases in TNF mRNA (54 and 14%, respectively) when compared to cells cultured in complete medium alone. In serum-free, low endotoxin medium (less than 6 pg/ml), both copper and zinc failed to stimulate either TNF or IL-1β secretion. Under the same conditions, the addition of lipopolysaccharide (LPS), at concentrations above 0.01 µg/ml, induced a concentration-dependent release of both cytokines. When either copper or zinc was combined with 0.01 µg/ml LPS, a synergistic stimulation of TNF secretion resulted. IL-1β secretion, unlike TNF, was not synergistically stimulated by combining metals and LPS in serum-free medium. Combining copper and zinc with inhibitors of TNF secretion, TGF-β, prostaglandin E2, and plasma α-globulins, resulted in a reduction of the suppressive effects of each of these agents. Thus, trace metals copper and zinc may play important and possibly distinct roles in regulating leukocyte secretion of TNF, IL-1β, and IL-6.[108]

The fall in serum iron and zinc and the rise in serum copper in an acute phase response are brought about by changes in the concentration of specific tissue proteins controlled by cytokines, especially IL-1, TNF, and IL-6. These are generally believed to be beneficial aspects of the early acute phase response. One difficulty associated with these changes is that assessment of status for these elements is particularly difficult, because plasma concentration may bear little relationship to tissue status. Simultaneous assessment of the acute phase response — for example, serum C-reactive protein — together with trace elements and the monitoring of changes in concentrations may, however, permit interpretation of trace element requirements. Suggestions are made for the requirements for these and other essential elements during enteral or intravenous nutrition, together with proposed methods of interpreting laboratory tests.[109]

Zinc induces monokine secretion by monocytes; however, effects of zinc on T cells appear contradictory. Apart from enhanced lymphocyte proliferation in peripheral blood mononuclear cells (PBMCs), inhibitory properties of high zinc dosages have also been described. PBMCs failed to produce lymphokines like IFN-γ after stimulation with zinc in a serum- and LPS-free cell culture system, whereas monokine secretion (IL-1β) has occurred. Zinc-uptake studies with the zinc-specific fluorescent probe zinquin revealed that zinc is taken up by PBMCs within a few minutes, reaching nearly equal levels in PBMCs, isolated monocytes, and T cells. However, if zinc was depleted 1 h after monocyte induction, zinc-free precultured T cells were stimulated to secrete IFN-γ by zinc-induced monokines. Furthermore, the necessity for a cell–cell interaction between monocytes and T cells for IFN-γ induction has been elucidated. Zinc ions inhibited the proliferation of the IL-1-dependent T cell line D 10N in a dose-dependent manner, suggesting a direct inhibitory effect of zinc. By immunoprecipitation, a specific inhibition of IL-1 receptor-associated protein kinase (IRAK) by zinc ions was shown. Therefore, in contrast to an indirect stimulation of T cells due to zinc-induced monokines, higher concentrations of zinc directly inhibit T cell functions by means of specific inhibition of IRAK and subsequent signaling events, such as NFκB activation. The divergent effects of zinc on different cell populations, depending on the zinc concentration, could explain contradictory results of zinc stimulation.[110]

Zinc deficiency can change immune functions prematurely from predominantly cellular T helper cell (Th1) responses to humoral Th2 responses. Th1 cells produce cytokines such as IL-2 and IFN-γ, thereby controlling viral infections and other intracellular pathogens more effectively than Th2 responses through cytokines such as IL-4, IL-5, IL-6, and IL-10. The accelerated shift from the production of extra Th1 cells during these cellular immune activities to more Th2 cells with their predominantly humoral immune functions, caused by such a zinc deficiency, adversely influences the course of diseases such as leprosy, schistosomiasis, leishmaniasis, and AIDS, and can result in allergies. It is noteworthy that AIDS viruses (HIVs) do not replicate in Th1 cells, which probably contain more zinc, but preferentially in the Th0 and Th2 cells; all the more so because zinc and copper ions are known to inhibit intracellular HIV replication. Considering the above Th1/Th2 switch, real prospects seem to be offered of vaccination against such parasites as leishmania and against HIVs.[111]

The nutritional status and needs of older people are associated with age-related biological and often socioeconomic changes. Decreased food intake, a sedentary lifestyle, and reduced energy expenditure in older adults become critical risk factors for malnutrition, especially protein and micronutrients. Surveys indicate that older people are particularly at risk for marginal deficiency of vitamins and trace elements.[112] This may explain why aging is associated with impaired immune responses and increased infection-related morbidity.[113]

The T lymphocyte is more susceptible to aging than the B lymphocyte, for which *in vitro* functions are almost preserved. All functions of cell-mediated immunity are decreased in older adults. T lymphocytes are less mature and present decreased T helper and T suppressive functions, decreased T proliferative ability responses to stimuli, and lower interleukin synthesis. T-dependent antibody responses are also decreased: primary responses are diminished, and secondary responses are less specific. Nevertheless, in healthy older adults such immune deficiency remains minor. When undernutrition occurs in aged individuals, a profound immunodeficit rapidly follows. Prevention of prompt treatment of all undernutrition states is a major concern in geriatrics.[114]

TRACE ELEMENT AND PROLIFERATION PHASE IMPLICATIONS

Numerous studies report the role of interactions between keratinocytes and fibroblasts, but the relationship between wound healing myofibroblasts and keratinocytes is not clear, even though these two cell types coexist during healing. To determine the speed and quality of epithelialization, the influence of myofibroblasts on keratinocyte growth and differentiation was studied using an *in vitro* skin model. When the dermis was populated with fibroblasts, a continuous epidermis was formed in 7 to 10 d. In contrast, with wound healing myofibroblasts or without cell in dermis, the complete reepithelialization never occurred over the 10 d period studied. After 7 further days of epidermal differentiation, histology showed a more disorganized epidermis, and the expression of basement membrane constituents was reduced when wound healing myofibroblasts or no cells were added in the dermis instead of fibroblasts. Results suggest that wound healing myofibroblasts are not efficient to stimulate keratinocyte growth and differentiation. Treatment of fibroblasts with TGF-β1 induced an increase of epidermal cell differentiation as seen when myofibroblasts were present. However, this cytokine did not change the reepithelialization rate and induced an increase of basement membrane matrix deposition in opposition to myofibroblasts. Thus TGF-β1 action is not sufficient to explain all the different keratinocyte reactions toward fibroblasts and wound healing myofibroblasts. Myofibroblasts, in contrast to fibroblasts, seem to have a limited role in the reepithelialization process and might be more associated with the increased extracellular matrix secretion.[115]

Some integrins that are modulated by trace elements and expressed by basal layer keratinocytes play an essential part in healing, notably α2β1, α3β1, α6β4, and αVβ5, whose expression and distribution in epidermis are modified during the reepithelialization phase. Integrin expression was studied in proliferating keratinocytes in monolayer cultures and in reconstituted skin that included a differentiation state. The expression of α6 was induced by zinc, copper, and manganese. The inductive effect of zinc was particularly notable on integrins affecting cellular mobility in the proliferation phase of wound healing (α3, α6, αV) and that of copper on integrins expressed by suprabasally differentiated keratinocytes during the final healing phase (α2, β1, and α6), but manganese had a mixed effect.[116]

Selenium is an essential trace element, and it is well known that selenium is necessary for cell culture. However, the mechanism underlying the role of selenium in cellular proliferation and survival is still unknown. Investigators using Jurkat cells showed that selenium deficiency in a serum-free medium decreased the selenium-dependent enzyme activity (glutathione peroxidases and thioredoxin reductase) within cells and cell viability. To understand the mechanism of this effect of selenium, the effect of other antioxidants, the act by different mechanisms was examined. Vitamin E, a lipid-soluble radical-scavenging antioxidant, completely blocked selenium deficiency-induced cell death, although α-tocopherol (biologically the most active form of vitamin E) could not preserve selenium-dependent enzyme activity. Other antioxidants, such as different isoforms and derivatives of vitamin E, BO-653, and deferoxamine mesylate, also exerted an inhibitory effect. However, the water-soluble antioxidants, such as ascorbic acid, N-acetyl cysteine, and glutathione, displayed no such effect. Dichlorodihydrofluorescein (DCF) assay revealed that cellular ROS increased before cell death, and sodium selenite and -tocopherol inhibited ROS increase in a dose-dependent manner. The generation of lipid hydroperoxides was observed by fluorescence probe diphenyl-1-pyrenylphosphine (DPPP) and high-performance liquid chromatography (HPLC) chemiluminescence only in selenium-deficient cells. These results suggest that the ROS, especially lipid hydroperoxides, are involved in the cell death caused by selenium deficiency and that selenium and vitamin E cooperate in the defense against oxidative stress upon cells by detoxifying and inhibiting the formation of lipid hydroperoxides.[117]

Zinc is not only an important nutrient and cofactor of numerous enzymes and transcription factors, but it also acts as an intracellular mediator, similarly to calcium. The recent discovery of its intracellular molecular pathways opens the door to new fields of drug design. Zinc homeostasis results from a coordinated regulation by different proteins involved in uptake excretion and intracellular storage/trafficking of zinc. These proteins are membranous transporters, belonging to the ZIP and ZnT families, and MTs. Their principal function is to provide zinc to new synthesized proteins important for several functions such as gene expression, immunity, reproduction, or protection against free radicals damage. Zinc intracellular concentration is correlated to cell fate (i.e., proliferation, differentiation, or apoptosis), and modifications of zinc homeostasis are observed in several pathologies affecting humans at any stage of life. Two zinc-related diseases, acrodermatitis enteropathica and lethal milk syndrome, have recently been related to mutations in zinc transporters SLC39A4 and ZnT-4, respectively. Zinc acts as an inhibitor of apoptosis, while its depletion induces programmed cell death in many cell lines. However, excess zinc can also be cytotoxic, and zinc transporters as well as MTs serve as zinc detoxification systems. Several zinc channels controlling the intracellular zinc movements and the free form of the metal maintain the intracellular zinc homeostasis and thus the balance between life and cell death. Apart from these general activities, zinc has particular biological roles in some specialized cells. It acts as a paracrine regulator in pancreatic cell, neuron, or neutrophil activity by a mechanism of vesicles-mediated metal excretion and uptake.[118]

Keratinocyte growth factor (KGF) stimulates epithelial cell differentiation and proliferation in animals and promises to be of major importance for wound healing. Local protein administration, however, has been shown to be ineffective due to enzymes and proteases in the wound fluid. Liposomes containing the KGF cDNA gene constructs were effective in improving epidermal and dermal regeneration. KGF gene transfer to acute wounds may represent a new therapeutic strategy to enhance wound healing.[119]

Finally, proliferation of keratinocytes has been demonstrated in toxic epidermal necrolysis, a rare disease observed as a consequence of adverse reactions to drugs. γIFN-γ, soluble αTNF-α, and soluble Fas ligand (sFas-L) are present in much higher concentrations in the blister fluids of patients with toxic epidermal necrolysis (TEN). IFN-γ and to a lesser extent IL-18 were produced by mononuclear cells present in the fluid. Other cytokines (TNF-α, sFas-L, IL-10) originated from activated keratinocytes. Fas-L was overexpressed on the membranes of keratinocytes in lesional skin *in situ*. The Th1 profile of T-lymphocyte activation found in the blister fluid of patients with TEN is consistent with a key role for drug-specific cytotoxic T lymphocytes (CTL) as previously reported — the activation of keratinocytes by IFN-γ, making them sensitive to cell-mediated cytolysis. It was proposed that the production of Fas-L, TNF-α, and IL-10 by keratinocytes could be a defense mechanism against CTL rather than a way of propagating apoptosis among epidermal cells.[120]

Thus, keratinocyte proliferation and migration are essential for the reconstruction of the cutaneous barrier after skin injury. Interestingly, thermal waters rich in trace elements (e.g., boron and manganese) are known to be able to improve wound healing. In order to understand the mechanism of action of this effect, investigators have studied the *in vitro* modulation of keratinocyte migration and proliferation by boron and manganese salts, which are present in high concentrations in thermal water (Saint Gervais). *In vitro* study has demonstrated that incubating keratinocytes for 24 h with boron salts at concentrations between 0.5 and 10 mcg/ml or manganese salts at concentrations between 0.1 and 1.5 mcg/ml accelerated wound closure compared with control medium (+20%). As this acceleration was not related to an increase in keratinocyte proliferation, it was suggested that boron and manganese act on wound healing mainly by increasing the migration of keratinocytes.[121]

TRACE ELEMENT AND REMODELING PHASE IMPLICATIONS

Wound healing encompasses coagulation, inflammation, angiogenesis, fibroplasia, contraction, epithelialization, and remodeling. Granulation tissue is produced following incision of tissue, such as skin, abdominal wall, or the gastrointestinal tract, and the strength of the wound is determined primarily by the collagen content early in the healing course.[122]

Zinc (Zn) retains insulin-like growth factor binding proteins (IGFBPs) on the surface of cultured cells, lowers the affinity of cell-associated IGFBPs, and increases the affinity of the cell surface insulin-like growth factor (IGF)-type 1 receptor (IGF-1R). Investigators have characterized a mechanism by which the trace micronutrient Zn could regulate IGF activity.[123] Another study showed that zinc decreases IGF binding to fibroblast-associated IGFBPs by lowering the affinity of the IGF–IGFBP interaction.[124]

The addition of copper and zinc salts to human peripheral blood leukocytes cultured in complete medium containing endotoxin and fetal calf serum stimulated TNF secretion in a concentration-dependent manner. The secretion of IL-1β (IL–1β) and IL-6 was inhibited by copper under the same culture conditions, while zinc stimulated IL-1β secretion in a concentration-dependent manner and had no effect on leukocyte IL-6 release. Both copper and zinc induced increases in TNF mRNA (54 and 14%, respectively) when compared to cells cultured in complete medium alone. In serum-free, low endotoxin medium (less than 6 pg/ml), both copper and zinc failed to stimulate either TNF or IL-1β secretion. Under the same conditions, the addition of lipopolysaccharide (LPS) at concentrations above 0.01 μg/ml induced a concentration-dependent release of both cytokines. When either copper or zinc was combined with 0.01 μg/ml LPS, a synergistic stimulation of TNF secretion resulted. IL-1β secretion, unlike TNF, was not synergistically stimulated by combining metals and LPS in serum-free medium. Combining copper and zinc with inhibitors of TNF secretion, TGF-β, prostaglandin E2, and plasma α-globulins resulted in a reduction of the suppressive effects of each of these agents. This suggests that the trace metals copper and zinc may play important and possibly distinct roles in regulating leukocyte secretion of TNF, IL-1β, and IL-6.[125]

To evaluate the modulatory effects of trace metals on lymphocyte growth and maturation, thymidine uptake (TU), protein, ATP, Fe, Cu, Zn, ferritin, CD3, CD4, CD8 antigens, surface transferrin receptors (TFR), and interleukin-2 receptors (IL-2R) were assessed in normal and T-cell leukemia human lymphocytes (ALL), cultured in media with varying Fe, Cu, and Zn concentrations [Me]. The response of normal lymphocytes to stimuli is sensitive to variation in trace metals, whereas this response, absent in ALL lymphocytes, reappears only in media with low [Me] and is independent from TFR.[126]

Zinc induces monocytes to produce IL-1, IL-6, and TNF-α in peripheral blood mononuclear cells and separated monocytes. This effect is higher in serum-free medium. However, only in the presence of serum does zinc also induce T cells to produce lymphokines. This effect on T cells is mediated by cytokines produced by monocytes. Stimulation also requires cell-to-cell contact of monocytes and T cells.[127] INF-α and INF-α 2β may also reduce scar formation. These cytokines decrease the proliferation rate of fibroblasts.[128] Zinc is an essential trace element that also increases osteoblast numbers and bone formation.[129] In addition, other trace elements play important roles in regulating the metabolism of the extracellular matrix.[130]

Free radicals prevent wound healing. Findings suggest that collagen is denatured by scavenging the hydroxyl radical before fibroblasts are damaged, so that the radical may influence the remodeling of collagen.[131]

The state of excessive fibroblastic proliferation for wound healing results in hypertrophic and keloid scars. The levels of zinc (Zn), copper (Cu), manganese (Mn), and selenium (Se) in serum, normal skin, and scar tissue of 40 patients with keloid and hypertrophic scars were assessed. There was a significant increase in manganese (Mn) levels in the skin of patients with burns, trauma, and surgical incisions compared to controls. Furthermore, the zinc, copper, and selenium contents of the skin in patients with incisions were decreased significantly when compared to other groups. No significant changes occurred regarding serum levels of zinc, copper, manganese, and selenium in the different groups.[132]

In a study aimed at testing human skin wound healing improvement with a 21 d supplementation of 1 g ascorbic acid (AA) and 0.2 g pantothenic acid (PA), 49 patients undergoing surgery for tattoos by the successive resections procedure entered a double-blind, prospective, and randomized study. Tests performed on both skin and scars determined hydroxyproline concentrations, number of fibroblasts, trace element contents, and mechanical properties. In the 18 patients who received supplementation, it was shown that in skin (day 8), Fe increased ($p < 0.05$) and Mn decreased ($p < 0.05$); in scars (day 21), Cu ($p = 0.07$) and Mn ($p < 0.01$) decreased, and Mg ($p < 0.05$) increased; the mechanical properties of scars in group A were significantly correlated to their contents in Fe, Cu, and Zn, whereas no correlation was shown in group B. In blood, AA increased after surgery with supplementation, whereas it decreased in controls. Although no major improvement of the wound healing process could be documented in this study, results suggested that the benefit of AA and PA supplementation could be due to the variations of the trace elements, as they are correlated to mechanical properties of the scars.[133]

Normal wound healing is a complex, highly regulated dynamic process that requires coordinate responses of both epidermal and dermal compartments. To accomplish the healing process, several growth factors, chemokines, and matrix elements signal both cell proliferation and migration during the inflammatory and reparative phases and limit these responses during the remodeling phase. A stimulated keratinocyte/target cell coculture system revealed that IFN-γ inducible protein 9 acts as a soluble keratinocyte-derived paracrine factor for both fibroblasts and keratinocytes. Further, it was found that in both fibroblasts and undifferentiated keratinocytes, IFN-γ inducible protein 9 exerted its action through modulation of a cytosolic protease, calpain. Interestingly, IFN-γ inducible protein 9 increased calpain activity in undifferentiated keratinocytes, whereas the same chemokine inhibited the calpain activity in fibroblasts. This provides for a model whereby redifferentiated basal keratinocytes could limit fibroblast repopulation of the dermis underlying healed wounds while simultaneously promoting reepithelialization of the remaining provisional wound.[134]

Finally, the interaction of other micronutrients such as electrolytes with the actions of trace elements may impact on successful wound healing. Signal transduction of many intracellular events is initiated by a minute influx of calcium ions into the cells, resulting in the formation of a calcium–calmodulin complex and cAMP. There is reciprocity between epidermal calmodulin and cAMP levels, which may be modulated by external factors such as zinc.[135]

RECOMMENDATIONS FOR SUPPLEMENTATION AND AVOIDING TOXICITY

Although trace elements are micronutrients, there are major roles in wound healing that are carried out with adequate supplementation. Dosing for wound healing will be contingent on sampling fluid/tissue, comorbidity, salt, bioabsorption to target sites, and current/historical intake/excretion. To provide the recommended daily dietary allowances, 1 to 1.5 l of most commercially available enteral formulas will be needed. Injectable products will be dosed lower than enteral products because most products will be given intravenously, which will provide enhanced bioavailability. Deficiencies are best determined by recognition, then supplementation, and subsequent serial monitoring of signs and symptoms. From a pragmatic perspective, chromium (Cr), copper (Cu), iron (Fe), selenium (Se), and zinc (Zn) inadequacies are likely respectively manifested by hyperglycemia (Cr), neutropenia (associated with microcytic/hypochromic anemia), as well as kinky hair (Cu), microcytic/hypochromic anemia (Fe), muscle pain/cardiomyopathy (Se), and diarrhea/alopecia/delayed wound healing (Zn) phenomena.

Similarly, signs and symptoms are often associated with micronutrient overdosing. Chromium, copper, iron, selenium, and zinc toxicities are likely respectively manifested by hypoglycemia (Cr), Wilson's Disease (Cu), hyperferritinemia (Fe), dermatitis/garlic breath (Se), and hyperamylasemia (Zn).

FUTURE DIRECTIONS

Despite many years of study and a substantial knowledge base of the specific processes and factors involved, wound healing phenomenon remains puzzling. There is still much to learn about the wound-specific nutritional interventions that are available to improve wound healing.

Nutrition, foundationally and profoundly, adds to this confounding clinical enigma. Nutritional depletion may exert inhibitory effects, while sound nutritional supplementation, macronutrients, and micronutrients can contribute to positive wound amelioration. Within this paradigm, the clinician should be able to recognize patients who may be expected to have wound healing difficulties and offer early nutritional intervention, respecting micronutrient nutriture, and especially trace elements, to avoid wound failure.

Future research will further define the role of trace elements in all macronutrient (protein, carbohydrate, and lipid) and micronutrient (electrolyte and vitamin) *in vivo* reactions as they relate to wound care.

REFERENCES

1. Mathus-Vliegen, E.M., Old age, malnutrition, and pressure sores: an ill-fated alliance, *J. Gerontol. A Biol. Sci. Med. Sci.*, 59(4), 355, 2004.
2. Langer, G. et al., Nutritional interventions for preventing and treating pressure ulcers, *Cochrane Database Syst. Rev.*, (4), CD003216, 2003.
3. Wellinghausen, N., Martin, M., and Rink, L., Zinc inhibits interleukin-1-dependent T cell stimulation, *Eur. J. Immunol.*, 27, 2529, 1997.
4. Driessen, C. et al., Induction of cytokines by zinc ions in human peripheral blood mononuclear cells and separated monocytes, *Lymphokine Cytokine Res.*, 13, 15, 1994.
5. Frechette, J.P., Martineau, I., and Gagnon, G., Platelet-rich plasmas: growth factor content and roles in wound healing, *J. Dent. Res.*, 84, 434, 2005.
6. Diegelmann, R.F. and Evans, M.C., Wound healing: an overview of acute, fibrotic and delayed healing, *Front. Biosci.*, 9, 283, 2004.
7. Komarcevic, A., The modern approach to wound treatment, *Med. Pregl.*, 53, 363, 2000.
8. Curtis, G.E. et al., The effect of nutritional status on the cytokine and acute phase protein responses to elective surgery, *Cytokine*, 7, 380, 1995.
9. Russell, L., The importance of patients' nutritional status in wound healing, *Br. J. Nurs.*, 10(6 Suppl.), S42, S44, 2001.
10. Haydock, G.A. and Hill, G.L., Impaired wound healing in surgical patients with varying degrees of malnutrition, *J. Parenter. Enteral Nutr.*, 10, 550, 1986.
11. Williamson, M.B. and Fromm, H.J., The incorporation of sulfur amino acids into protein of regenerating wound tissue, *J. Biol. Chem.*, 212, 705, 1955.

12. Localio, S.A., Morgan, M.E., and Hintown, R., The biological chemistry of wound healing: the effect of di-methionine on healing of wounds in protein depleted animals, *Surg. Gynecol. Obstet.*, 86, 582, 1948.

13. Liu, A.J. and Richardson, M.A., Effects of N-acetyl cysteine on experimentally induced esophageal lye injury, *Ann. Otol. Rhinol. Laryngol.*, 94, 477, 1985.

14. Cerra, F.B. et al., Branched chains support postoperative protein synthesis, *Surgery*, 92, 192, 1982.

15. Cerra, F.B. et al., Enteral feeding in sepsis: a prospective, randomized double blind trial, *Surgery*, 98, 632, 1985.

16. Sax, H.C., Talamini, M.A., and Fischer, J.E., Clinical use of branched chain amino acids in liver disease, trauma, sepsis and burns, *Arch. Surg.*, 121, 358, 1986.

17. Cerra, F.B. et al., Septic auto cannibalism: a failure of exogenous nutritional support, *Ann. Surg.*, 192, 570, 1980.

18. Hedden, M.P. and Buse, M.G., General stimulation of muscle protein synthesis by branched chain amino acids *in vitro*, *Proc. Soc. Exp. Biol. Med.*, 160, 410, 1979.

19. Buse, M.G. and Reid, S.S., Leucine, a possible regulator of protein turnover in muscles, *J. Clin. Invest.*, 56, 1250, 1975.

20. Freund, H.R., Lapidot, A., and Fischer, J.E., The use of branched chain amino acids in the injured-septic patient, in *Metabolism and Clinical Implications of Branch Chain Amino and Keto Acids*, Walser, M. and Williamson, J.R., Eds., Elsevier, New York, 1981, p. 527.

21. Aquilani, R. et al., Branched-chain amino acids enhance the cognitive recovery of patients with severe traumatic brain injury, *Arch. Phys. Med. Rehabil.*, 86, 1729, 2005.

22. McCauley, R. et al., Influence of branched chain amino acid solutions on wound healing, *Aust. N.Z. J. Surg.*, 60, 471, 1990.

23. Dudrick, S.J. et al., Effect of enriched branched chain amino acid solutions in traumatized rats, *J. Parenter. Enteral Nutr.*, 8, 86, 1984.

24. Demling, R.H. and Desanti, L., Involuntary weight loss and the nonhealing wound: the role of anabolic agents, *Adv. Wound Care*, 12(Suppl.), 1, 1999.

25. Bergstrom, J. et al., Intracellular free amino acid concentration in human muscle tissue, *J. Appl. Physiol.*, 36, 693, 1974.

26. Zetterberg, A. and Engstrom, W., Glutamine and the regulation of DNA replication and cell multiplication in fibroblasts, *J. Cell. Physiol.*, 108, 365, 1981.

27. Zielke, H.R. et al., Growth of human diploid fibroblasts in the absence of glucose utilization. *Proc. Natl. Acad. Sci. U.S.A.*, 73, 4110, 1976.

28. Ardawi, M.S.M. et al., Glutamine metabolism in lymphocytes of the rat, *Biochemistry*, 212, 835, 1983.

29. Newsholme, E.A. and Newsholme, P., A role for muscle in the immune system and its importance in surgery, trauma, sepsis and burns, *Nutrition*, 4, 261, 1988.

30. Demling, R.H. and Desanti, L., Involuntary weight loss and the nonhealing wound: the role of anabolic agents, *Adv. Wound Care*, 12(Suppl.), 1, 1999.

31. Askanazi, J. et al., Muscle and plasma amino acids following injury: influence of intercurrent infection, *Ann. Surg.*, 92, 78, 1980.

32. Roth, E. and Funovics, J., Metabolic disorders in severe abdominal sepsis: glutamine deficiency in skeletal muscle, *Clin. Nutr.*, 1, 25, 1982.

33. Ziegler, T.R. et al., Clinical and metabolic efficacy of glutamine-supplemented parenteral nutrition after bone marrow transplant. A randomized, double-blind, controlled study, *Ann. Intern. Med.*, 116, 821, 1992.

34. McCauly, R. et al, Effects of glutamine on colonic strength anastamosis in the rat, *J. Parenter. Enteral Nutr.*, 15, 437, 1991.

35. Barbul, A., Biochemistry, physiology and therapeutic implications, *J. Parenter. Enteral Nutr.*, 10, 227, 1986.

36. Kowalewski, K. and Young, S., Effect of growth hormone and an anabolic steroid on hydroxyproline in healing dermal wounds in rats, *Acta. Endocrinol.*, 59, 53, 1968.

37. Jorgensen, P.H. and Andreassen, T.T., Influence of biosynthetic human growth hormone on biochemical properties of rat skin incisional wounds, *Acta. Chir. Scand.*, 154, 623, 1988.

38. Herndon, D.N. et al., Effects of recombinant human growth hormone on donor site-healing in severely burned children, *Ann. Surg.*, 212, 424, 1990.

39. Schaffer, M.R. et al., Inhibition of nitric oxide synthesis in wounds: pharmacology and effect on accumulation of collagen in wounds in mice, *Eur. J. Surg.*, 165, 262, 1999.

40. Efron, D.T. et al., Expression and function of inducible nitric oxide synthase during rat colon anastomotic healing, *J. Gastrointest. Surg.*, 3, 592, 1999.

41. Shi, H.P. et al., Supplemental dietary arginine enhances wound healing in normal but not inducible nitric oxide synthase knockout mice, *Surgery*, 128, 374, 2000.

42. Marletta, M.A. and Spiering, M.M., Trace elements and nitric oxide function, *J. Nutr.*, 133(5 Suppl. 1), 1431S, 2003.

43. Burgess, P. et al., The effect of total parenteral nutrition on hepatic drug oxidation, *J. Parenter. Enteral Nutr.*, 11, 540, 1987.

44. Levenson, S.M., Seifter, E., and VanWinkle, W., Nutrition, in *Fundamentals of Wound Management in Surgery*, Hunt, T.K. and Dunphy, J.E., Eds., Appleton-Century-Crofts, New York, 1979, p. 286.

45. Demling, R.H. and DeBiasse, M., Micronutrients in critical illness, *Crit. Care Clin.*, 11, 651, 1995.

46. Rayssiguier, Y. and Mazur, A., Magnesium and inflammation: lessons from animal models, *Clin. Calcium*, 15, 245, 2005.

47. Demetriou, A.A. et al., Vitamin A and retinoic acid: induced fibroblast differentiation *in vitro*, *Surgery*, 98, 931, 1985.

48. Jetten, A.M., Modulation of cell growth by retinoids and their possible mechanisms of action, *Fed. Proc.*, 43, 134, 1984.

49. Moody, B.J., Changes in the serum concentrations of thyroxine-binding prealbumin and retinol binding protein following burn injury, *Clin. Chim. Acta*, 118, 87, 1982.

50. Rai, K. and Coutemanche, A.J., Vitamin A assay in burned patients, *J. Trauma*, 15, 419, 1975.

51. Ramsden, D.B. et al., The interrelationship of thyroid hormones, vitamin A and the binding proteins following stress, *Clin. Endocrinol.*, 8, 109, 1978.

52. Goodson, III, W.H. and Hunt, T.K., Wound healing and nutrition, in *Nutrition and Metabolism in Patient Care*, Kinney, J.M., Jeejeebhoy, K.N., and Hill, G.L., Eds., W.B. Saunders, Philadelphia, 1988, p. 635.

53. Demling, R.H. and DeBiasse, M., Micronutrients in critical illness, *Crit. Care Clin.*, 11, 651, 1995.

54. Hunt, T.K., Vitamin A and wound healing, *J. Am. Acad. Dermatol.*, 15, 817, 1986.

55. Baxter, C.R., Immunologic reactions in chronic wounds, *Am. J. Surg.*, 167, 12, 1994.

56. Shukla, A., Rasik, A.M., and Patnaik, G.K., Depletion of reduced glutathione, ascorbic acid, and vitamin E and antioxidant defense enzymes in a healing cutaneous wound, *Free. Radic. Res.*, 26, 93, 1997.

57. Demling, R.H. and DeBiasse, M., Micronutrients in critical illness, *Crit. Care Clin.*, 11, 651, 1995.

58. Prasad, A.S., Acquired zinc deficiency and immune dysfunction in sickle cell anemia, in *Nutrient Modulation of the Immune Response*, Cunningham-Rundles, S., Ed., Marcel Dekker, New York, 1993, p. 393.

59. Braunschweig, C.L. et al., Parenteral zinc supplementation in adult humans during the acute phase response increases the febrile response, *J. Nutr.*, 127, 70, 1997.

60. Jackson, M.J., Diagnosis and detection of deficiencies of micronutrients: minerals, *Br. Med. Bull.*, 55, 634, 1995.

61. Mayland, C. et al., Micronutrient concentrations in patients with malignant disease: effect of the inflammatory response, *Ann. Clin. Biochem.*, 41, 138, 2004.

62. Horne, B.D. et al., Intermountain Heart Collaborative Study Group, Which white blood cell subtypes predict increased cardiovascular risk? *J. Am. Coll. Cardiol.*, 45, 1638, 2005, E-pub, April 25, 2005.

63. Baumgartner, T.G., Trace elements in clinical nutrition, *Nutr. Clin. Pract.*, 8, 251, 1993.

64. Perry, Jr., H.M., Perry, E.F., and Hixon, B.B., Trace-metal concentrations in normal human liver: methods to cope with marked variability, *Sci. Total Environ.*, 9, 125, 1978.

65. Selmanpakoglu, A.N. et al., Trace element (Al, Se, Zn, Cu) levels in serum, urine and tissues of burn patients, *Burns*, 20, 99, 1994.

66. Nutrition Advisory Group, American Medical Association, Guidelines for essential trace element preparations for parenteral use, *J. Parenter. Enteral Nutr.*, 3, 263, 1979.

67. Chebassier, N. et al., *In vitro* induction of matrix metalloproteinase-2 and matrix metalloproteinase-9 expression in keratinocytes by boron and manganese, *Exp. Dermatol.*, 13, 484, 2004.

68. Vincent, J.B., Recent advances in the nutritional biochemistry of trivalent chromium, *Proc. Nutr. Soc.*, 63, 41, 2004.

69. Ryan, G.J. et al., Chromium as adjunctive treatment for type 2 diabetes, *Ann. Pharmacother.*, 37, 876, 2003.

70. Vincent, J.B., The potential value and toxicity of chromium picolinate as a nutritional supplement, weight loss agent and muscle development agent, *Sports Med.*, 33, 213, 2003.

71. Reading, S.A., Chromium picolinate. *J. Fla. Med. Assoc.*, Jan., 83 (1), 29–31, 1996.

72. Anon., A scientific review: the role of chromium in insulin resistance, *Diabetes Educ.*, 14 (2), 2004.

73. Shrivastava, R. et al., Effects of chromium on the immune system. *FEMS Immunol. Med. Microbiol.*, 34, 1, 2002.

74. Gunton, J.E. et al., Chromium supplementation does not improve glucose tolerance, insulin sensitivity, or lipid profile: a randomized, placebo-controlled, double-blind trial of supplementation in subjects with impaired glucose tolerance, *Diabetes Care*, 28, 712, 2005.

75. Althuis, M.D. et al., Glucose and insulin responses to dietary chromium supplements: a meta-analysis, *Am. J. Clin. Nutr.*, 76, 148, 2002.

76. Elkoubi, P., Copper, *J. Chir. (Paris)*, 126, 248, 1989.

77. Holtzman, N.A., Menkes' kinky hair syndrome: a genetic disease involving copper, *Fed. Proc.*, 35, 2276, 1976.

78. Horwitt, M.K., Harvey, C.C., and Dahm, Jr., C.H., Relationship between levels of blood lipids, vitamins C, A, and E, serum copper compounds, and urinary excretions of tryptophan metabolites in women taking oral contraceptive therapy, *Am. J. Clin. Nutr.*, 28, 403, 1975.

79. Gosling, P. et al., Serum copper and zinc concentrations in patients with burns in relation to burn surface area, *J. Burn Care Rehabil.*, 16, 481, 1995.

80. Gaetke, L.M. and Chow, C.K., Copper toxicity, oxidative stress, and antioxidant nutrients, *Toxicity*, 189, 47, 2003.

81. Menkes, J.H., Kinky hair disease: twenty five years later, *Brain Dev.*, 10, 77, 1988.

82. Prodan, C.I. et al., CNS demyelination associated with copper deficiency and hyperzincemia, *Neurology*, 59, 1453, 2002.

83. Uriu-Adams, J.Y. and Keen, C.L., Copper, oxidative stress, and human health, *Mol. Aspects Med.*, 26, 268, 2005.

84. Sen, C.K., Copper-induced vascular endothelial growth factor expression and wound healing, *Am. J. Physiol. Heart Circ. Physiol.*, 282, H1821, 2002.

85. Tapiero, H., Townsend, D.M., and Tew, K.D., Trace elements in human physiology and pathology, Copper, *Biomed. Pharmacother.*, 57, 386, 2003.

86. Shetty, K.R. and Duthie, Jr., E.H., Thyrotoxicosis induced by topical iodine application, *Arch. Intern. Med.*, 150, 2400, 1990.

87. Dobson, A.W., Erikson, K.M., and Aschner, M., Manganese neurotoxicity, *Ann. N.Y. Acad. Sci.*, 1012, 115, 2004.

88. Alissa, E.M., Bahijri, S.M., and Ferns, G.A., The controversy surrounding selenium and cardiovascular disease: a review of the evidence, *Med. Sci. Monit.*, 9, RA9, 2003.

89. Petrie, H.T., Klassen, L.W., and Kay, H.D., Selenium and the immune response: modulation of alloreactive human lymphocyte functions *in vitro*, *J. Leukoc. Biol.*, 45, 207, 1989.

90. Carlisle, E.M., Silicon as a trace nutrient, *Sci. Total Environ.*, 73, 95, 1988.

91. Monafo, W. and Moyer, C., The treatment of extensive thermal burns with 0.5% silver nitrate solution in early treatment of severe burns, *Ann. N.Y. Acad. Sci.*, 50, 937, 1968.

92. Prasad, A.S., Clinical, endocrinological and biochemical effects of zinc deficiency, *Clin. Endocrinol. Metab.*, 14, 567, 1985.

93. Rostan, E.F. et al., Evidence supporting zinc as an important antioxidant for skin, *Int. J. Dermatol.*, 41, 606, 2002.

94. Ilback, N.G. et al., Metallothioneins induced and trace element balance changed in target organs of a common viral infection, *Toxicology*, 199, 241, 2004.

95. Lansdown, A.B., Sampson, B., and Rowe, A., Sequential changes in trace metal, metallothionein and calmodulin concentrations in healing skin wounds, *J. Anat.*, 195, 375, 1999.

96. Mocchegiani, E. et al., Metallothioneins/PARP-1/IL-6 interplay on natural killer cell activity in elderly: parallelism with nonagenarians and old infected humans. Effect of zinc supply, *Mech. Aging Dev.*, 124, 459, 2003.

97. Ravanti, L. and Kahari, V.M., Matrix metalloproteinases in wound repair, *Int. J. Mol. Med.*, 6, 391, 2000.

98. Diegelmann, R.F. and Evans, M.C., Wound healing: an overview of acute, fibrotic and delayed healing, *Front. Biosci.*, 9, 283, 2004.

99. Grimble, R.F., Nutritional antioxidants and the modulation of inflammation: theory and practice, *New Horiz.*, 2, 175, 1994.

100. Bryant, R.E., Crouse, R., and Deagen, J.T., Zinc, iron, copper, selenium, lactoferrin, and ferritin in human pus, *Am. J. Med. Sci.*, 327, 73, 2004.

101. Chandra, R.K. and Grace, A., Goldsmith Award lecture. Trace element regulation of immunity and infection, *J. Am. Coll. Nutr.*, 4, 5, 1984.

102. Ferencik, M. and Ebringer, L., Modulatory effects of selenium and zinc on the immune system, *Folia. Microbiol. (Praha)*, 48, 417, 2003.

103. Kim, S.H. et al., Selenium attenuates lipopolysaccharide-induced oxidative stress responses through modulation of p38 MAPK and NF-B signaling pathways, *Exp. Biol. Med. (Maywood)*, 229, 203, 2004.

104. Gartner, R., Albrich, W., and Angstwurm, M.W., The effect of a selenium supplementation on the outcome of patients with severe systemic inflammation, burn and trauma, *Biofactors*, 14, 199, 2001.

105. Gazdik, F., Kadrabova, J., and Gazdikova, K., Decreased consumption of corticosteroids after selenium supplementation in corticoid-dependent asthmatics, *Bratisl. Lek. Listy.*, 103, 22, 2002.

106. Gartner, R. and Angstwurm, M., Significance of selenium in intensive care medicine. Clinical studies of patients with SIRS/sepsis syndrome, *Med. Klin. (Munich)*, 94(Suppl. 3), 54, 1999.

107. Srinivas, U. et al., Trace element alterations in infectious diseases, *Scand. J. Clin. Lab. Invest.*, 48, 495, 1988.

108. Scuderi, P., Differential effects of copper and zinc on human peripheral blood monocyte cytokine secretion, *Cell. Immunol.*, 126, 391, 1990.

109. Shenkin, A., Trace elements and inflammatory response: implications for nutritional support, *Nutrition*, 11(1 Suppl.), 100, 1995.

110. Wellinghausen, N., Martin, M., and Rink, L., Zinc inhibits interleukin-1-dependent T cell stimulation, *Eur. J. Immunol.*, 27, 2529, 1997.

111. Sprietsma, J.E., Zinc-controlled Th1/Th2 switch significantly determines development of diseases, *Med. Hypothese.*, 49, 1, 1997.

112. Meydani, M., Nutrition interventions in aging and age-associated disease, *Ann. N.Y. Acad. Sci.*, 928, 226, 2001.

113. Chandra, R.K., Effect of vitamin and trace-element supplementation on immune responses and infection in elderly subjects, *Lancet*, 340, 1124, 1992.

114. Lesourd, B.M., Immunologic aging. Effect of denutrition, *Ann. Biol. Clin. (Paris)*, 48, 309, 1990.

115. Moulin, V. et al., Role of wound healing myofibroblasts on re-epithelialization of human skin, *Burns*, 26, 3, 2000.

116. Tenaud, I. et al., *In vitro* modulation of keratinocyte wound healing integrins by zinc, copper and manganese, *Br. J. Dermatol.*, 140, 26, 1999.

117. Saito, Y. et al., Cell death caused by selenium deficiency and protective effect of antioxidants, *J. Biol. Chem.*, 278, 39428, 2003.

118. Chimienti, F. et al., Zinc homeostasis-regulating proteins: new drug targets for triggering cell fate, *Curr. Drug Targets*, 4, 323, 2003.

119. Jeschke, M.G. et al., Non-viral liposomal keratinocyte growth factor (KGF) cDNA gene transfer improves dermal and epidermal regeneration through stimulation of epithelial and mesenchymal factors, *Gene Ther.*, 9, 1065, 2002.

120. Nassif, A. et al., Evaluation of the potential role of cytokines in toxic epidermal necrolysis, *J. Invest. Dermatol.*, 123, 850, 2004.

121. Chebassier, N. et al., Stimulatory effect of boron and manganese salts on keratinocyte migration, *Acta. Derm. Venereol.*, 84, 191, 2004.

122. Jorgensen, L.N., Collagen deposition in the subcutaneous tissue during wound healing in humans: a model evaluation, *APMIS*, Suppl.(115), 1, 2003.

123. McCusker, R.H. and Novakofski, J., Zinc partitions insulin-like growth factors (IGFs) from soluble IGF binding protein (IGFBP)-5 to the cell surface receptors of BC3H-1 muscle cells, *J. Cell. Physiol.*, 197 (3), 388, 2003.

124. Sackett, R.L. and McCusker, R.H., Multivalent cations depress ligand affinity of insulin-like growth factor-binding proteins-3 and -5 on human GM-10 fibroblast cell surfaces, *J. Cell. Biochem.*, 69, 364, 1998.

125. Scuderi, P., Differential effects of copper and zinc on human peripheral blood monocyte cytokine secretion, *Cell Immunol.*, 126, 391, 1990.

126. Carpentieri, U. et al., Trace metals, surface receptors and growth of human normal and leukemic lymphocytes, *Anticancer Res.*, 8, 1393, 1988.

127. Rink, L. and Kirchner, H., Zinc-altered immune function and cytokine production, *J. Nutr.*, 130(5S Suppl.), 1407S, 2000.

128. Scott, G.M. et al., Effects of cloned interferon 2 in normal volunteers: febrile reactions and changes in circulating corticosteroids and trace metals, *Antimicrob. Agents Chemother.*, 23, 589, 1983.

129. Wu, X. et al., Zinc-induced sodium-dependent vitamin C transporter 2 expression: potent roles in osteoblast differentiation, *Arch. Biochem. Biophys.*, 420, 114, 2003.

130. Miao, M., Qin, Z.L., and Niu, X.T., Trace elements and extracellular matrix, *Zhongguo Xiu Fu Chong Jian Wai Ke Za Zhi.*, 15, 188, 2001.

131. Arisawa, S. et al., Effect of the hydroxyl radical on fibroblast-mediated collagen remodelling *in vitro*, *Clin. Exp. Pharmacol. Physiol.*, 23, 222, 1996.

132. Bang, R.L. and Dashti, H., Keloid and hypertrophic scars: trace element alteration, *Nutrition,* 11(5 Suppl.), 527, 1995.

133. Vaxman, F. et al., Effect of pantothenic acid and ascorbic acid supplementation on human skin wound healing process. A double-blind, prospective and randomized trial, *Eur. Surg. Res.*, 27, 158, 1995.

134. Satish, L., Yager, D., and Wells, A., Glu-Leu-Arg-negative CXC chemokine interferon inducible protein-9 as a mediator of epidermal-dermal communication during wound repair, *J. Invest. Dermatol.*, 120, 1110, 2003.

135. Heng, M.K., Song, M.K., and Heng, M.C., Reciprocity between tissue calmodulin and cAMP levels: modulation by excess zinc, *Br. J. Dermatol.*, 129, 280, 1993.

11 Nutrition and Wound Healing in Burns, Trauma, and Sepsis

Corilee A. Watters, Edward E. Tredget, and Carmelle Cooper

CONTENTS

A   B

Survival Without Inhalation Injury   Survival With An Inhalation Injury

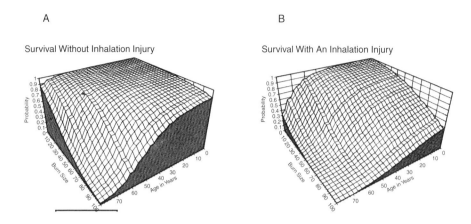

FIGURE 11.1 Relationship between age, total body surface area burn, inhalation injury, and mortality.

NUTRITION AND METABOLISM IN BURNS, TRAUMA, AND SEPSIS

Trauma, burns, and sepsis are characterized by severe metabolic and inflammatory disturbances. In burns, the extent of the injury, cardiopulmonary status, and age of the patient are key factors in determining the probability of survival [1] (Figure 11.1). Improvements in the resuscitation of the burn and trauma victims have allowed patients to survive into a postinjury hypermetabolic phase during which subsequent wound care and other operative interventions are required [2,3]. For such post-resuscitative survivors, the principal causes of subsequent morbidity and mortality are sepsis and uncontrolled inflammation. Profound alterations in immunometabolic regulation in traumatized individuals are becoming better understood [2,4]. Nutrition is one component of the care of a critically ill patient that influences wound healing and survival.

PATHOPHYSIOLOGY AND METABOLIC RESPONSE TO INJURY AND STRESS

As described originally by Cuthbertson [5], the metabolic response to injury includes an immediate shock or ebb phase and is associated with decreased intravascular volume, reduced tissue perfusion, low cardiac output, and relative hypometabolism, where total oxygen consumption is below normal levels [6]. Profound hypovolemia during this stage of injury may predispose or prime such patients for exacerbated hemodynamic and metabolic responses to subsequent injury after a second insult, such as endotoxemia, surgery, or further hypovolemia [7].

As successful restoration of adequate tissue perfusion is achieved, a physiologic state (the flow phase) of increased oxygen consumption and cardiac output is accompanied by increased muscle catabolism, erosion of lean body mass, and loss of body weight due to mobilization of fixed tissue stores of amino acids and other nutrients for biologic processes of seemingly higher biologic priority with inflammation that can last from days to weeks [2,3,6]. In patients with wounds, the catabolic phase gives way to a proliferative phase and maturation or remodeling of the wound. In the proliferative phase, fibroblasts are recruited to the inflammatory site, and extracellular matrix and collagen deposition occurs. Finally, in the maturation or remodeling phase, matrix metalloproteinases control extracellular matrix composition and facilitate cell migration to the epithelium.

CYTOKINE RESPONSE TO TRAUMA AND SURGERY

Thrombocytosis that occurs during the first hours after tissue injury aids in hemostasis, and platelets release many growth factors, such as transforming growth factor beta (TGF-β) and insulin-like growth factor (IGF-1), which regulate inflammation, immune response, and cell migration. In the inflammatory phase, the local effects of inflammation can be amplified to a systemic level due to production of cytokines, such as tumor necrosis factor (TNF), interferon-γ, interleukin-1 (IL-1), IL-6, IL-8, and IL-12 associated with a Th1 proinflammatory pathway, or cytokines with anti-inflammatory type 2 helper cell (Th2), including IL-4 and IL-10, which may contribute to the immunosuppression in sepsis and burns (Table 11.1). Thus critically ill patients have a biphasic immunological response. An initial excessive systemic inflammatory response syndrome (SIRS) with increased TNF, IL-1, and IL-10, interferon (IFN)-γ or an inadequate compensatory anti-inflammatory response syndrome (CARS) is

---

TABLE 11.1
Metabolic Effects of Cytokines in Burns, Trauma, and Sepsis

Proinflammatory Cytokines

TNF	Primary mediator in inflammatory response, increase in acute phase proteins, reduction in skeletal muscle and diaphragm contractility
IL-1	Activation of T cells, iNOS expression, prostaglandin production, inhibition of lipoprotein lipase, procoagulant activity, increase in acute phase proteins
IL-6	Key later role in inflammatory cascade, activation of lymphocytes, increase in acute phase proteins, endogenous pyrogen
IL-8	Key later role in inflammatory cascade, regulates neutrophil activity

Anti-inflammatory Cytokines

IL-10	Feedback role in limiting inflammatory response; may lessen neutrophil activation; potent inhibitor of TNF-α, IL-1β, IL-6, and IL-8 production/release
TGF-β	Downregulates proinflammatory cytokine production, lessens lymphocyte activation, stimulates extracellular matrix synthesis
IL-1ra	IL-1 receptor antagonist

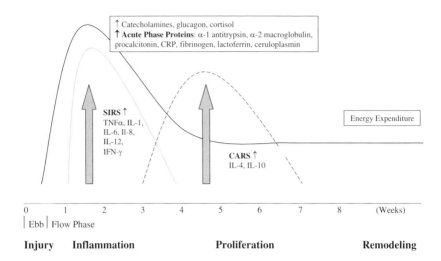

↑ Catecholamines, glucagon, cortisol
↑ **Acute Phase Proteins**: α-1 antitrypsin, α-2 macroglobulin, procalcitonin, CRP, fibrinogen, lactoferrin, ceruloplasmin

SIRS ↑
TNFα, IL-1,
IL-6, Il-8,
IL-12,
IFN-γ

Energy Expenditure

CARS ↑
IL-4, IL-10

| 0 | 1 | 2 | 3 | 4 | 5 | 6 | 7 | 8 | (Weeks) |

| Ebb | Flow Phase

Injury   Inflammation   Proliferation   Remodeling

FIGURE 11.2 Metabolic response to burns, trauma, and sepsis.

followed by immunodepression (Figure 11.2) with increased IL-4 and IL-10, reduced IL-2 [8], and decreased natural killer (NK) cell toxicity. This biphasic immune response may explain why the systemic inflammatory response occurs immediately after surgery, whereas infections occur later [9]. The immunosuppression that occurs post-burn or post-trauma increases with age. As shown in an animal model, there is an increase in the production of Th2 cytokines, particularly IL-4 and IL-10, and a reduction in Th1 cytokine IL-2 with advancing age [10].

Independent co-identification of a small polypeptide molecule present in the plasma of rabbits infected with *Trypanosoma brucei* which led to hypertriglyceridemia, hyperglycemia, and cachexia (hence, cachectin) [11] with the same molecule that induces hemorrhagic necrosis of tumors in animals after exposure of macrophages to endotoxin (tumor necrosis factor) has rapidly increased the understanding of metabolism following injury [12,13]. In healthy individuals, plasma TNF levels are less than 35 pg/ml; however, in both animals and humans, peak levels of TNF (240 pg/ml) occur after 90 to 120 min of exposure to endotoxin or Gram-negative bacteria and are positively correlated with mortality [14–16]. TNF induces hypertriglyceridemia, weight loss, and cachexia, in part by inhibition of endothelial lipoprotein lipase, but also by increased lipolysis and mobilization of fat stores. Administration of TNF to animals and humans induces proteolysis, hepatocyte amino acid uptake, by increasing the number of transport protein molecules in the plasma membrane for amino acids, including glutamine and arginine, negative nitrogen balance, and suppressed dietary intake [17,18]. However, control of dietary intake in pair-fed animals exposed to TNF demonstrated that depletion of whole body protein stores is independent of nutritional intake. Studies in adrenalectomized animals given corticosterone suggest that glucocorticoids are involved in mediating the effects of TNF on muscle proteolysis [19,20].

Similar to TNF, IL-1 is produced by a wide variety of cell types as IL-1 or IL-1 with a somewhat slower rate of appearance and onset of action after bacteremia or endotoxin [21–23]. Both TNF and IL-1 can induce the production of the other [24] and can act synergistically in producing hypotension, thrombocytopenia, metabolic acidosis with increased lactate, anaerobic glycolysis, hyperglycemia, and hypertriglyceridemia [25]. There are beneficial effects of IL-1, however. Taros and colleagues [26] showed in an animal model that administration of IL-1α lessened the mesenteric ischemia and reperfusion injury and reduced bacterial translocation after burn and sepsis.

Alterations of hepatic protein synthesis, such as reduction in albumin, transferrin, and pre-albumin production and dramatic rises in the acute phase proteins, α-1 antitrypsin, α-2 macroglobulin, procalcitonin, C-reactive protein (CRP), and fibrinogen were originally considered effects of IL-1 and TNF [27,28]. However, IL-6 has also been demonstrated to be a mediator of the hepatic acute phase response to trauma and infection [29–31]. Unlike TNF and IL-1, sustained elevations of IL-6 plasma levels have been found following major burn injury [32,33], sepsis [17,34–36], and trauma [37]. Other acute phase response proteins include lactoferrin leading to depressed serum iron concentration, which is inhibitory for growth of microorganisms [38], and ceruloplasmin and metallothionien with reduced serum zinc and copper in trauma and sepsis [38–42]. Serial measurement of prealbumin and CRP can be used to monitor nutritional status. For example, if prealbumin is not increasing and CRP is not decreasing, a low prealbumin may be due to inadequate nutrition vs. stress response [302].

Subsequently, glucagon, cortisol, and insulin are increased after major trauma, such as thermal injury [23,43]. Also, in the acute phase of the stress response, there is a tenfold increase in the catecholamines epinephrine and norepinephrine produced endogenously [23]. During shock, catecholamines dopamine, dobutamine, epinephrine, and norepinephrine are also administered exogenously as vasopressors to restore arterial pressure, with differential effects on metabolism. Dobutamine [44] and norepinephrine [45] result in greater improvements in splanchnic blood flow than other catecholamines, and dopamine and dobutamine have less of an inhibitory effect on intestinal motility than do norepinephrine and epinephrine [46]. Epinephrine in comparison to norepinephrine is associated with increased lactate levels (an indicator of tissue hypoxia), decreased pH, and higher blood glucose levels [47], and it is an immunosuppressant. Based on an animal model of the effects of catecholamines on small bowel peristalsis, Fruhwald [48] indicated that epinephrine, especially in combination with the anesthetic, sufentanil, should not be used in the intensive care setting. Furthermore, administration of a vasoconstrictor, such as epinephrine, without sufficient volume therapy can lead to temporary reduction of skin perfusion and progression of burn necrosis [49]. Dopamine impairs mucosal blood flow, worsens reduced gastric motility, and suppresses the secretion of anterior pituitary hormones, increasing catabolism and immune dysfunction [50]. Given the potential deleterious effects of large amounts of vasopressors, studies are investigating the potential to reduce vasopressor requirements by administering corticosteriods [51].

Sepsis is the systemic response to infection. Early studies suggested that sepsis and, subsequently, multiple organ dysfunction syndrome (MODS) were caused by uncontrolled infection and bacteria or endotoxins. However, some patients with adequately controlled infection and those without sepsis develop MODS and signs of systemic inflammation. This discrepancy led to investigations of systemic activation of inflammation by a wider variety of biological modulators than just infection. Activators of the inflammatory response include surgical trauma, blood loss or trans-fusion, and hypothermia. Despite the apparent involvement of biological modulators and cytokines such as TNF, and IL-1 receptor in MODS, agents that neutralize these modulators have failed to attenuate the progression of sepsis, septic shock, and organ failure. The failure of anti-cytokine therapy may be due to the complexity of septic shock, the heterogeneity of patients with septic shock, the timing of interventions, and interventions that reduce the immune response and may reduce clearance of the primary infection and exacerbate the immunosuppression [52]. In contrast, more success has been found manipulating the clotting cascade as compared with the immune system in ameliorating sepsis. Recombinant human activated protein C, an anticoagulant that inactivates clotting factors Va and VIIIa, preventing the formation of thrombin, resulted in a 16% decrease in mortality in patients with sepsis [53].

As part of the inflammatory phase of wound healing, the complement cascade and immune cells such as neutrophils are involved in the removal of debris and bacteria. In burn patients and trauma patients with wounds, it is important to limit the extent and duration of the inflammatory process by early debridement and removing infected and necrotic material as soon as possible to minimize inflammation by early closure of wounds [54]. Debridement of wounds removes burn eschar and can prevent invasive wound infections. Hydrotherapy should not be used due to the propensity for contam-ination with *Pseudomonas aeruginosa* and subsequent increased mortality [1].

ENERGY REQUIREMENTS

Thermal injury is among the most hypermetabolic conditions encountered in clinical practice, and investigations of metabolism in burn patients have demonstrated energy expenditure increases with the extent of body surface area injured to about 60% total body surface area (TBSA), where increases up to twice the basal energy expenditure (BEE) can occur [55–59].

FACTORS INFLUENCING ENERGY REQUIREMENTS

There are many factors that influence energy expenditure (Table 11.2). Because many critically ill patients are mechanically ventilated and receive sedatives and narcotics for pain control, energy expenditure may be reduced by 24 to 33% [60] with an increase in depth of sedation progressively decreasing resting energy expenditure [61]. In patients with head injuries receiving neuromuscular blockade with pancuronium, energy expen-diture was reduced by 20% from 29 kcal/kg to 24 kcal/kg [62]. In pediatric burn patients, oral propranolol, a β-adrenergic receptor blocker, reduced energy expenditure by 25% and improved net muscle protein balance by 82% [63]. β-Blockade also reduces triglyceride-free fatty acid (TG-FFA) cycling from the lipolytic effects of catecholamines [64] and decreases hepatic steatosis by limiting fatty acid delivery [65].

Energy requirements are also affected by temperature changes both internally and externally. Gore [66] reported in a study of 84 burn-injured children, that during febrile episodes, resting energy expenditure (REE)/predicted BEE increased from 1.39 to 1.68 for patients with severe fever (> 40°C) and increased muscle protein

---

TABLE 11.2
Factors Influencing Energy Expenditure

Increasing Energy Expenditure
- Pain, anxiety
- Tachycardia
- Ventilator weaning versus assisted ventilation
- Activity
- Fever, infection
- Increased with trauma, injury, and total body surface area burn
- Reduced ambient temperature in burn-injured patients

Reducing Energy Expenditure
- Analgesia for pain control, sedation, anesthetics
- Neuromuscular blockade
- β-Blockade
- Obesity (reduced caloric requirements per actual body weight)
- Warmer ambient temperature in burn-injured patients

---

catabolism occurred. Pruitt and colleagues [67] reported in a study of 44 burn injured adults that energy expenditure increased significantly when the ambient temperature was reduced to 22°C due to increased heat loss through the burn wound and nonshivering thermogenesis. In contrast to burn injured patients, Bardutzky [68] reported that in ten patients with acute ischemic stroke, basal energy expenditure decreased by 30% with moderate hypothermia, from a mean daily total energy expenditure of 1549 kcal/d with a body temperature of 37°C to 1099 kcal/d with 33°C. Thus, the presence of fever or hypothermia and ambient temperatures are important factors influencing energy expenditure, emphasizing the need to measure actual energy expenditure.

METHODS FOR DETERMINING ENERGY REQUIREMENTS

It is important to measure REE by indirect calorimetry, because many of the equations used to predict energy requirements, such as the Harris–Benedict equation or the Curreri formula, can overestimate energy needs by as much as 44% and can lead to overfeeding [60]. Indirect calorimetry is especially important in underweight and obese patients, where estimation of energy expenditure is difficult [69]. An indirect calorimeter is used to measure heat and energy production indirectly through measurement of oxygen consumption and carbon dioxide production and calculation of REE using the Weir equation. The recommended practice for performing indirect calorimetry is to measure REE while patients are receiving continuous enteral feeding in a thermoneutral environment. This accounts for the thermic effect of feeding and any shivering/nonshivering themogenesis, with the remainder being stress or activity. The usual practice in critically ill patients is to add up to 10% to the measured REE to account for the activity/stress of patient care and in burn patients, 20 to 30% of REE. Swinamer reported in 1987 [70] that in critically ill patients activities such as weighing, repositioning, and chest physiotherapy increased energy expenditure above resting levels by 20 to 30%, but the actual contribution of these activities to total energy expenditure was small (1 to 3.6%) resulting in a mean total 24 h energy expenditure only 6.9% above the measured resting energy expenditure, and that an activity factor of no greater than 10% above resting energy expenditure is appropriate. However, McClave [71] reported that the addition of 10% to the measured REE in critically ill patients reduces the accuracy by which the "snapshot" REE correlates to the 24 h total energy expenditure (TEE) and should not be done. Hart [72] indicated that overfeeding burn patients with calories greater than 20% beyond measured REE is not beneficial and results in increased carbon dioxide production as well as increased fat deposition rather than lean body mass.

In the past, the respiratory quotient (RQ) value obtained from indirect calorimetry was used to assess substrate utilization, since theoretically metabolism of fat should result in a RQ of 0.7, protein 0.8, and 1.00 for carbohydrate. However, the body's ability to use individual nutrient substrates may be altered by the stress response and overall disease process [71]. McClave also cautions against the use of RQ to diagnose overfeeding (RQ is increased) or underfeeding (RQ is reduced), because the specificity and sensitivity are low, and the measured RQ does not correlate to under- or overfeeding in all patients. However, the RQ value is useful to confirm that results are within the physiologic range of 0.67 to 1.3.

Although measurement of energy expenditure via indirect calorimetry is the most accurate method of determining energy requirements, indirect calorimetry may not be available or appropriate in many circumstances. It should not be performed when FiO_2 is greater than 60% in ventilated patients, in patients with air leaks from chest tubes or bronchopleural fistulas, during hemodialysis or continuous renal replacement therapy, within 24 h following general anesthetic, and with cases where it has not been possible to achieve "steady state" (where VO_2 and VCO_2 change by less than 10). In critically ill patients, it is recommended that patients with a BMI < 20 kg/m2 receive approximately 37 kcal/kg actual body weight (ABW); patients with a BMI between 20 to 30 kg/m^2 25 to 30 kcal/kg; and for obese patients with a BMI > 30 kg/m^2 approximately 20 kcal/kg [69]. In patients with burns, there are over 40 published predictive equations for assessing energy requirements; however, the Harris–Benedict equation multiplied by a stress factor 1.5 to 2.0, depending on burn size, is commonly used. In obese patients, adjusting the actual weight by 50% has shown to improve correlation of Harris–Benedict from 0.39 to 0.42 with measured REE [73].

Underweight and overweight critically ill patients may be at increased risk. Severely obese (BMI > 40 kg/m^2) critically ill patients are at increased risk of morbidities, such as prolonged ventilator dependence, increased incidence of multiorgan failure, and intensive care unit (ICU) length of stay, and depressed left ventricular ejection fraction [74]. Gottschlich and colleagues in a prospective study of 15 obese patients matched to nonobese patients reported that obese burn patients are at increased risk of morbidities, such as of infection, sepsis, longer ventilation, and greater requirements for exogenous insulin [75]. Anesthetists have shown in patients undergoing abdominal surgery that intraoperative subcutaneous tissue oxygen tension is significantly less in obese patients (BMI > 30 kg/m^2) even with supplemental oxygen administration, predisposing to a significantly increased risk of infection [76]. In over 500 patients undergoing colorectal surgery randomly assigned to received 30 or 80% oxygen during and for 2 h after surgery, the arterial and subcutaneous partial pressure of oxygen was higher and the incidence of wound infection was halved in the high oxygen group [77]. However, in regards to mortality, in a retrospective analysis of 63,646 patient data sets from a multi-institutional ICU database, Tremblay [78] reported increased mortality only in underweight patients (BMI < 20 kg/m²), not in overweight, obese, or severely obese patients.

RISKS OF UNDERFEEDING

In critically ill patients, underfeeding can result in depressed ventilatory drive, decreased respiratory muscle function, impaired immune function, and increased infection. Recently, Rubinson and colleagues [79] reported that in a prospective cohort analysis of 138 patients, patients who were underfed (6 kcal/kg) had significantly increased risk of developing nosocomial bloodstream infections. Burn patients are at even greater risk of underfeeding due to their hypermetabolism and requirements for wound healing.

Providing nutrition support after underfeeding can result in refeeding syndrome. Refeeding syndrome includes the metabolic and physiologic changes in glucose and electrolytes occurring from providing nutrients after a period of starvation or low caloric intake. The presence of nutrients stimulates insulin and anabolism resulting in the intracellular uptake of potassium, phosphorus, and magnesium, expansion of extracellular fluid space, and subsequent reduction in circulating levels of potassium, phosphorus, and magnesium to deleterious levels, leading to cardiac arrhythmias and congestive heart failure.

RISKS OF OVERFEEDING

Overfeeding can be associated with increased carbon dioxide production, requiring increased ventilation, and can lead to hyperglycemia, hypertriglyceridemia, hepatic steatosis, refeeding syndrome, azotemia, hypertonic dehydration, and metabolic acidosis [80]. Overfeeding complications were more common in the past when critically ill patients were receiving hyperalimentation and excessive glucose calories by total parenteral nutrition (TPN) [81]. Jeejeebhoy and colleagues [82] showed that in an animal model of sepsis (TNF-α treated rats), increasing energy intake was not beneficial due to increased stabilization and prolongation of the effects of TNF activity with increased morbidity; however, increasing protein was beneficial [83].

Krishnan and colleagues report in a prospective cohort study of 187 critically ill adults (excluding trauma and burns) with a mean BMI of 25 kg/m² that feeding more than 66% of goal intake (18 kcal/kg) was associated with increased morbidity and mortality [84]. In particular, obese patients may be at increased risk of overfeeding, and Dickerson and colleagues [85] indicated that in a retrospective analysis of 40 critically ill, overweight patients (> 125% of ideal body weight), those who received hypocaloric enteral nutrition (< 20 kcal/kg) had a shorter ICU stay and no difference in prealbumin or nitrogen balance. Thus in critically ill patients, permissive underfeeding may be helpful in overweight patients.

TABLE 11.3
Consequences of Nutrient Deficiency or Excess

Nutrient Deficiency
- Decreased respiratory muscle strength, hypoventilation, failure to wean from mechanical ventilation
- Alkalosis
- Ketosis
- Immunosuppression, increased risk of nosocomial infection
- Poor wound healing: decreased fibroblast proliferation, diminished collagen synthesis, remodeling of previously healed wounds, development of decubitus ulcers
- Risk of refeeding syndrome
- Reduction in lean body mass, increased mortality

Nutrient Excess
- Failure to wean from mechanical ventilation, hyperventilation
- Hyperglycemia
- Azotemia
- Metabolic acidosis
- Hypertriglyceridemia
- Hepatic steatosis
- Hypertonic dehydration
- Overfeeding of previously malnourished patients can lead to refeeding syndrome
- Mortality

Meeting nutritional requirements in burn patients is important; however, additional nutritional support beyond requirements will not prevent the marked hypermetabolism and elevation in energy expenditure that remains for 40 to 50 d following injury [86]. In critically ill patients, it is important to monitor actual energy intake as a percentage of goal requirements to ensure that requirements are being met while avoiding the complications associated with under- and overfeeding (Table 11.3).

PROTEIN AND AMINO ACID METABOLISM

Posttraumatic hypermetabolism is associated with increased catabolism and loss of lean body mass in proportion to the severity of the injury. It is well established that an increased intake of protein is required for wound healing and achievement of nitrogen balance. Patients with sepsis can lose up to 250 g of lean body mass per day if unfed [87]. Muscle proteolysis, a hallmark of protein metabolism in sepsis and trauma, can result in compromised respiratory function and further immunosuppression. Animal studies have shown that protein deficiency leads to decreased fibroblast proliferation, diminished collagen synthesis, remodeling of previously healed wounds [88], and increased TNF [89]. Compared to other trauma, thermal injury represents a severe form of trauma, where loss of as much as 20% of the body protein may occur following the insult. The severity of loss of lean body mass is closely related to the increased risk of morbidity and mortality in the acute phase of injury [90–92]. It is recommended that burn patients receive 1.5 to 2.5 g protein per kilogram actual body weight per day or approximately 20 to 25% of calories as protein [93,94]. Assessment of protein status through monitoring of prealbumin, transferrin, and nitrogen balance should be done on a regular basis. However, nitrogen balance studies need to be interpreted carefully in view of factors affecting results, such as reliance on accurate 24-h urine collection and normal renal function. In addition, fluid status, blood urea nitrogen, and creatinine should be monitored on an ongoing basis to assess tolerance to the high nitrogen renal solute load.

In nonseptic severely burned children, Jahoor et al. found that the rate of proteolysis was elevated after injury and remained high throughout the entire acute or flow phase of injury as well as the convalescent phase, which lasted 40 to 90 d after the burn [95]. However, the net protein loss, as demonstrated by the urea kinetics, was elevated only during the first 2 weeks after injury. This suggests that aggressive nutritional therapy in burn patients may increase protein synthesis but cannot ameliorate the prolonged elevation of protein breakdown.

Stable isotope turnover studies in 33 severely burned adults and 8 pediatric patients (range 2 to 15 yr) using either methionine [96] or leucine tracers [96–98] further confirmed that during the flow phase of injury, nutrition support improved whole body net protein balance by increasing the rate of protein synthesis but not by reducing the rate of protein breakdown, findings that also resemble those of Claugue et al. in postoperative surgical patients [99]. Similarly, in endotoxin-induced sepsis, reductions in protein synthesis were combined with an increased rate of protein breakdown [100,101]. Recognition of these fundamental alterations in amino acid and nitrogen metabolism has led to a number of strategies to improve recovery and limit morbidity in the hypermetabolic and catabolic patient.

Thus many investigators have attempted to increase or optimize protein synthesis by providing the "ideal" compositions of both energy and protein which can be maximally utilized by patients to replenish tissue proteins despite the prolonged proteolysis. More recently, attention has focused on the role of specific amino acids in contributing to wound healing — in particular, glutamine and arginine.

GLUTAMINE

Glutamine is the most abundant free amino acid in the body, comprising 69% of the total muscle free amino acid pool [102], where it serves as an important modulator or intermediate in a number of metabolic pathways. Studies have demonstrated a direct inhibitory effect of glutamine on protein degradation in cultured muscle tissue [103]. A correlation between intracellular glutamine level and muscle protein synthesis has also been shown both *in vitro* and *in vivo* [104–106].

In healthy humans, glutamine has been recognized as a nonessential amino acid, because it can be synthesized by glutamine synthetase from glutamate via α-ketoglutarate. It functions in the synthesis of nucleotides, is a precursor for the antioxidant glutathione, and like most other amino acids is gluconeogenic. However, glutamine is more important than other amino acids in gluconeogenesis in the postabsorptive state [107]. Glutamine is a major transporter of nitrogen in the form of ammonia from glutamate; it functions in acid–base homeostasis and is present in blood and muscle in higher concentrations than other amino acids.

During stress and burn injury, synthesis of glutamine is inadequate to meet metabolic demands [108], and it becomes conditionally essential. Parry-Billings [109] found in patients with major burn injury that plasma glutamine concentration was 58% lower than normal controls, and it remained low for at least 21 d postinjury. Although plasma concentrations of all amino acids were decreased after burn injury, glutamine levels did not return to normal, whereas concentrations of alanine and branched-chain amino acids did [109]. The authors postulated that the decrease in glutamine concentration may be a contributing factor to the immunosuppression that occurs after major burn injury. Because glutamine is needed for lymphocyte prolif-eration, and because it is the main energy source for enterocytes, it may be important in the maintenance of gut barrier function [110]. The effect of glutamine deficiency is also seen when *in vitro* glutamine supplementation of neutrophils isolated from burn patients results in increased bactericidal function [111]. In addition, due to glutamine's role via citrulline as a precursor of arginine, some of the effects of deficiency in catabolic states may possibly be due to a reduction in arginine synthesis [112].

Studies by Newsholme and his colleagues have also shown an important role of glutamine in the immune system, where it is an extremely important fuel for macrophages and lymphocytes, as well as other immune system cells [113,114]. These cells possess high proliferation rates, resembling enterocytes and tumor cells, which also have high glutamine utilization rates. Newsholme et al. [115–118] revealed that utilization of glu-cose and glutamine by the cells of the immune system proceeds at a very high rate, estimated at 25% of the rate of the glucose utilized by the maximally working perfused heart [114]. Most glucose and glutamine metabolized by immune cells appears to undergo partial oxidation in these tissues, which involves only the "left hand" of the Kreb's citric acid cycle (i.e., from α-ketoglutarate to oxaloacetate), despite possessing all the enzymes necessary for complete oxidation in the Kreb's cycle [114]. In this way, the tricarboxylic acid (TCA) cycle is operated at a higher rate with a relatively lower level of citric acid concentration, which would otherwise inhibit glycolysis via a feedback mechanism. Therefore by utilizing glutamine as a fuel, both glycolysis and the TCA cycle can be maintained at a constantly higher rate to meet the high demand of energy for these actively proliferating cells. Thus the high uptake rate and partial oxidation of glucose and glutamine result in the partial metabolization of glucose to lactate and the conversion of glutamine to lactate, aspartate, and alanine. The physiological significance is that it may afford cells of the immune system a rapid and immediate response to the immune challenge (such as invasion of bacteria or endotoxin). Partial oxidation of these substrates may also provide intermediates for the biosynthesis of other substrates that are important for cell proliferation and immune function, for example, the product of glycolysis, glucose 6-phosphate, can be used for the formation of 5-ribose-phosphate, which is required for DNA and RNA synthesis. Similarly, glycerol 3-phosphate is necessary for phospholipid synthesis; glutamine itself and the products of its degradation, aspartate and ammonia, serve as direct precursors for purine and pyrimidine synthesis; and the amide nitrogen of glutamine is also utilized for the formation of glucosamine, GTP, and NAD^+. Therefore, any significant decrease in glutamine and glucose utilization could be expected to decrease the rate of proliferation of these cells and impair the immune function of the host. Based on the factors regulating glutamine released from the muscle, it was proposed that the transport of glutamine out of the muscle acts as the flux-generating step for its utilization by the cells of the immune system [119], and it was suggested that burn and other trauma patients may require supplementation of glutamine to spare its loss from muscle tissue and to preserve host immune function. Although subsequent research has shown failure of glutamine supplementation to influence muscle protein metabolism [120], its effects on immune function remain promising [121].

Research has been done on the effects of glutamine supplementation in surgical and critically ill patients. Unfortunately, glutamine is not stable in solution and converts to the cyclic product, pyroglutamic acid (pGlu) and ammonia [122]. This difficulty has been overcome by supplementing glutamine in its dipeptide form with other amino acids [123–125]. Clinical trials have confirmed the efficiency of dipeptide utilization by different tissues within the body [123,124]. Furthermore, in a series of dose response tests it was found that glutamine is readily metabolized and cleared from the bloodstream and no evidence was found of clinical toxicity or generation of toxic metabolites of glutamine in patients receiving continuous glutamine-containing parenteral feeding for up to 6 weeks [126–129]. These observations support the safety of glutamine in nutritional support formula.

The first studies were done with glutamine supplemented total parenteral nutrition, first with free glutamine and later with dipeptide glutamine [130]. Improvements in nitrogen balance, immune function, infection reduction, and maintenance of total body water were noted [130]. Supplementation of parenteral nutrition with glutamine in 84 critically ill patients reduced mortality from 67 to 43% at 6 months [131,132]. In a study of 26 burn patients fed enterally and parenterally, intravenous (IV) supplementation with 0.57 g/kg glutamine (40 g/70 kg man) resulted in a significant reduction in Gram-negative bacteria and improvement in serum transferrin and prealbumin at 14 d post-burn in comparison with isonitrogenous controls [133]. In a study of 41 burn patients fed enterally and parenterally, Garrel and colleagues found that enterally administered glutamine, 26 g/d (0.4 g/kg for a 70 kg man) from the beginning of enteral feeding until wounds were healed, resulted in a significant reduction in blood infection, *Pseudomonas aeruginosa* infection, and mortality [134]. The higher amount of enteral glutamine in Garrel's study may explain the positive result in contrast to previous studies of glutamine administered enterally to critically ill patients in amounts of 10 g/d with no effect [133]. Due to the positive effects of glutamine and no documentation of adverse effects [135], it is recommended that enteral glutamine be considered in burn and trauma patients [136].

Arginine

In adults, arginine is classified as a nonessential amino acid that becomes conditionally essential during growth, trauma, and wound healing. In healthy adults fed an Arg-free diet for 6 to 7 d, *de novo* arginine synthesis is not affected, unlike nutritionally essential amino acids [137]. Arginine stimulates the secretion of insulin, glucagon, prolactin, catecholamines, corticosteroids, somatostatin, and growth hormone. Increased amounts of arginine are needed for growth for synthesis of collagen and connective tissue proteins [138]. Collagen is composed primarily of glycine, proline, and hydroxyproline. The high arginase level found in wound tissues converts arginine to ornithine, which is a substrate for collagen synthesis (via proline) and polyamines (via ornithine decarboxylase), which are important for tissue growth and wound repair. Arginine can also be converted via nitric oxide synthase (NOS) to nitric oxide (NO).

Fibroblasts, which are important in the proliferative phase of wound healing, can take up citrulline from the circulation and convert it to arginine [139]. In turn, fibroblasts can convert arginine to nitric oxide by both the constitutive and inducible pathways [140]. This indicates that nitric oxide production and, thus, arginine, could be important in the proliferation stages of wound healing. Supplemental arginine was only effective in enhancing wound healing in normal but not knockout mice with the inducible nitric oxide synthase pathway removed, indicating that the production of nitric oxide is one mechanism by which arginine improves wound healing [141]. Nitric-oxide-releasing nonsteroidal anti-inflammatory drugs (NSAIDs) significantly enhance collagen deposition at a wound site in comparison to regular NSAIDs [142]. In hypertrophic scars, where excessive fibrosis has occurred, there is a reduced expression of nitric oxide synthase [143]. Because nitric oxide has a role in vasodilation and inhibition of cell proliferation, it is thought that a lack of nitric oxide and perhaps its precursor arginine might be a contributing factor to the increased cellularity of abnormally healed hypertrophic scars [143]. Vasodilation or increased blood flow to the wound is important, because collagen synthesis requires increased oxygen (PO_2 of 200 torr) as compared with normal cell replication (PO_2 of 40 torr) [144]. While local vasodilation may be beneficial for immune defense and wound healing, the release of large quantities of NO may cause systemic vasodilation and hypotension and may be deleterious in a patient with sepsis.

Possible benefits of arginine supplementation in trauma patients may include promotion of wound healing [138,145] and improved patient immunity [145]. Additionally, a beneficial effect of arginine on nitrogen metabolism has also been reported in clinical and laboratory experiments [146]. Saito et al. [147] fed burned guinea pigs with different amounts of arginine in enteral diets and found that arginine supplementation at 2% of the total dietary energy intake reduced the mortality of the burn injury. Based on a series of laboratory experiments on thermally injured animals, Alexander et al. [148] proposed the composition of an "optimal" diet for burn patients, in which 2% of the dietary energy is derived from arginine. The diet was found to reduce the rate of wound infection, hospital length of stay, and mortality when compared to other "standard" enteral formulations. In surgical patients, a randomized, prospective trial conducted by Daly et al. [149] revealed that supplying 16 g/d of arginine to cancer patients undergoing major surgery resulted in enhancement of various parameters of the T-lymphocyte response, compared to a group of similar patients receiving isonitrogenous glycine supplements (25 g/d). Other studies also demonstrated improved thymic function in injured patients with an enhanced arginine supply ranging from 15 to 30 g/d [149–153].

In burn-injured animals, elevated NO production has been found to last for months [154]. Under these circumstances, inducible NO synthase (iNOS) is induced, and prolonged overproduction of NO [154–156] may contribute to hypotension and shock [157,158], free-radical-mediated tissue damage, and subsequent organ malfunction [159,160] and, thus, multiple organ dysfunction syndrome (MODS).

From a nutritional perspective, it is important to determine if the NO production can be modulated by arginine supply. A number of studies have demonstrated that a bolus IV injection of arginine to healthy [161,162] and septic human subjects [163] at a level above 0.2 g/kg resulted in an increased level of NO in the expired air [162] and increased urinary excretion of nitrite, nitrate, and cyclic GMP [161]. In some cases, such increased production of NO was accompanied by immediate but transient vasodynamic changes [161]. Because NO is a short-lived paracrine mediator, regulation of its production is potentially important for burn and trauma patients. Merely enhancing the arginine content in the nutritional support may not be sufficient, and a combined nutritional–pharmacological approach with arginine as well as combinations of NOS agonist and antagonist may be required. The design of highly selective inhibitors of NO production [164] will likely improve the understanding of the function of NO and lead to the development of therapeutic strategies for manipulating NO synthesis for the benefit of severely injured patients. The reported "therapeutic" dose of arginine is from 0.2 to 0.5 g/kg/d of oral intake [149,151–153] or parenteral feeding [146], and the reported bolus arginine infusion that exerts an effect on modulating NO production and hemodynamic change in human subjects are similar (above 0.2 g/kg) [161,162]. Such amounts of arginine given chronically via enteral or parenteral feeding may benefit trauma patients; however, the same dose given by rapid IV infusion or bolus injection would cause an immediate "surge" of NO production and subsequent hemodynamic change in human subjects. However, Beaumier et al. [165] did not demonstrate an increase in urinary nitrate excretion or the conversion of plasma L-$[^{15}N_2$-guanidino] arginine to NO_3 in healthy human subjects receiving a therapeutic intake of arginine 0.56 g/kg/d in the diet for 6 d.

NO has also been shown to be important in healing tendons and fractures, with increased NOS activity following injury [166,167]. Studies done in rats indicate that all three NOS isoforms are expressed in a coordinated sequence [168] during healing [168,169], and suppression of NOS impairs fracture healing [169].

Due to the possible role of NO in the pathogenesis of septic shock syndrome and the role of NO in mediating the hypotensive effect of TNF [170], there has been concern that arginine supplementation might not be indicated in critically ill patients [171]. A study of the metabolic effects of supplementing enterally fed critically ill patients with arginine indicated that arginine is mainly metabolized into ornithine by the arginase enzyme rather than into NO [172,173]. In a study of 50 burn patients Saffle et al. [173] reported no differences in mortality in patients randomized to receive an immune-enhancing enteral formula containing arginine as compared with patients received a standard high-protein formula. However, in a review of immunonutrition in critically ill patients, there was increased mortality with immunonutrition, especially in patients with sepsis [174]. In a randomized multicenter clinical trial, mortality was 44% in patients with severe sepsis receiving enteral nutrition (containing additional L-arginine, omega-3 fatty acids) as compared to 14% in those given parenteral nutrition resulting in ending the recruitment of patients with severe sepsis [175].

It was postulated that providing an arginine-containing immunoenhancing formula during compensatory anti-inflammatory response syndrome (CARS) and immunosuppression might stimulate the immune system and be beneficial, whereas in sepsis and systemic inflammatory response syndrome (SIRS), arginine-containing enteral products should not be used [176]. This remains an area for further investigation, and although arginine is important for wound healing, routine supplementation of arginine in critically ill patients cannot be recommended at this time [177].

Research has also been done on the effects of ornithine α-ketoglutarate, a precursor to glutamine, arginine, and proline. In a prospective, double-blind randomized trial of 47 patients with 25 to 95% total body surface area burns, 20 g of ornithine α-ketoglutarate added to enteral feeding significantly reduced wound healing time and improved nutritional status [178].

LIPID METABOLISM

Although fat is a necessary component of nutritional support, providing excessive lipid is not beneficial. Clinical studies of burn patients have shown an improved outcome when patients are enterally fed lower amounts of fat. Burn patients fed a diet containing 15 to 20% fat (in comparison with a 37 to 50% fat diet) had reduced incidence of pneumonia and wound infections and reduced length of hospital stay [179,180]. Gottschlich [181] also reported an association between dietary lipid content and diarrhea and recommended a low fat diet to promote tolerance to enteral feeds. Following burn injuries and in critical care, prolonged elevation of triglycerides may be associated with increased mortality [182], although it is not clear whether the increase in triglycerides is due to increased lipid administration with propofol or an indication of hypermetabolism. Propofol, a widely used sedative due to its rapid onset and quick recovery, is based in a 10% lipid emulsion and can provide a significant amount of calories from IV lipid that needs to be accounted for in the provision of nutrition support to prevent overfeeding and elevation of serum triglycerides.

Absorbed triacylglycerol (TAG) from the systemic circulation may be stored as fat or alternatively oxidized as an energy source depending on the physiological state of the host. However, utilization of circulating TAG is dependent on the enzyme lipoprotein lipase, which is bound to the endothelial surface of capillaries in all but central nervous system tissues [183], and if its capacity to hydrolyze circulating TAG is exceeded, clinical lipemia develops [183–185]. Inhibition of lipoprotein lipase is known to occur after endothelial exposure to the cytokine TNF or cachectin, which appears to limit TAG metabolism in sepsis, severe inflammatory states including trauma, and in cancer cachexia [11,186], whereas heparin stimulates lipoprotein lipase activity in relatively low doses [186,187]. Mobilization of TAG represents an important endogenous source of stored energy in adipocytes, hepatocytes, and other tissues. Intracellularly, hormone-sensitive lipase metabolizes stored TAG into free fatty acids (FFAs) and glycerol. Using stable isotope tracers of glycerol and FFA [188,189], this process has been found to be sensitive to stimulation by circulating epinephrine or inhibition by insulin via signal transduction through their respective receptors on the cell surface of adipocytes [190–192]. The synthesis of TAG by FFA esterification requires energy. Therefore, the accelerated lipolysis–TAG synthesis cycle is part of the substrate recycling in severe burn patients, which contributes to increased energy expenditure in the hypermetabolic state.

During trauma and sepsis, the catabolic hormones epinephrine, norepinephrine, and glucagons stimulate lipase, resulting in lipolysis of stored triglycerides and increased FFAs. The intracellular transport of long-chain FFAs into mitochondria via carnitine is impaired. FFA accumulate and inhibit pyruvate dehydrogenase and glycolysis, resulting in anaerobic metabolism and increased lactate, pyruvate, and acidosis [193].

Based on investigations by Mildred and George Burr [194], it is now recognized that normally a group or family of polyunsaturated fatty acids essential for growth and development cannot be synthesized in humans but instead must be present in the diet [195–197], and these FFA are defined as essential fatty acids (EFAs). With the introduction of IV nutrition, Collins [198] and Holman [199] described clinical features of EFA deficiency, which occurs in adults and infants after prolonged feeding of a diet deficient in EFA. EFA deficiency occurs not only due to the lack of exogenous supply of EFA from the diet, but also due to elevated plasma insulin levels stimulated by high glucose intakes, which inhibit the release of fatty acids from the adipose tissue stores within the body. Lineolenic, linoleic, and arachidonic acids are recognized precursors of the prostanoid family, important diverse fatty acids involved in cell signal transduction in many immunometabolic functions. Eczematous skin lesions, sparse hair growth, poor wound healing, thrombocytopenia, and hypermetabolism are recognized clinical features of EFA deficiency, described initially by Holman [199]. Subsequently, IV lipid emulsions have been formulated with very high proportions of arachidonic and other EFA between 50 and 70% of total FFA, whereas normally, EFAs comprise only 8 to 10% of adipose tissue [193,200]. Thus, only small amounts of linoleic acid in the form of 500 ml per week of 20% IV fat emulsions will prevent EFA deficiency (EFAD) [201,202]. Conversely, adverse changes in membrane fluidity [203], stimulation of nonphysiologic prostaglandin synthesis [187,204], and impairment of reticuloendothelial clearance of bacteria due to the release of a nonphysiologic lipoprotein X carrier [205,206] are important, potentially deleterious effects of excessive EFA provision in the diet.

Fatty acid levels vary much more widely than glucose in normal uninjured man (0.1 mM in the fed state to 1.0 to 1.5 mM in nonstressed starvation) [184,207,208]. Similarly, FFA concentrations in plasma following major trauma, such as thermal injury, are highly variable; however, FFA turnover measured by ^{13}C palmitate is significantly elevated in proportion to the severity of the injury, as is the release of FFA from stored TAG (lipolysis) [188]. However, as in carbohydrate metabolism, burn and trauma victims demonstrate substantial futile cycling in lipid metabolism, in that a larger proportion of FFA turnover is recycled through resynthesis of TAG (reesterification), both intracellularly and by interorgan transfer via lipolysis and reesterification [64,209]. Increases of 450% in TAG–FFA recycling in burn patients appear to be due to the lipolytic effects of high circulating catecholamines that are partially attenuated by β-blockade [64,209]. This increase in FFA released by lipolysis appears to be well in excess of their oxidation rate, and as much as 70% of the FFA released undergo reesterification [189,201]. Although increased plasma glucose increases the rate of glucose oxidation, the oxidation of FFA is reduced and reesterification increased by increased glucose availability, a nonmetabolic cycle described by Randle as the glucose–fatty acid cycle [210]. The principal site of plasma FFA clearance and reesterification is the liver, where TAG in the form of very low-density lipoprotein (VLDL) is synthesized and released into the plasma normally for storage in peripheral adipocytes or as an energy source for other tissues. In critically ill patients, secretion of VLDL by the liver appears limited by impaired lipoprotein synthesis (apoprotein B), representing another mechanism by which accumulation of intracellular hepatic TAG may occur, in addition to excessive carbohydrate feeding as discussed earlier [189,211]. Clinically, hepatic steatosis appears most closely correlated with the severity of illness and, to a lesser extent, the nature of the nutritional support [212].

In addition, the eicosanoid family of fatty acids exerts diverse effects in modulating the inflammatory and metabolic response in traumatized patients. Attempts have been made to attenuate the untoward inflammatory effects of some eicosanoids by altering the type of exogenous FFA supply. Provision of TAG containing n-3 FFA, in which the first double bond is located at the third carbon from the methyl end of the FFA, was found to reduce the extent of weight loss, skeletal muscle wasting, and energy expenditure in a burned guinea pig model [213]. Dietary augmentation of fish-oil-derived n-3 FFA has reduced monocyte production of the cytokines, IL-1, and TNF in normal human subjects [214] and has led to similar approaches in the burn and trauma population [179,213]. Attempts to provide structured lipids as TAG manufactured with both medium-chain fatty acids and n-3 FFA have been shown to improve hepatic protein synthesis, reduce protein catabolism, and decrease TEE in animal models of thermal injury [215]. Reductions in infection rate and immunosuppressive eicosanoids have been demonstrated by others [216,217].

Dietary fatty acids can also affect lymphocyte function through changes in the membrane phospholipid composition and function as well as a precursor for eicosanoids. In burn patients receiving enteral formula containing 29% fat (mainly MCT and 18:2 n-6 fatty acids), there was a reduction in arachadonic acid in lymphocyte phospholipids early after burn injury, indicating either increased metabolism of arachidonic acid metabolites involved with the inflammatory process or inhibition of the δ-6-desaturase enzyme slowing conversion of 18:2 n-6 to 20:4 n-6, and was associated with reduced NK cytotoxicity [218]. Because n-3 fatty acids compete with n-6 fatty acids for composition of cell membranes and for metabolism, and n-3 produce anti-inflammatory metabolites, n-3 fatty acids are less inflammatory.

Patients with acute respiratory distress syndrome (ARDS) randomized to receive a 55% fat enteral formula rich in omega-3 fatty acids (40% of fat source as borage and fish oil) or a formula rich in omega-6 fatty acids (97% corn oil) had significant improvements in oxygenation, lower ventilation requirements, reduced length of stay in the ICU, and decreased pulmonary inflammation [219]. In healthy humans, supplementation of the diet with 18 g of fish-oil-derived omega-3 fatty acids daily for 6 weeks reduced IL-1 and TNF-α production by monocytes *ex vivo* [214] up to 50% of controls and persisted for up to 4 months following supplementation. Similar reductions in IL-1, TNF, and IL-6 found in women whose diets were supplemented with eicosapentaenoic and docosahexaenoic acid [220] have led to dietary formulations enriched in omega-3 fatty acids for burn patients [179]. In 24 elective abdominal surgery patients randomized to receive perioperative parenteral nutrition supplemented with 10 g fish oil or regular parenteral nutrition support, there was a reduction in inflammatory response and IL-6 levels [221]. Also, in 21 critically ill patients intolerant of enteral nutrition randomized to received n-3 vs. n-6 lipid infusion, a reduction in proinflammatory cytokines TNF-α and IL-1 was seen [222]. In an animal model of pancreatitis, n-3 fatty acid supplementation increased IL-10, anti-inflammatory cytokine [223]. In 23 adult burn patients, there was an improvement in insulin-like growth factor (IGF) when patients were enterally fed formula containing of 15% fat (rich in omega-3 fatty acids, 50% of the fat source was fish oil), in comparison to patients fed 15% fat (mainly omega-6 fatty acids), or 35% fat, mainly omega-6 fatty acids [224]. It is thought that higher levels of IGF-1 promote wound healing and protein balance [224].

In contrast to beneficial effects on inflammation, in rats fed a diet high in menhaden oil (omega-3 fatty acids) in comparison to those fed corn oil (omega-6 fatty acids) for 30 d, there was a significant reduction in wound strength, indicating that omega-3 fatty acids may adversely change the maturational phases of wound healing [225]. Thus, providing a formula with n-3 fatty acids may be appropriate during the inflammatory phase and may not be beneficial during the proliferative and maturation phase [176].

CARBOHYDRATE METABOLISM

Isotopic tracer studies have shown that glucose is oxidized as an energy substrate up to a rate of about 5 mg/kg/min. In hypermetabolic states, a large portion of oxidized glucose is derived from endogenous lipid and amino acid substrates via gluconeogensis, providing approximately 2 mg/kg/min. Excess glucose is used for lipogenesis and results in increased CO_2 production and RQ. The RQ for the oxidation of glucose is 1, whereas lipogenesis results in an RQ greater than 1. Theoretically, RQ could be as high as 8 with lipogenesis; however, physiologically, RQs rarely exceed 1.3, perhaps due to the stress response preventing lipogenesis [71]. It has been thought that the hypercapnic effect of excess glucose calories was due to an excess proportion of carbohydrates. However, a study by Talpers and colleagues in 1992 showed that total calories affect CO_2 production more than the proportion of carbohydrate. In this study, 20 stable mechanically ventilated patients were randomized to receive isocaloric TPN as 40% CHO/40% fat/20% protein, 60% CHO/20% fat/20% protein, and 75% CHO/5% fat/20% protein. The VCO_2 did not change with increasing CHO proportion (205, 203, and 211 ml/min, respectively); however, the VCO_2 did increase when the patients received increased total calories (1.0, 1.5, and 2.0 times REE) from 181 to 244 ml/min ($p < 0.01$). Thus, although the proportion of carbohydrates is important, it is more important to avoid overfeeding critically ill patients, because the respiratory workload will be increased and may interfere with ventilator weaning.

Glucose is the principal carbohydrate fuel source with plasma levels that vary normally within a narrow range [207]. Its storage form, glycogen, is in limited supply, with 80 to 100 g total stored in liver and muscle, and it is depleted quickly after injury, within 24 to 48 h, by tissues that are predominately carbohydrate utilizing (brain, kidney, heart, red blood cells, and muscle) and that metabolize up to 300 g/d of glucose [27,29,30]. As illustrated in Figure 11.3, glucose undergoes anaerobic or oxygen-independent metabolism in the cytoplasm at a cellular level.

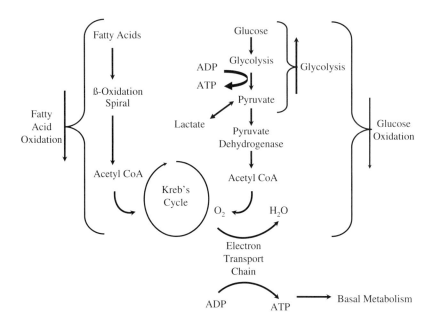

FIGURE 11.3 Glucose and free fatty acid metabolism.

After injury, considerable glycolytic metabolism occurs despite the presence of seemingly adequate oxygen supply, resulting in efflux of lactate measured in the arteriovenous differences across the extremity of injured animals or patients [226,227]. Additionally, using the stable isotope ^{13}C at various locations in the six-carbon glucose ring to differentiate recycling at the allosteric steps in glycolysis, abundant apparently futile recycling appears to occur after thermal trauma [64] (Figure 11.3), in sharp contrast to the hypometabolic state of hypothyroidism, where recycling is reduced below normal [228]. Burn and trauma patients appear to benefit from substrate cycling by the use of ATP to generate heat or thermogenesis [64,189].

Using stable and radioactive glucose isotopes, independent investigators have established that in humans, after-injury provision of glucose calories to spare amino acid oxidation for energy purposes increases glucose oxidation up to about 5 mg/kg/min, beyond which protein synthesis minimally improves, and increases in CO_2 production and RQ occur, consistent with the intrahepatic synthesis of long-chain fatty acids [25,229,230]. Clinically, the consequences of the provision of excessive carbohydrates appear to be a marked increase in minute ventilation (VO_2) and CO_2 production (VCO_2), which is deleterious to pulmonary function and weaning from mechanical ventilation. Similarly, the provision of excessive carbohydrate has been associated with intrahepatic steatosis and cholestatic jaundice [193,228].

After thermal trauma, regional glucose metabolism occurs primarily by glyco-lysis, despite adequate oxygen, particularly in inflamed tissues with the release of lactate into the venous effluent and systemic circulation [189,227,231]. Hepatic formation of new glucose (gluconeogenesis) can occur from amino acids, principally alanine, after transamination of pyruvate in skeletal muscle [232–234], from glycerol released from lipolysis of esterified FFAs in triacylglycerides (TAG) [64] (see below), and from lactate as a result of glycolysis of glucose in muscle and wound tissue [64,235]. Quantitatively, gluconeogenesis from lactate is the most important and completes the Cori cycle, which normally represents 10 to 15% of total glucose production in a fasting human and is greatly accelerated by injury. In part, the recycling of lactate released by injured peripheral tissues into glucose by the liver requires 2 H^+ for each mole of glucose (2 lactate + 2 H^+ → 1 glucose) [230,236]. This process serves, in part, to buffer the systemic pH, the importance of which has become more greatly appreciated intraoperatively during liver transplantation. Clinically, local lactate production in wounds may regulate collagen synthesis by increased transcription of collagen genes and posttranslational hydroxylation by prolyl hydroxylase through reductions in intracellular ADP ribose and its polymer [237]. During sepsis, increased plasma glucose (hyperglycemia) appears to signal marked increases in glycolytic glucose metabolism, lactate production, and hepatic compensation of the acidosis by gluconeogenesis [190].

Following injury, chronic elevations of glucose accompanied by increased plasma insulin concentrations suggest that for both septic and burn patients, a state of tissue resistance to the normal effects of insulin exists [190], blunting the normal increase in cellular uptake of glucose, as well as the insulin-mediated uptake of amino acids by skeletal muscle for protein synthesis [119]. Black et al. [190] and Shangraw et al. [238] employed the euglycemic hyperinsulinemic clamp technique in human patients *in vivo* to maintain constant plasma glucose concentrations by supraphysiologic infusions of insulin. They found evidence for a postreceptor or intracellular defect in the metabolism of glucose, which exists in burn, trauma, and sepsis [6,238,239]. By maintaining the patients eukalemic during their study, Shangraw provided *in vivo* evidence for increased insulin-induced clearance of potassium in sepsis and burn stress, suggesting that cellular uptake of potassium occurring principally in the liver and mediated through the interactions of insulin with its receptor were intact despite the stress [238]. Additionally, Shaw et al. demonstrated insulin-mediated suppression of lipolysis in septic patients, which further supports the view that insulin binding to its receptor is unimpaired [239]. However, deuterated glucose isotopic kinetics confirmed that increased glucose turnover, plasma clearance, and oxidation are typical of uncomplicated stress and sepsis in an injured human as compared to bed-rested normal controls. Further, exogenous insulin infusions in burn and septic patients to supraphysiologic ranges (up to 2000 uU/ml) beyond the maximal endogenous insulin range (300 uU/ml) appear capable of suppressing hepatic gluconeogenesis but did not increase the proportion of glucose oxidized (approximately 40 to 50%) or the percent energy derived from glucose oxidation (53% and 65% in burns and sepsis, respectively) [238]. Similarly, Jahoor et al. used the euglycemic insulin clamp technique in burn patients to pharmacologically stimulate glucose/energy substrate availability in order to counteract a potential cellular energy deficit through enhanced glucose utilization, either via pyruvate entry in the tricarboxylic acid cycle through pyruvate dehydrogenase or by a reduction in amino acid oxidation (Figure 11.3). Small reductions in protein breakdown and oxidation were possible. However, the magnitude of improvement in protein kinetics by the provision of excessive amounts of substrates, such as glucose, or hormonal stimulation via insulin at supraphysiologic doses was small and insufficient to correct the excessive protein breakdown and glucose turnover characteristic of this form of trauma. Collectively, these isotopic turnover studies *in vivo* following burn trauma and sepsis point to intracellular derangements in carbohydrate and intermediary metabolism. Insulin regulates at least 100 different genes through insulin response sequences (IRSs) [240] in critical genes, such as phosphoenolpyruvate [241], apoprotein CIII [242], and tyrosine aminotransferase [243].

A recent study [244] indicated that high carbohydrate enteral feeding (3% fat, 82% carbohydrate, 15% protein) in pediatric patients with burns greater than 40% total body surface area resulted in decreased muscle protein degradation as compared with a high-fat diet (44% fat, 42% carbohydrates, 14% protein). The authors attributed the protein sparing effect of the high-carbohydrate diet to the anabolic effect of insulin. Previous and recent work by this group has shown significantly greater skeletal muscle protein synthesis in burn patients receiving insulin [66,245,246].

A common finding in hospitalized patients, whether due to surgery, critical illness, inactivity, or aging, is insulin resistance and stress hyperglycemia with increased glycogenolysis and gluconeogenesis. In addition to glycosylation of hemoglobin, elevated blood glucose can result in glycosylation of various immunoglobins and lymphocytes impairing their function [247]. Chronic hyperglycemia can affect wound healing by impairing the transport of vitamin C into cells, including leukocytes and fibroblasts [88], and inhibiting the proliferation of fibroblasts [248].

In a landmark study, Van den Berghe [249] studied critically ill patients randomized to receive conventional treatment (insulin given if the blood glucose level exceeded 12 mmol/l) or intensive insulin therapy (maintenance of blood glucose between 4 and 6 mmol/l). There was a 34% reduction in mortality from those receiving conventional therapy to those receiving intensive insulin therapy [249]. In the 1548 patients studied, there was a 46% reduction in bloodstream infections, 41% decrease in acute renal failure, 50% decrease in blood transfusions, and a 44% reduction in polyneuropathy [249]. Post-hoc analysis of the data indicated that it is the glucose control rather than the provision of insulin that contributed to the improved outcome [250]. In a retrospective study of burn patients, Gore et al. [251] found that despite similar age, burn size, caloric intake, and frequency of wound infection, patients with poor glucose control (> 7.8 mmol/l) had significantly greater incidence of positive blood cultures, less percentage of skin graft take, and increased mortality. These studies support the clinical observations of impaired wound healing in patients with diabetes and indicate the importance of euglycemia and the beneficial effects of insulin in reducing morbidity and mortality.

Increased evidence has accumulated on the importance of providing fiber as a gut fuel. Fibers such as pectin or inulin are not absorbed by the mucosal cells and reach the large intestine to be degraded by bacteria into metabolites, such as short-chain fatty acids (acetate, butyrate, and proprionate) that stimulate mucosal growth, reduce translocation, and stimulate the intestinal immune system. Rayes and coworkers in Germany [252] reported that enteral nutrition with fiber reduces the incidence of postoperative infection compared with a fiber-free enteral formula. Although enteral formulas containing fiber are commonly used for critical care patients [136], there is insufficient data to generate recommendations as part of the Canadian clinical practice guidelines for nutrition support in mechanically ventilated, critically ill adult patients [177]. However, it seems intuitive that fiber is necessary given the importance of fiber in the healthy population and the recommendations to consume 25 to 30 g of fiber each day, although patients at risk of small bowel obstruction/ischemia such as those undergoing duodenal surgery should be given fiber free formula [303]. In addition to fiber as a prebiotic or substrate for healthy bacteria, research is being done on the administration of nonpathogenic bacteria, utilizing strains of *Lactobacillus plantarum* that can adhere and colonize the gut. This remains an area under investigation [253].

PROVISION OF NUTRIENTS — GUT BARRIER FUNCTION

Following attempts by Dr. John Burke and colleagues [254] to isolate patients with massive burns in bacterially controlled nursing units, it became evident that burn victims can still acquire life-threatening infection; many of the organisms causing these infections appeared to arise from the host's own endogenous flora in the gastrointestinal (GI) tract. Animal models of bacterial translocation devised by Deitch and Berg [255] demonstrated that the intestinal mucosa in a healthy subject represents a barrier to bacteria, and with deprivation of nutrients in the GI tract along with an insult such as endotoxins or thermal injury, there is increased permeability to bacteria. However, intestinal atrophy with nutrient deprivation alone does not necessarily correlate with bacterial translocation [256], unless intestinal ischemia or endotoxins are present. In healthy humans given *Escherichia coli* endotoxin, intestinal permeability, measured by urinary excretion of nonmetabolizable sugars, lactulose, and mannitol, is increased [257]. In contrast to healthy humans, the measurement of intestinal permeability in critically ill patients by urinary recovery of enterally administered probes, such as lactulose and mannitol, yields invalid results due to changes in renal function and the presence of mannitol in banked blood given for blood transfusion [258]. However, there is indirect evidence of the human intestine becoming permeable to bacteria in patients with hemorrhagic shock assessed by association of positive blood cultures with hypotension [259]. Sedman and colleagues [260,261] also reported bacterial translocation (measured by bacterial analysis of intestinal serosa and mesenteric lymph node samples taken at time of surgery) in 15% of surgical patients, with 41% of patients with bacterial translocation developing sepsis as compared with 14% in patients with no bacteria. In animal models, after severe trauma and major burns, there is mesenteric vasoconstriction and splanchnic ischemia (determined by measurement of mesenteric O_2 delivery and intestinal mucosal pH), especially during the early phase after thermal injury, which is associated with increased bacterial translocation and endotoxin absorption from the gut [26,262].

A number of approaches have been investigated for the prevention of bacterial translocation. Barret [263] randomized 23 pediatric patients with burns greater than 30% TBSA to receive placebo or selective gut decontamination (SGD) of the digestive tract using a combination of antibiotics; however, there was no effect on colonization rates of the wound, sputum, nasogastric aspirates, cytokines, pneumonia, and sepsis, except for a higher incidence of diarrhea. A meta-analysis on the effect of antibiotics in critically ill patients indicated that although the incidence of pneumonia was significantly decreased, there was no effect on length of stay or mortality [263].

ENTERAL VS. PARENTERAL NUTRITION

Parenteral nutrition is usually referred to as "total parenteral nutrition" (TPN), because the total nutritional needs of a patient can be met by delivery of nutrients intravenously, bypassing the gastrointestinal tract. Due to the hyperosmolarity of the solution (1300 to 1800 mOsm/l), TPN must be delivered into a large-diameter vein, usually the superior vena cava. The American Society for Parenteral and Enteral Nutrition (ASPEN) suggests that TPN should be used when enteral nutrition is contraindicated or the intestinal tract has severely diminished function due to underlying disease or treatment, such as paralytic ileus, mesenteric ischemia, small bowel obstruction, or a GI fistula where enteral access cannot be placed distal to the fistula [264].

From reports of randomized trials, septic morbidity and infections are greater in patients receiving parenteral as compared with enteral nutrition. Herndon et al. reported in 1989 [304] that mortality was significantly greater (63% versus 26%) in 39 patients with burns > 50% TBSA randomized to receive parenteral supplementation of enteral support as compared with enteral support alone. Kudsk [265] also reported fewer infectious complications in trauma patients receiving enteral than those receiving parenteral nutrition. However, because fewer infections also occur with both standard care (oral diet) and enteral nutrition, it is not that enteral nutrition reduces infections, but rather that TPN increases infection risks [266]. It has been argued that the increased infections and sepsis seen with TPN are due to overfeeding and hyperglycemia [267–269]. In some centers, TPN continues to be given in standard TPN mixtures that contain 60 to 75% energy as dextrose (in comparison to 40 to 50% carbohydrate in standard enteral solutions); thus, patients may receive greater amounts of glucose, contributing to more complications than when TPN is tailored to each patient and carbohydrate not given in amounts greater than 5 mg/kg/min. Others state that TPN-associated sepsis is due to its immunosuppressive effects [270]. IV lipid emulsions available in North America contain only long-chain omega-6 fatty acids, which can be immunosuppressive [271], whereas most enteral formulations contain mixtures of long-chain and medium-chain triglyercides. In addition, studies have shown that lipid-containing TPN given to critically ill patients resulted in increased length of stay and ventilation compared to lipid-free TPN [272].

It should be noted that enteral nutrition is not without complications, and when TPN-related catheter sepsis is categorized as a nutrition support complication, the risk of complications from enteral compared to parenteral support is similar [266]. Overall, enteral nutrition is preferable to TPN in regards to lower risk of infections and should be used when possible.

ROUTE AND ACCESS OF ENTERAL FEEDING

Obtaining and maintaining enteral access is not always straightforward. Gastric tubes can be inserted nasally or orally in the case of multiple facial fractures. The tube should be marked at its entrance to the nares so that any migration can be detected. Smaller-diameter nasogastric tubes that are easier to insert and are associated with less sinusitis, aspiration, and airway obstruction are recommended [273]; however, smaller tubes clog more easily and make monitoring of residual volumes more difficult. It should be noted that diagnosis and treatment of sinusitis is important in reducing mortality in critically ill burn patients [274], and if there is a concern of sinusitis, the patient should be fed orogastrically. Radiographic confirmation of tube placement before initiation of feeding is necessary, and in some centers, tubes are advanced only 35 cm and a chest radiograph obtained to ensure the tube is not in the airway to prevent pneumothoraces before further advancing the tube, and this is then followed by a second chest radiograph if bedside fluoroscopy is not used [275]. Regular flushing and avoidance of administering medications via feeding tubes is important to maintain tube patency. Gastrostomy tubes placed surgically or endoscopically transverse the abdominal wall and are associated with more frequent and serious complications than nasoenteric tubes, including perforation of adjacent organs, infection of the insertion site, gastric bleeding, and further surgery required for replacement of displaced tubes [273].

Sefton and colleagues [276] recommend consideration of nasojejunal feeding in patients after the failure of nasogastric feeding. In critically ill patients receiving nasogastric tube feeding, high gastric aspirate volume is more frequent in patients receiving sedatives or catecholamines [277]. Also, after trauma and major metabolic insult, ileus is common and can be a significant contributor to underfeeding in patients with burns [278]. Ileus can last 24 to 48 h in the stomach but usually resolves in the small intestine within 12 to 24 h. Other arguments for postpyloric feeding include preservation of gastric pH and lowered microbial colonization as compared with gastric feeding [279]. High gastric residual volumes and associated gastroesophageal reflux may be reduced as well as aspiration pneumonia in patients fed jejunally. In a study of 54 critically ill patients, the aspiration rate was not significantly different between 7% in gastric as compared to 13% in transpylorically fed patients [280]; however, there is increased gastroesophageal regurgitation and microaspiration in patients fed into the stomach [281]. In critically ill patients randomized to gastric or small intestine enteral feeding, there was no difference in gastric microbial colonization [282] and ventilator-associated pneumonia, except that patients fed postpylorically received higher calorie and protein intakes [283,284]. It should be noted that variability in incidence of aspiration is likely due to the differences in definitions and assessment techniques [285].

POSITIONING DURING ENTERAL FEEDING

Semi-recumbency, with the head of the bed elevated to 30 to 45° from horizontal, is important in reducing reflux of gastric contents and possibly preventing pneumonia [286], which accounts for half of all infections in ICUs [287]. Recently, it was reported in critically ill patients with acute lung injury that there can be improved oxygenation when patients are in the prone position [288]. Researchers in the Netherlands report that in a study of 20 critically ill patients, enteral feeding can be continued when critically ill patients are in the prone position with no significant difference in gastric residual volume [289]; however, concerns remain regarding risk of aspiration. Patients with burns or open wounds on the face or ventral body surface, spinal instability, pelvic fractures, or life-threatening cardiac arrhythmias or hypotension should be fed in the supine position [290].

Timing of Enteral Feeding

Initiation of enteral feeding is recommended as soon as possible in a fluid-resuscitated and hemodynamically stable patient, usually within 24 to 48 h of injury or admission. Peng et al. [291] studied 15 burn patients (average 61% TBSA) receiving early (< 24 h) vs. delayed (> 48 h) nasogastric or oral feeding and reported increased gut permeability and TNF levels with delayed feeding. In contrast, Gottschlich and colleagues [292] studied 77 pediatric burn patients randomized to feeding within 24 h of injury compared to feeding at least 48 h post-burn and found increased adverse events and higher serum insulin levels with early feeding. They indicated that feeding within 24 h of injury does not improve morbidity or mortality. The increased complications with early feeding are not surprising given the mesenteric vasoconstriction and splanchnic ischemia that occurs early after thermal injury, which is associated with increased bacterial translocation and endotoxin absorption from the gut [26]. Some centers continue postpyloric enteral feeding during surgery [293]; however, the effects of anesthetics on intestinal motility and risks of enteral feeding during low splanchnic perfusion need to be considered.

Due to the risks of feeding a hypoperfused gut, resulting in small bowel ischemia and necrosis, it is recommended that in unstable critically ill patients who need catecholamine support, heavy sedation, or therapeutic neuromuscular blockade, or who develop sudden abdominal distension, enteral nutrition should be ceased and reevaluated [294]. Although the incidence of intestinal ischemia is low (0.2%), the incidence increases (to 3.8%) with jejunal feeding either via a jejunostomy or nasojejunal tube feeding [295]. Due to the high mortality rate of 80 to 100% associated with intestinal ischemia, hypotensive patients should be closely monitored for any GI intolerance, such as a sudden increase in nasogastric output, abdominal distention or pain, and cessation of bowel movements, and if present, enteral feedings should be promptly discontinued [296]. Radiographic demonstration of free air in the peritoneal space or clinical signs of an acute abdomen require immediate surgical intervention. Thus, the morbidity risks of underfeeding for a short period of time need to be balanced with the mortality risk of developing small bowel necrosis.

Continuous vs. Intermittent Feeding

Due to the association of continuous enteral feeding with decreased gastric acidity, and increased propensity for gastric colonization and pneumonia, effects of intermittent enteral feeding on pH have been investigated. In a study of 43 patients randomized to continuous or intermittent gastric feeding or continuous jejunal feeding, pH was highest in the gastric group at 5.0, followed by the intermittent gastric group at 4.0, and was lowest with jejunal feeding at 3.2. The authors estimated that the probability of colonization was lower in the jejunal group as compared with the gastric groups [279]. However, continuous feeding remains the preferred method due to the need to maximize caloric intake in patients with burns and minimize risk of aspiration in critically ill patients with reduced levels of consciousness.

Growth Factors

It has been known for some time that growth hormone can stimulate wound healing and improve nitrogen balance [297]. However, due to insulin resistance, hyperglycemia, and increased mortality, growth hormone is not recommended for critically ill patients [298]. In contrast, the testosterone analogue oxandrolone, has been shown to reduce weight loss, improve nitrogen balance, and improve wound healing in burn patients without an increase in hyperglycemia or other complications [299].

TGF-β is a local and circulating cytokine that can enhance wound healing [300]. However, excessive TGF-β can lead to the formation of hypertrophic scars [301]. Interferons have been used as antifibrogenic factors to modulate the excessive production of extracellular matrix associated with dermal fibroproliferative disorders by reducing type I collagen mRNA and histamine levels [301].

CURRENT RECOMMENDATIONS FOR NUTRITION SUPPORT OF THE BURN AND CRITICALLY ILL PATIENT

Based on current information, present recommendations for the nutrition support of burned and critically ill patients are summarized in Table 11.4. Patients with an intact gastrointestinal tract should be fed enterally via a nasogastric or orogastric tube within 24 to 48 h of admission. Given all the factors influencing energy requirements, indirect calorimetry is recommended to measure expenditure, and if unavailable the Harris–Benedict equation should be used in burn patients and empiric kcal/kg formulas based on BMI should be used in critically ill patients. Enteral formula containing arginine with glutamine added should be used in burn patients; however in critically ill patients

---

TABLE 11.4
Nutrition Support Recommendations for Critically Ill and Burn-Injured Patients

	Critically Ill	Burns
Energy — predictive equations	BMI < 20 kg/m²: 37 kcal/kg	Harris–Benedict equation: BEE × Injury/Activity Factor 1.5 to 2 depending on TBSA
	BMI 20–25 kg/m²: 30 kcal/kg	
	BMI 25–30 kg/m²: 25 kcal/kg	
	BMI > 30 kg/m² : 20 kcal/kg	
Energy — indirect calorimetry	Measured resting energy expenditure (REE)	Measured REE × Activity Factor 10 to 20%
Protein	1.5 to 2.0 g/kg	1.5 to 2.5 g /kg/d, depending on TBSA
	(actual body weight, unless obese, then adjusted body weight is used)	20 to 25% of total calories glutamine: 0.5 g/kg/d up to 40 g/d
Carbohydrate	Include fiber except in patients at risk of small bowel obstruction/ischemia	50 to 60% of total calories
Fat		20 to 25% of total calories

immune-modulating nutrition should not be used. Fiber-free enteral formulas should be used in patients at risk of small bowel obstruction. Positioning patients in an upright supine position is important in promoting gastric emptying and preventing aspiration pneumonia. In those who develop high gastric residuals, a promotility agent, such as metoclopramide, should be used [177], and if feeding intolerance continues, postpyloric access should be obtained. Concomitant use of parenteral nutrition should be avoided.

CONCLUSIONS

Nutrition is an integral component of the care for patients with burns, trauma, or sepsis, as it influences morbidity and mortality. Significant alterations in metabolism and immune function that occur and their interaction with nutrition support continue to be investigated. Continued progress in studying the roles of various nutrients and drug and treatment interventions in ameliorating the effects of burn injury and sepsis will result in improved wound healing and survival outcomes.

ACKNOWLEDGMENTS

The authors would like to thank Cathy Alberda, R.D., MSc for her review and comments, as well as Heather Shankowsky, R.N., for her assistance with organizing and formatting the references. This project was funded by the Alberta Heritage Foundation for Medical Research (AHFMR), Canadian Institutes of Health Research (CIHR), and the Firefighters' Burn Trust Fund of the University of Alberta (FFBTF).

REFERENCES

1. Tredget, E.E. and Y.M. Yu, The metabolic effects of thermal injury, *World J. Surg.*, 16(1): 68–79, 1992.
2. Feller, I., D. Tholan, and R.G. Cornell, Improvements in burn care, *JAMA*, 244(18), 2074–2078, 1980.
3. Department of Health, E.A.W., Reports of the Epidemiology and Surveillance of Injuries. Atlanta: Centers for Disease Control, DHEW Publication No. (HSM), 1982, pp. 73–10001.
4. Deitch, E.A., The management of burns, *N. Engl. J. Med.*, 323(18), 1249–1253, 1990.
5. Cuthbertson, D.P., The disturbance of metabolism produced by bony and non-bony injury, with notes on certain abnormal conditions of bone, *Biochem. J.*, 24(4), 1244–1247, 1930.
6. Kinney, J.M., Metabolic Responses of the Critically Ill Patient. Medical Clinics of North America, 11(Nutrition in the critically injured patient), 1995, pp. 569–585.
7. Deitch, E.A., Multiple organ failure — pathophysiology and potential future therapy, *Ann. Surg.*, 216, 117–134, 1992.
8. O'Riordain, D.S. et al., Interleukin-2 receptor expression and function following thermal injury, *Arch. Surg.*, 130(2), 165–170, 1995.
9. Franke, A. et al., Proinflammatory and antiinflammatory cytokines after cardiac operation: different cellular sources at different times, *Ann. Thorac. Surg.*, 74(2), 363–370; discussion 370–371, 2002.
10. Plackett, T.P. et al., Aging enhances lymphocyte cytokine defects after injury, *FASEB J.*, 17(6), 688–689, 2003.

11. Carswell, E.A. et al., An endotoxin induced serum factor that causes necrosis of tumors, *Proc. Natl. Acad. Sci. U.S.A.*, 72(9), 3666–3670, 1975.

12. Beutler, B.A. et al., Purification of cachectin: a lipoprotein lipase suppressing hormone secreted by endotoxin induced RAW 264.7 cells, *J. Exp. Med.*, 161, 989–994, 1985.

13. Beutler, B.A., D. Greenwald, and J.D. Hulmes, Identity of tumor necrosis factor and the macrophage-secreted factor cachectin, *Nature*, 316, 552–554, 1985.

14. Beutler, B.A., I.W. Milsark, and A. Cerami, Cachectin/tumor necrosis factor: production, distribution and metabolic rate *in vivo*, *J. Immunol.*, 135, 3972–3977, 1985.

15. Hesse, D.G., K.J. Tracey, and Y. Fong, Cytokine appearance in human endotoxemia and primate bacteremia, *Surg. Gynecol. Obstet.*, 166(2), 147–153, 1988.

16. Michie, H.R., K.R. Manogue, and D.R. Spriggs, Detection of circulating tumor necrosis factor after endotoxin administration, *N. Engl. J. Med.*, 318(23), 1481–1486, 1988.

17. Starnes, H.F. Jr., et al., Anti-IL-6 monoclonal antibodies protect against lethal *Escherichia coli* infection and lethal tumor necrosis factor- challenge in mice, *J. Immunol.*, 145(12), 4185–4191, 1990.

18. Flores, E.A. et al., Infusion of tumor necrosis factor/cachectin promotes muscle catabolism in the rat. A synergistic effect with interleukin 1, *J. Clin. Invest.*, 83(5), 1614–1622, 1989.

19. Hall-Angeras, M. et al., Interaction between corticosterone and tumor necrosis factor stimulated protein breakdown in rat skeletal muscle, similar to sepsis, *Surgery*, 108(2), 460–466, 1990.

20. Mealy, K. et al., Are the catabolic effects of tumor necrosis factor mediated by glucocorticoids? *Arch. Surg.*, 125(1), 42–47; discussion 47–48, 1990.

21. Dinarello, C.A., Biology of interleukin 1, *FASEB J.*, 2(2), 108–115, 1988.

22. Dinarello, C.A., Interleukin-1 and interleukin-1 antagonism, *Blood*, 77(8), 1627–1652, 1991.

23. Wilmore, D.W. et al., Catecholamines: mediator of the hypermetabolic response to thermal injury, *Ann. Surg.*, 180(4), 653–669, 1974.

24. Dinarello, C.A. et al., Tumor necrosis factor (cachectin) is an endogenous pyrogen and induces production of interleukin 1, *J. Exp. Med.*, 163(6), 1433–1450, 1986.

25. Tredget, E.E. et al., Role of interleukin 1 and tumor necrosis factor on energy metabolism in rabbits, *Am. J. Physiol.*, 255(6 Pt. 1), E760–E768, 1988.

26. Tadros, T. et al., Effects of interleukin-1 administration on intestinal ischemia and reperfusion injury, mucosal permeability, and bacterial translocation in burn and sepsis, *Ann. Surg.*, 237(1), 101–109, 2003.

27. Warren, R.S. et al., The acute metabolic effects of tumor necrosis factor administration in humans, *Arch. Surg.*, 122(12), 1396–1400, 1987.

28. Fong, Y. et al., Cachectin/TNF or IL-1 induces cachexia with redistribution of body proteins, *Am. J. Physiol.*, 256(3 Pt. 2), R659–R665, 1989.

29. Castell, J.V. et al., Interleukin-6 is the major regulator of acute phase protein synthesis in adult human hepatocytes, *FEBS Lett.*, 242(2), 237–239, 1989.

30. Castell, J.V. et al., Acute-phase response of human hepatocytes: regulation of acute-phase protein synthesis by interleukin-6, *Hepatology*, 12(5), 1179–1186, 1990.

31. Gauldie, J. et al., Interferon 2/B-cell stimulatory factor type 2 shares identity with monocyte-derived hepatocyte-stimulating factor and regulates the major acute phase protein response in liver cells, *Proc. Natl. Acad. Sci. U.S.A.*, 84(20), 7251–7255, 1987.

32. Guo, Y. et al., Increased levels of circulating interleukin 6 in burn patients, *Clin. Immunol. Immunopathol.*, 54(3), 361–371, 1990.

33. de Bandt, J.P. et al., Cytokine response to burn injury: relationship with protein metabolism, *J. Trauma*, 36(5), 624–628, 1994.

34. Ertel, W. et al., The complex pattern of cytokines in sepsis. Association between prostaglandins, cachectin, and interleukins, *Ann. Surg.*, 214(2), 141–148, 1991.

35. Fearon, K.C. et al., Elevated circulating interleukin-6 is associated with an acute-phase response but reduced fixed hepatic protein synthesis in patients with cancer, *Ann. Surg.*, 213(1), 26–31, 1991.

36. Hack, C.E. et al., Increased plasma levels of interleukin-6 in sepsis, *Blood*, 74(5), 1704–1710, 1989.

37. Ayala, A. et al., Differential alterations in plasma IL-6 and TNF levels after trauma and hemorrhage, *Am. J. Physiol.*, 260(1 Pt. 2), R167–R171, 1991.

38. Souba, W.W., Cytokine control of nutrition and metabolism in critical illness, *Curr. Probl. Surg.*, 31(7), 577–643, 1994.

39. Cousins, R.J. and A.S. Leinart, Tissue-specific regulation of zinc metabolism and metallothionein genes by interleukin 1, *FASEB J.*, 2(13), 2884–2890, 1988.

40. Huber, K.L. and R.J. Cousins, Maternal zinc deprivation and interleukin-1 influence metallothionein gene expression and zinc metabolism of rats, *J. Nutr.*, 118(12), 1570–1576, 1988.

41. Helyar, L. and A.R. Sherman, Iron deficiency and interleukin 1 production by rat leukocytes, *Am. J. Clin. Nutr.*, 46(2), 346–352, 1987.

42. Prasad, A.S. et al., Serum thymulin in human zinc deficiency, *J. Clin. Invest.*, 82(4), 1202–1210, 1988.

43. Bessey, P.Q. et al., Combined hormonal infusion simulates the metabolic response to injury, *Ann. Surg.*, 200(3), 264–281, 1984.

44. Levy, B. et al., Dobutamine improves the adequacy of gastric mucosal perfusion in epinephrine-treated septic shock, *Crit. Care Med.*, 25(10), 1649–1654, 1997.

45. Marik, P.E. and M. Mohedin, The contrasting effects of dopamine and norepinephrine on systemic and splanchnic oxygen utilization in hyperdynamic sepsis, *JAMA*, 272(17), 1354–1357, 1994.

46. Fruhwald, S. et al., Low potential of dobutamine and dopexamine to block intestinal peristalsis as compared with other catecholamines, *Crit. Care Med.*, 28(8), 2893–2897, 2000.

47. Trager, K., P. Radermacher, and X. Leverve, The adrenergic coin: perfusion and metabolism, *Intensive Care Med.*, 29(2), 150–153, 2003.

48. Fruhwald, S. et al., Sufentanil potentiates the inhibitory effect of epinephrine on intestinal motility, *Intensive Care Med.*, 28(1), 74–80, 2002.

49. Knabl, J.S. et al., Progression of burn wound depth by systemical application of a vasoconstrictor: an experimental study with a new rabbit model, *Burns*, 25(8), 715–721, 1999.

50. Debaveye, Y.A. and G.H. Van den Berghe, Is there still a place for dopamine in the modern intensive care unit? *Anesth. Analg.*, 98(2), 461–468, 2004.

51. Winter, W. et al., Hydrocortisone improved haemodynamics and fluid requirement in surviving but not non-surviving of severely burned patients, *Burns*, 29(7), 717–720, 2003.

52. Astiz, M.E. and E.C. Rackow, Septic shock, *Lancet*, 351(9114), 1501–1505, 1998.

53. Bernard, G.R. et al., Efficacy and safety of recombinant human activated protein C for severe sepsis, *N. Engl. J. Med.*, 344(10), 699–709, 2001.

54. Barret, J.P. and D.N. Herndon, Modulation of inflammatory and catabolic responses in severely burned children by early burn wound excision in the first 24 hours, *Arch. Surg.*, 138(2), 127–132, 2003.

55. Cunningham, J.J. et al., Measured and predicted calorie requirements of adults during recovery from severe burn trauma, *Am. J. Clin. Nutr.*, 49(3), 404–408, 1989.

56. Gump, F.E. and J.M. Kinney, Energy balance and weight loss in burned patients, *Arch. Surg.*, 103(4), 442–448, 1971.

57. Ireton, C.S. et al., Evaluation of energy expenditures in burn patients, *J. Am. Diet. Assoc.*, 86(3), 331–333, 1986.

58. Saffle, J.R. et al., Use of indirect calorimetry in the nutritional management of burned patients, *J. Trauma*, 25(1), 32–39, 1985.

59. Phang, P.T., T. Rich, and J. Ronco, A validation and comparison study of two metabolic monitors, *J. Parenter. Enteral Nutr.*, 14(3), 259–261, 1990.

60. Barton, R.G. et al., Chemical paralysis reduces energy expenditure in patients with burns and severe respiratory failure treated with mechanical ventilation, *J. Burn Care Rehabil.*, 18(5), 461–468; discussion 460, 1997.

61. Terao, Y. et al., Quantitative analysis of the relationship between sedation and resting energy expenditure in postoperative patients, *Crit. Care Med.*, 31(3), 830–833, 2003.

62. McCall, M. et al., Effect of neuromuscular blockade on energy expenditure in patients with severe head injury, *J. Parenter. Enteral Nutr.*, 27(1), 27–35, 2003.

63. Herndon, D.N. et al., Reversal of catabolism by -blockade after severe burns, *N. Engl. J. Med.*, 345(17), 1223–1229, 2001.

64. Wolfe, R.R. et al., Effect of severe burn injury on substrate cycling by glucose and fatty acids, *N. Engl. J. Med.*, 317(7), 403–408, 1987.

65. Barrow, R.E., R.R Wolfe, et al. The use of beta-adrenergic blockage in preventing trauma-induced hepatomegaly. *Ann. Surg.*, 243(1), 115–120, 2006.

66. Gore, D.C. et al., Influence of fever on the hypermetabolic response in burn-injured children, *Arch. Surg.*, 138(2), 169–174; discussion 174, 2003.

67. Kelemen, J.J., III et al., Effect of ambient temperature on metabolic rate after thermal injury, *Ann. Surg.*, 223(4), 406–412, 1996.

68. Bardutzky, J. et al., Energy expenditure in ischemic stroke patients treated with moderate hypothermia, *Intensive Care Med.*, 30(1), 151–154, 2004.

69. Alberda, C. et al., Energy requirements in critically ill patients: how close are our estimates? *Nutr. in Clin. Prac.*, 17(1), 38–42, 2002.

70. Swinamer, D.L. et al., Twenty-four hour energy expenditure in critically ill patients, *Crit. Care Med.*, 15(7), 637–643, 1987.

71. McClave, S.A. et al., Clinical use of the respiratory quotient obtained from indirect calorimetry, *J. Parenter. Enteral Nutr.*, 27(1), 21–26, 2003.

72. Hart, D.W. et al., Energy expenditure and caloric balance after burn: increased feeding leads to fat rather than lean mass accretion, *Ann. Surg.*, 235(1), 152–161, 2002.

73. Barak, N., E. Wall-Alonso, and M.D. Sitrin, Evaluation of stress factors and body weight adjustments currently used to estimate energy expenditure in hospitalized patients, *J. Parenter. Enteral Nutr.*, 26(4), 231–238, 2002.

74. El-Solh, A. et al., Morbid obesity in the medical ICU, *Chest*, 120(6), 1989–1997, 2001.

75. Gottschlich, M.M. et al., Significance of obesity on nutritional, immunologic, hormonal, and clinical outcome parameters in burns, *J. Am. Diet. Assoc.*, 93(11), 1261–1268, 1993.

76. Kabon, B. et al., Obesity decreases perioperative tissue oxygenation, *Anesthesiology*, 100(2), 274–280, 2004.

77. Greif, R. et al., Supplemental perioperative oxygen to reduce the incidence of surgical-wound infection. Outcomes Research Group, *N. Engl. J. Med.*, 342(3), 161–167, 2000.

78. Tremblay, A. and V. Bandi, Impact of body mass index on outcomes following critical care, *Chest*, 123(4), 1202–1207, 2003.

79. Rubinson, L. et al., Low caloric intake is associated with nosocomial bloodstream infections in patients in the medical intensive care unit, *Crit. Care Med.*, 32(2), 350–357, 2004.

80. Klein, C.J., G.S. Stanek, and C.E. Wiles, III, Overfeeding macronutrients to critically ill adults: metabolic complications, *J. Am. Diet. Assoc.*, 98(7), 795–806, 1998.

81. Schloerb, P.R. and J.F. Henning, Patterns and problems of adult total parenteral nutrition use in US academic medical centers, *Arch. Surg.*, 133(1), 7–12, 1998.

82. Raina, N. et al., Effect of nutrition on tumor necrosis factor receptors in weight-gaining and -losing rats, *Am. J. Physiol.*, 277(3 Pt. 1), E464–E473, 1999.

83. Raina, N. and K.N. Jeejeebhoy, Effect of low-protein diet and protein supplementation on the expressions of TNF-α, TNFR-I, and TNFR-II in organs and muscle of LPS-injected rats, *Am. J. Physiol. Endocrinol. Metab.*, 286(3), E481–E487, 2004.

84. Krishnan, J.A. et al., Caloric intake in medical ICU patients: consistency of care with guidelines and relationship to clinical outcomes, *Chest*, 124(1), 297–305, 2003.

85. Dickerson, R.N. et al., Hypocaloric enteral tube feeding in critically ill obese patients, *Nutrition*, 18(3), 241–246, 2002.

86. Noordenbos, J. et al., Enteral nutritional support and wound excision and closure do not prevent postburn hypermetabolism as measured by continuous metabolic monitoring, *J. Trauma*, 49(4), 667–671; discussion 671–672, 2000.

87. Chang, Y.H. and M.D. Peck, Nutrition in sepsis and infection, in *The Science and Practice of Nutrition Support: A Case-Based Core Curriculum*, Gottschlich, M.M., Ed., Dubuque, IA; Kendall/Hunt, 2001, p. 469.

88. Levenson, S.M. and A.A. Demetrious, Metabolic Factors, in *Wound Healing: Biochemical and Clinical Aspects*, I.K. Cohen, R.F. Diegelmann, and W.J. Lindblad, Eds., Toronto: W.B. Saunders, 1992, p. 250.

89. Raina, N. and K.N. Jeejeebhoy, Effect of low protein diet and protein supplementation on the expressions of TNF-α, TNFR-1 and TNFR-11 in organs and muscle of LPS injected rats, *Am. J. Physiol. Endocrinol. Metab.*, 286(3), E481–487, 2004.

90. Kinney, J.M. and D.H. Elwyn, Protein metabolism and injury, *Annu. Rev. Nutr.*, 3, 433–466, 1983.

91. Mullen, J.L., Consequences of malnutrition in the surgical patient, *Surg. Clin. North Am.*, 61(3), 465–487, 1981.

92. Moore, F.D. and M.F. Brennan, Surgical injury, in *Manual of Surgical Nutrition*, F.D. Bellinger, Ed., Philadelphia: Saunders, 1975.

93. Alexander, J.W. et al., Beneficial effects of aggressive protein feeding in severely burned children, *Ann. Surg.*, 192(4), 505–517, 1980.

94. Bell, S.J. et al., Adequacy of a modular tube feeding diet for burned patients, *J. Am. Diet. Assoc.*, 86(10), 1386–1391, 1986.

95. Jahoor, F. et al., Dynamics of the protein metabolic response to burn injury, *Metabolism*, 37(4), 330–337, 1988.

96. Yu, Y.M. et al., Comparative evaluation of the quantitative utilization of parenterally and enterally administered leucine and L-[1-13C,15N]leucine within the whole body and the splanchnic region, *J. Parenter. Enteral Nutr.*, 19(3), 209–215, 1995.

97. Yu, Y.M. et al., Plasma arginine and leucine kinetics and urea production rates in burn patients, *Metabolism*, 44(5), 659–666, 1995.

98. Yu, Y.M. et al., Relations among arginine, citrulline, ornithine, and leucine kinetics in adult burn patients, *Am. J. Clin. Nutr.*, 62(5), 960–968, 1995.

99. Clague, M.B. et al., The effects of nutrition and trauma on whole-body protein metabolism in man, *Clin. Sci. (London)*, 65(2), 165–175, 1983.

100. Jurasinski, C.V. and T.C. Vary, Insulin-like growth factor I accelerates protein synthesis in skeletal muscle during sepsis, *Am. J. Physiol.*, 269(5 Pt. 1), E977–E981, 1995.

101. Breuille, D. et al., Pentoxifylline decreases body weight loss and muscle protein wasting characteristics of sepsis, *Am. J. Physiol.*, 265(4 Pt. 1), E660–E666, 1993.

102. Bergstrom, J. et al., Intracellular free amino acid concentration in human muscle tissue, *J. Appl. Physiol.*, 36(6), 693–697, 1974.

103. Smith, R.J., Regulation of protein degradation in differentiated skeletal muscle cells in monolayer culture, in *Intracellular Protein Catabolism, Progress in Clinical and Biological Research*, Vol. 180, E.A. Khairallah, J.S. Bond, and J.W.C. Bird, Eds., New York: A.R. Liss, 1984, pp. 633–635.

104. Rennie, M.J. et al., Characteristics of a glutamine carrier in skeletal muscle have important consequences for nitrogen loss in injury, infection, and chronic disease, *Lancet*, 2(8514), 1008–1012, 1986.

105. Jepson, M.M. et al., Relationship between glutamine concentration and protein synthesis in rat skeletal muscle, *Am. J. Physiol.*, 255(2 Pt. 1), E166–E172, 1988.

106. MacLennan, P.A., R.A. Brown, and M.J. Rennie, A positive relationship between protein synthetic rate and intracellular glutamine concentration in perfused rat skeletal muscle, *FEBS Lett.*, 215(1), 187–191, 1987.

107. Stumvoll, M. et al., Role of glutamine in human carbohydrate metabolism in kidney and other tissues, *Kidney Int.*, 55(3), 778–792, 1999.

108. Mittendorfer, B. et al., Accelerated glutamine synthesis in critically ill patients cannot maintain normal intramuscular free glutamine concentration, *J. Parenter. Enteral Nutr.*, 23(5), 243–250; discussion 250–252, 1999.

109. Parry-Billings, M. et al., Does glutamine contribute to immunosuppression after major burns? *Lancet*, 336(8714), 523–525, 1990.

110. Ardawi, M.S., Glutamine and glucose metabolism in human peripheral lymphocytes, *Metabolism*, 37(1), 99–103, 1988.

111. Ogle, C.K. et al., Effect of glutamine on phagocytosis and bacterial killing by normal and pediatric burn patient neutrophils, *J. Parenter. Enteral Nutr.*, 18(2), 128–133, 1994.

112. Houdijk, A.P. et al., Glutamine-enriched enteral diet increases renal arginine production, *J. Parenter. Enteral Nutr.*, 18(5), 422–426, 1994.

113. Newsholme, E.A. et al., A role for muscle in the immune system and its importance in surgery, trauma, sepsis and burns, *Nutr. Int.*, 4, 261–268, 1988.

114. Newsholme, E.A. and E.A. Leech, Regulation of glucose and fatty acid oxidation in relation to energy demand in muscle, in *Biochemistry for the Medical Sciences*, Newsholme, E.A. and E.A. Leech, Eds., Chichester: John Wiley & Sons, 1983, pp. 99–113.

115. Newsholme, E.A., B. Crabtree, and M.S. Ardawi, Glutamine metabolism in lymphocytes: its biochemical, physiological and clinical importance, *Q. J. Exp. Physiol.*, 70(4), 473–489, 1985.

116. Newsholme, E.A., P. Newsholme, and R. Curi, The role of the citric acid cycle in cells of the immune system and its importance in sepsis, trauma and burns, *Biochem. Soc. Symp.*, 54, 145–162, 1987.

117. Newsholme, E.A., B. Crabtree, and M.S. Ardawi, The role of high rates of glycolysis and glutamine utilization in rapidly dividing cells, *Biosci. Rep.*, 5(5), 393–400, 1985.

118. Newsholme, E.A. and M. Parry-Billings, Properties of glutamine release from muscle and its importance for the immune system, *J. Parenter. Enteral Nutr.*, 14(4 Suppl.), 63S–67S, 1990.

119. Jahoor, F. et al., Role of insulin and glucose oxidation in mediating the protein catabolism of burns and sepsis, *Am. J. Physiol.*, 257(3 Pt. 1), E323–E331, 1989.

120. Gore, D.C. and R.R. Wolfe, Metabolic response of muscle to alanine, glutamine, and valine supplementation during severe illness, *J. Parenter. Enteral Nutr.*, 27(5), 307–314, 2003.

121. Exner, R. et al., Perioperative GLY-GLN infusion diminishes the surgery-induced period of immunosuppression: accelerated restoration of the lipopolysaccharide-stimulated tumor necrosis factor-α response, *Ann. Surg.*, 237(1), 110–115, 2003.

122. Dimarchi, R.D. et al., Weak acid-catalyzed pyrrolidone carboxylic acid formation from glutamine during solid phase peptide synthesis. Minimization by rapid coupling, *Int. J. Pept. Protein Res.*, 19(1), 88–93, 1982.

123. Stehle, P., I. Ratz, and P. Furst, *In vivo* utilization of intravenously supplied L-alanyl-L-glutamine in various tissues of the rat, *Nutrition*, 5(6), 411–415, 1989.

124. Adibi, S.A., Experimental basis for use of peptides as substrates for parenteral nutrition: a review, *Metabolism*, 36(10), 1001–1011, 1987.

125. Furst, P., S. Albers, and P. Stehle, Glutamine-containing dipeptides in parenteral nutrition, *J. Parenter. Enteral Nutr.*, 14(4 Suppl.), 118S–124S, 1990.

126. Hammarqvist, F. et al., Addition of glutamine to total parenteral nutrition after elective abdominal surgery spares free glutamine in muscle, counteracts the fall in muscle protein synthesis, and improves nitrogen balance, *Ann. Surg.*, 209(4), 455–461, 1989.

127. Stehle, P. et al., Effect of parenteral glutamine peptide supplements on muscle glutamine loss and nitrogen balance after major surgery, *Lancet*, 1(8632), 231–233, 1989.

128. Ziegler, T.R. et al., Safety and metabolic effects of L-glutamine administration in humans, *J. Parenter. Enteral Nutr.*, 14(4 Suppl.), 137S–146S, 1990.

129. Grant, J.P. and P.J. Snyder, Use of L-glutamine in total parenteral nutrition, *J. Surg. Res.*, 44(5), 506–513, 1988.

130. Boelens, P.G. et al., Glutamine alimentation in catabolic state, *J. Nutr.*, 131(9 Suppl.), p. 2569S–2577S; discussion 2590S, 2001.

131. Griffiths, R.D., C. Jones, and T.E. Palmer, Six-month outcome of critically ill patients given glutamine-supplemented parenteral nutrition, *Nutrition*, 13(4), 295–302, 1997.

132. Griffiths, R.D., Outcome of critically ill patients after supplementation with glutamine, *Nutrition*, 13(7–8), 752–754, 1997.

133. Wischmeyer, P.E. et al., Glutamine administration reduces Gram-negative bacteremia in severely burned patients: a prospective, randomized, double-blind trial versus isonitrogenous control, *Crit. Care Med.*, 29(11), 2075–2080, 2001.

134. Garrel, D.R. and J. Bernier, Decreased mortality and infectious morbidity in adult burn patients with enteral glutamine supplements, *Clin. Nutr.*, 22(S1), S78, 2003.

135. Garlick, P.J., Assessment of the safety of glutamine and other amino acids, *J. Nutr.*, 131(9 Suppl.), 2556S–2561S, 2001.

136. Heyland, D.K. et al., Nutrition support in the critical care setting: current practice in canadian ICUs — opportunities for improvement? *J. Parenter. Enteral Nutr.*, 27(1), 74–83, 2003.

137. Castillo, L. et al., Plasma arginine kinetics in adult man: response to an arginine-free diet, *Metabolism*, 43(1), 114–122, 1994.

138. Seifter, E. et al., Arginine: an essential amino acid for injured rats, *Surgery*, 84(2), 224–230, 1978.

139. Kirk, S.J. and A. Barbul, Role of arginine in trauma, sepsis, and immunity, *J. Parenter. Enteral Nutr.*, 14(5 Suppl.), 226S–229S, 1990.

140. Wang, R. et al., Human dermal fibroblasts produce nitric oxide and express both constitutive and inducible nitric oxide synthase isoforms, *J. Invest. Dermatol.*, 106(3), 419–427, 1996.

141. Shi, H.P. et al., Supplemental dietary arginine enhances wound healing in normal but not inducible nitric oxide synthase knockout mice, *Surgery*, 128(2), 374–378, 2000.

142. Muscara, M.N. et al., Wound collagen deposition in rats: effects of an NO-NSAID and a selective COX-2 inhibitor, *Br. J. Pharmacol.*, 129(4), 681–686, 2000.

143. Wang, R. et al., Nitric oxide synthase expression and nitric oxide production are reduced in hypertrophic scar tissue and fibroblasts, *J. Invest. Dermatol.*, 108(4), 438–444, 1997.

144. Cohen, P.R., Y.D. Eliezri, and D.N. Silvers, Athlete's nodules: sports-related connective tissue nevi of the collagen type (collagenomas), *Cutis*, 50(2), 131–135, 1992.

145. Barbul, A., Arginine: biochemistry, physiology, and therapeutic implications, *J. Parenter. Enteral Nutr.*, 10(2), 227–238, 1986.

146. Barbul, A. et al., Metabolic and immune effects of arginine in postinjury hyperalimentation, *J. Trauma*, 21(11), 970–974, 1981.

147. Saito, H. et al., Metabolic and immune effects of dietary arginine supplementation after burn, *Arch. Surg.*, 122(7), 784–789, 1987.

148. Alexander, J.W. and M.M. Gottschlich, Nutritional immunomodulation in burn patients, *Crit. Care Med.*, 18(2 Suppl.), S149–S153, 1990.

149. Daly, J.M. et al., Immune and metabolic effects of arginine in the surgical patient, *Ann. Surg.*, 208(4), 512–523, 1988.

150. Barbul, A. et al., Optimal levels of arginine in maintenance intravenous hyperalimentation, *J. Parenter. Enteral Nutr.*, 8(3), 281–284, 1984.

151. Barbul, A. et al., Arginine stimulates thymic immune function and ameliorates the obesity and the hyperglycemia of genetically obese mice, *J. Parenter. Enteral Nutr.*, 5(6), 492–495, 1981.

152. Daly, J.M. et al., Enteral nutrition with supplemental arginine, RNA, and omega-3 fatty acids in patients after operation: immunologic, metabolic, and clinical outcome, *Surgery*, 112(1), 56–67, 1992.

153. Elsair, J., J. Poey, and H. Isaad, Effect of arginine chlohydrate on nitrogen balance during the three days following routine surgery in man, *Biomed. Press*, 29, 312–317, 1978.

154. Carter, E.A. et al., Nitric oxide production is intensely and persistently increased in tissue by thermal injury, *Biochem. J.*, 304 (Pt. 1), 201–204, 1994.

155. Goode, H.F. et al., Nitric oxide synthase activity is increased in patients with sepsis syndrome, *Clin. Sci. (London)*, 88(2), 131–133, 1995.

156. Ochoa, J.B. et al., Nitrogen oxide levels in patients after trauma and during sepsis, *Ann. Surg.*, 214(5), 621–626, 1991.

157. Szabo, C., Alterations in nitric oxide production in various forms of circulatory shock, *New Horiz.*, 3(1), 2–32, 1995.

158. Persson, M.G. et al., Endogenous nitric oxide as a probable modulator of pulmonary circulation and hypoxic pressor response *in vivo*, *Acta Physiol. Scand.*, 140(4), 449–457, 1990.

159. Moncada, S. and A. Higgs, The L-arginine-nitric oxide pathway, *N. Engl. J. Med.*, 329(27), 2002–2012, 1993.

160. Harbrecht, B.G. et al., Inhibition of nitric oxide synthesis during endotoxemia promotes intrahepatic thrombosis and an oxygen radical-mediated hepatic injury, *J. Leukoc. Biol.*, 52(4), 390–394, 1992.

161. Bode-Boger, S.M. et al., L-arginine infusion decreases peripheral arterial resistance and inhibits platelet aggregation in healthy subjects, *Clin. Sci. (London)*, 87(3), 303–310, 1994.

162. Kharitonov, S.A. et al., L-arginine increases exhaled nitric oxide in normal human subjects, *Clin. Sci. (London)*, 88(2), 135–139, 1995.

163. Lorente, J.A. et al., L-arginine pathway in the sepsis syndrome, *Crit. Care Med.*, 21(9), 1287–1295, 1993.

164. Kelly, E., S.M. Morris, Jr., and T.R. Billiar, Nitric oxide, sepsis, and arginine metabolism, *J. Parenter. Enteral Nutr.*, 19(3), 234–238, 1995.

165. Beaumier, L. et al., Urea cycle intermediate kinetics and nitrate excretion at normal and "therapeutic" intakes of arginine in humans, *Am. J. Physiol.*, 269(5 Pt. 1), E884–E896, 1995.

166. Murrell, G.A. et al., Modulation of tendon healing by nitric oxide, *Inflamm. Res.*, 46(1), 19–27, 1997.

167. Diwan, A.D. et al., Nitric oxide modulates fracture healing, *J. Bone Miner. Res.*, 15(2), 342–351, 2000.

168. Zhu, W. et al., Nitric oxide synthase isoforms during fracture healing, *J. Bone Miner. Res.*, 16(3), 535–540, 2001.

169. Lin, J. et al., The cell specific temporal expression of nitric oxide synthase isoforms during achilles tendon healing, *Inflamm. Res.*, 50(10), 515–522, 2001.

170. Logothetis, C.J. et al., Escalated therapy for refractory urothelial tumors: methotrexate-vinblastine-doxorubicin-cisplatin plus unglycosylated recombinant human granulocyte-macrophage colony-stimulating factor, *J. Natl. Cancer Inst.*, 82(8), 667–672, 1990.

171. Cynober, L., Can arginine and ornithine support gut functions? *Gut*, 35(1 Suppl.), S42–S45, 1994.

172. Preiser, J.C. et al., Metabolic effects of arginine addition to the enteral feeding of critically ill patients, *J. Parenter. Enteral Nutr.*, 25(4), 182–187, 2001.

173. Saffle, J.R. et al., Randomized trial of immune-enhancing enteral nutrition in burn patients, *J. Trauma*, 42(5), 793–800; discussion 800–802, 1997.

174. Heyland, D.K. and F. Novak, Immunonutrition in the critically ill patient: more harm than good? *J. Parenter. Enteral Nutr.*, 25(2 Suppl.), S51–S55; discussion S55–S56, 2001.

175. Bertolini, G. et al., Early enteral immunonutrition in patients with severe sepsis: results of an interim analysis of a randomized multicentre clinical trial, *Intensive Care Med.*, 29(5), 834–840, 2003.

176. Jabbar, A. et al., Gut immunology and the differential repsonse to feeding and starvation, *Nutr. in Clin. Prac.*, 18, 461–482, 2003.

177. Heyland, D.K. et al., Canadian clinical practice guidelines for nutrition support in mechanically ventilated, critically ill adult patients, *J. Parenter. Enteral Nutr.*, 27(5), 355–373, 2003.

178. Coudray-Lucas, C. et al., Ornithine α-ketoglutarate improves wound healing in severe burn patients: a prospective randomized double-blind trial versus isonitrogenous controls, *Crit. Care Med.*, 28(6), 1772–1776, 2000.

179. Gottschlich, M.M. et al., Differential effects of three enteral dietary regimens on selected outcome variables in burn patients, *J. Parenter. Enteral Nutr.*, 14(3), 225–236, 1990.

180. Garrel, D.R. et al., Improved clinical status and length of care with low-fat nutrition support in burn patients, *J. Parenter. Enteral Nutr.*, 19(6), 482–491, 1995.

181. Gottschlich, M.M. et al., Diarrhea in tube-fed burn patients: incidence, etiology, nutritional impact, and prevention, *J. Parenter. Enteral Nutr.*, 12(4), 338–345, 1988.

182. Kamolz, L.P. et al., Treatment of patients with severe burn injuries: the impact of schizophrenia, *Burns*, 29(1), 49–53, 2003.
183. Mayes, P.A., Metabolism of lipids in *Harper's Review of Biochemistry*, 18th ed., D.W. Martin, P.A. Mayes, and V.W. Rodwell, Eds., Los Altos: Lange, 1981.
184. Blackburn, G.L. and S.D. Phinney, Lipid metabolism in injury, in *Surgical Physiology*, J.F. Burke, Ed., Philadelphia: Saunders, 1983.
185. Reaven, G.M. et al., Kinetics of triglyceride turnover of very low density lipoproteins of human plasma, *J. Clin. Invest.*, 44(11), 1826–1833, 1965.
186. Boberg, J., L.A. Carlson, and L. Normell, Production of lipolytic activity by the isolated, perfused dog liver in response to heparin, *Life Sci.*, 18 (3), 1011–1019, 1964.
187. Krauss, R.M. et al., Selective measurement of two different triglyceride lipase activities in rat postheparin plasma, *J. Lipid Res.*, 14(3), 286–295, 1973.
188. Galster, A.D. et al., Plasma palmitate turnover in subjects with thermal injury, *J. Trauma*, 24(11), 938–945, 1984.
189. Wolfe, R.R., Metabolic response to burn injury: nutritional implications, *Semin. Nephrol.*, 13(4), 382–390, 1993.
190. Black, P.R. et al., Mechanisms of insulin resistance following injury, *Ann. Surg.*, 196(4), 420–435, 1982.
191. Hales, C.N., J.P. Luzio, and K. Siddle, Hormonal control of adipose-tissue lipolysis, *Biochem. Soc. Symp.*, (43), 97–135, 1978.
192. Steinberg, D., Interconvertible enzymes in adipose tissue regulated by cyclic AMP-dependent protein kinase, *Adv. Cyclic Nucleotide Res.*, 7, 157–198, 1976.
193. Tredget, E.E. and J.F. Burke, Caloric and substrate requirements in trauma and sepsis, in *Trauma, Sepsis and Shock*, G.H.A. Clowes, Ed., New York: Marcel Dekker, 1988, pp. 269–305.
194. Burr, G.O. and M.M. Burr, A new deficiency disease produced by the rigid exclusion of fat from the diet, *J. Biol. Chem.*, 243, 14705–14709, 1968.
195. Ziboh, V.A. and S.L. Hsia, Effects of prostaglandin E 2 on rat skin: inhibition of sterol ester biosynthesis and clearing of scaly lesions in essential fatty acid deficiency, *J. Lipid Res.*, 13(4), 458–467, 1972.
196. Holman, R.T., Essential fatty acid deficiency in humans, in *Dietary Lipids and Postnatal Development*, C. Galli, Ed., New York: Raven Press, 1973, p. 127.
197. Rivers, J.P., A.J. Sinclair, and M.A. Craqford, Inability of the cat to desaturate essential fatty acids, *Nature*, 258(5531), 171–173, 1975.
198. Collins, F.D. et al., Plasma lipids in human linoleic acid deficiency, *Nutr. Metab.*, 13(3), 150–167, 1971.
199. Holman, R.T., Esstential fatty acid deficiency, in *Progress in the Chemistry of Fats and other Lipids*, Vol. 9, Part 2, R.T. Holman, Ed., Oxford: Pergamon Press, 1968, pp. 329–334.
200. Barr, L.H., G.D. Dunn, and M.F. Brennan, Essential fatty acid deficiency during total parenteral nutrition, *Ann. Surg.*, 193(3), 304–311, 1981.
201. Sinclair, H.M., Essential fatty acids in perspective, *Hum. Nutr. Clin. Nutr.*, 38(4), 245–260, 1984.
202. Gazzaniga, A.B., A.T. Day, and H. Sankary, The efficacy of a 20 per cent fat emulsion as a peripherally administered substrate, *Surg. Gynecol. Obstet.*, 160(5), 387–392, 1985.
203. Kinsella, J.E. et al., Dietary polyunsaturated fatty acids and eicosanoids: potential effects on the modulation of inflammatory and immune cells: an overview, *Nutrition*, 6(1), 24–44; discussion 59–62, 1990.
204. Hageman, J.R. et al., Intralipid alterations in pulmonary prostaglandin metabolism and gas exchange, *Crit. Care Med.*, 11(10), 794–798, 1983.

205. Griffin, E. et al., Appearance and characterization of lipoprotein X during continuous intralipid infusions in the neonate, *J. Clin. Invest.*, 64(6), 1703–1712, 1979.

206. Untracht, S.H., Intravascular metabolism of an artificial transporter of triacylglycerols. Alterations of serum lipoproteins resulting from total parenteral nutrition with Intralipid, *Biochim. Biophys. Acta*, 711(1), 176–192, 1982.

207. Newsholme, E.A. and E.A. Leech, Catabolism of carbohydrates, in *Biochemistry for the Medical Sciences*, Newsholme, E.A. and E.A. Leech, Eds., Chichester: John Wiley & Sons, 1983, pp. 167–177.

208. Passmore, R. and Y.E. Swindells, Observations on the respiratory quotients and weight gain of man after eating large quantities of carbohydrate, *Br. J. Nutr.*, 17, 331–339, 1963.

209. Wolfe, R.R. et al., Regulation of lipolysis in severely burned children, *Ann. Surg.*, 206(2), 214–221, 1987.

210. Randle, P.J. et al., The glucose fatty-acid cycle. Its role in insulin sensitivity and the metabolic disturbances of diabetes mellitus, *Lancet*, 1, April 13, 785–789, 1963.

211. Wolfe, R.R. and J.H. Shaw, Glucose and FFA kinetics in sepsis: role of glucagon and sympathetic nervous system activity, *Am. J. Physiol.*, 248(2 Pt. 1), E236–E243, 1985.

212. Wolfe, B.M. et al., Effect of total parenteral nutrition on hepatic histology, *Arch. Surg.*, 123(9), 1084–1090, 1988.

213. Alexander, J.W. et al., The importance of lipid type in the diet after burn injury, *Ann. Surg.*, 204(1), 1–8, 1986.

214. Endres, S. et al., The effect of dietary supplementation with n-3 polyunsaturated fatty acids on the synthesis of interleukin-1 and tumor necrosis factor by mononuclear cells, *N. Engl. J. Med.*, 320(5), 265–271, 1989.

215. DeMichele, S.J. et al., Enteral nutrition with structured lipid: effect on protein metabolism in thermal injury, *Am. J. Clin. Nutr.*, 50(6), 1295–1302, 1989.

216. Bell, S.J. et al., Alternative lipid sources for enteral and parenteral nutrition: long- and medium-chain triglycerides, structured triglycerides, and fish oils, *J. Am. Diet. Assoc.*, 91(1), 74–78, 1991.

217. Ling, P.R. et al., Structured lipid made from fish oil and medium-chain triglycerides alters tumor and host metabolism in Yoshida-sarcoma-bearing rats, *Am. J. Clin. Nutr.*, 53(5), 1177–1184, 1991.

218. Pratt, V.C. et al., Alterations in lymphocyte function and relation to phospholipid composition after burn injury in humans, *Crit. Care Med.*, 30(8), 1753–1761, 2002.

219. Gadek, J.E. et al., Effect of enteral feeding with eicosapentaenoic acid, -linolenic acid, and antioxidants in patients with acute respiratory distress syndrome. Enteral Nutrition in ARDS Study Group, *Crit. Care Med.*, 27(8), 1409–1420, 1999.

220. Meydani, S.N., Dietary modulation of cytokine production and biologic functions, *Nutr. Rev.*, 48(10), 361–369, 1990.

221. Weiss, G. et al., Immunomodulation by perioperative administration of n-3 fatty acids, *Br. J. Nutr.*, 87 Suppl. 1, S89–S94, 2002.

222. Mayer, K. et al., Short-time infusion of fish oil-based lipid emulsions, approved for parenteral nutrition, reduces monocyte proinflammatory cytokine generation and adhesive interaction with endothelium in humans, *J. Immunol.*, 171(9), 4837–4843, 2003.

223. Foitzik, T. et al., Omega-3 fatty acid supplementation increases anti-inflammatory cytokines and attenuates systemic disease sequelae in experimental pancreatitis, *J. Parenter. Enteral Nutr.*, 26(6), 351–356, 2002.

224. Abribat, T. et al., Decreased serum insulin-like growth factor-I in burn patients: relationship with serum insulin-like growth factor binding protein-3 proteolysis and the influence of lipid composition in nutritional support, *Crit. Care Med.*, 28(7), 2366–2372, 2000.

225. Albina, J.E., P. Gladden, and W.R. Walsh, Detrimental effects of an omega-3 fatty acid-enriched diet on wound healing, *J. Parenter. Enteral Nutr.*, 17(6), 519–521, 1993.

226. Wilmore, D.W. et al., Influence of the burn wound on local and systemic responses to injury, *Ann. Surg.*, 186(4), 444–458, 1977.

227. Goodwin, C.W., Metabolism and nutrition in the thermally injured patient, *Crit. Care Clin.*, 1(1), 97–117, 1985.

228. Shulman, G.I. et al., Substrate cycling between gluconeogenesis and glycolysis in euthyroid, hypothyroid, and hyperthyroid man, *J. Clin. Invest.*, 76(2), 757–764, 1985.

229. Burke, J.F. et al., Glucose requirements following burn injury. Parameters of optimal glucose infusion and possible hepatic and respiratory abnormalities following excessive glucose intake, *Ann. Surg.*, 190(3), 274–285, 1979.

230. Wolfe, R.R. et al., Investigation of factors determining the optimal glucose infusion rate in total parenteral nutrition, *Metabolism*, 29(9), 892–900, 1980.

231. Aulick, L.H. et al., Influence of the burn wound on peripheral circulation in thermally injured patients, *Am. J. Physiol.*, 233(4), H520–H526, 1977.

232. Hers, H.G. and L. Hue, Gluconeogenesis and related aspects of glycolysis, *Annu. Rev. Biochem.*, 52, 617–653, 1983.

233. Felig, P., The glucose–alanine cycle, *Metabolism*, 22(2), 179–207, 1973.

234. Felig, P., Amino acid metabolism in man, *Annu. Rev. Biochem.*, 44, 933–955, 1975.

235. Cori, C.F., Mammalian carbohydrate metabolism, *Physiol. Rev.*, 11, 143, 1931.

236. Kreisberg, R.A., Pathogenesis and management of lactic acidosis, *Ann. Rev. Med.*, 35, 181–193, 1931.

237. Laugness, U. and S. Udenfriend, Collagen proline hydroxylase activity and anaerobic metabolism, in *Biology of the Fibroblast*, E. Kulonen and J. Pikkarainen, Eds., New York: Academic Press, 1973, p. 373.

238. Shangraw, R.E. et al., Differentiation between septic and postburn insulin resistance, *Metabolism*, 38(10), 983–989, 1989.

239. Shaw, J.H., S. Klein, and R.R. Wolfe, Assessment of alanine, urea, and glucose interrelationships in normal subjects and in patients with sepsis with stable isotopic tracers, *Surgery*, 97(5), 557–568, 1985.

240. O'Brien, R.M. and D.K. Granner, Regulation of gene expression by insulin, *Biochem. J.*, 278 (Pt. 3), 609–619, 1991.

241. O'Brien, R.M. et al., Identification of a sequence in the PEPCK gene that mediates a negative effect of insulin on transcription, *Science*, 249(4968), 533–537, 1990.

242. Li, W.W. et al., Common genetic variation in the promoter of the human apo CIII gene abolishes regulation by insulin and may contribute to hypertriglyceridemia, *J. Clin. Invest.*, 96(6), 2601–2605, 1995.

243. Ganss, R., F. Weih, and G. Schutz, The cyclic adenosine 3,5-monophosphate- and the glucocorticoid-dependent enhancers are targets for insulin repression of tyrosine aminotransferase gene transcription, *Mol. Endocrinol.*, 8(7), 895–903, 1994.

244. Hart, D.W. et al., Determinants of blood loss during primary burn excision, *Surgery*, 130(2), 396–402, 2001.

245. Ferrando, A.A. et al., A submaximal dose of insulin promotes net skeletal muscle protein synthesis in patients with severe burns, *Ann. Surg.*, 229(1), 11–18, 1999.

246. Gore, D.C. et al., Extremity hyperinsulinemia stimulates muscle protein synthesis in severely injured patients, *Am. J. Physiol. Endocrinol. Metab.*, 286(4), E529–E534, 2004.

247. Geerlings, S.E. and A.I. Hoepelman, Immune dysfunction in patients with diabetes mellitus (DM), *FEMS Immunol. Med. Microbiol.*, 26(3–4), 259–265, 1999.

248. Hehenberger, K. et al., Inhibited proliferation of fibroblasts derived from chronic diabetic wounds and normal dermal fibroblasts treated with high glucose is associated with increased formation of l-lactate, *Wound Repair Regen.*, 6(2), 135–141, 1998.

249. van den Berghe, G. et al., Intensive insulin therapy in the critically ill patients, *N. Engl. J. Med.*, 345(19), 1359–1367, 2001.

250. Van den Berghe, G. et al., Outcome benefit of intensive insulin therapy in the critically ill: insulin dose versus glycemic control, *Crit. Care Med.*, 31(2), 359–366, 2003.

251. Gore, D.C. et al., Association of hyperglycemia with increased mortality after severe burn injury, *J. Trauma*, 51(3), 540–544, 2001.

252. Rayes, N. et al., Early enteral supply of lactobacillus and fiber versus selective bowel decontamination: a controlled trial in liver transplant recipients, *Transplantation*, 74(1), 123–127, 2002.

253. Bengmark, S., Probiotics, prebiotics and synbiotics in the intensive care unit, in *Nutritional Conisderations in the ICU: Science, Rationale, and Practice*, S.A. Shikora, R.G. Martindale, S.D. Swaitzberg, Eds., American Society for Parenteral and Enteral Nutrition and Kendall/Hunt, Dubuque, IA, 2002.

254. Burke, J.F. et al., The contribution of a bacterially isolated environment to the prevention of infection in seriously burned patients, *Ann. Surg.*, 186(3), 377–387, 1977.

255. Deitch, E.A., J. Winterton, and R. Berg, Effect of starvation, malnutrition, and trauma on the gastrointestinal tract flora and bacterial translocation, *Arch. Surg.*, 122(9), 1019–1024, 1987.

256. Lipman, T.O., Bacterial translocation and enteral nutrition in humans: an outsider looks in, *J. Parenter. Enteral Nutr.*, 19(2), 156–165, 1995.

257. O'Dwyer, S.T. et al., A single dose of endotoxin increases intestinal permeability in healthy humans, *Arch. Surg.*, 123(12), 1459–1464, 1988.

258. Oudemans-van Straaten, H.M. et al., Pitfalls in gastrointestinal permeability measurement in ICU patients with multiple organ failure using differential sugar absorption, *Intensive Care Med.*, 28(2), 130–138, 2002.

259. Rush, B.F., Jr. et al., Endotoxemia and bacteremia during hemorrhagic shock. The link between trauma and sepsis? *Ann. Surg.*, 207(5), 549–554, 1988.

260. O'Boyle, C.J. et al., Microbiology of bacterial translocation in humans, *Gut*, 42(1), 29–35, 1998.

261. Sedman, P.C. et al., The prevalence of gut translocation in humans, *Gastroenterology*, 107(3), 643–649, 1994.

262. Tokyay, R. et al., Postburn gastrointestinal vasoconstriction increases bacterial and endotoxin translocation, *J. Appl. Physiol.*, 74(4), 1521–1527, 1993.

263. Barret, J.P., M.G. Jeschke, and D.N. Herndon, Selective decontamination of the digestive tract in severely burned pediatric patients, *Burns*, 27(5), 439–445, 2001.

264. American Society for Parenteral and Enteral Nutrition, Guidelines for the use of parenteral and enteral nutrition in adult and pediatric patients, *J. Parenter. Enteral Nutr.*, 17(4 Suppl.), 1SA–52SA, 1993.

265. Kudsk, K.A. et al., Enteral versus parenteral feeding. Effects on septic morbidity after blunt and penetrating abdominal trauma, *Ann. Surg.*, 215(5), 503–511; discussion 511–513, 1992.

266. Braunschweig, C.L. et al., Enteral compared with parenteral nutrition: a meta-analysis, *Am. J. Clin. Nutr.*, 74(4), 534–542, 2001.

267. Bistrian, B.R., Update on total parenteral nutrition, *Am. J. Clin. Nutr.*, 74(2), 153–154, 2001.

268. Jeejeebhoy, K.N., Total parenteral nutrition: potion or poison? *Am. J. Clin. Nutr.*, 74(2), 160–163, 2001.

269. MacFie, J., Enteral versus parenteral nutrition: the significance of bacterial translocation and gut-barrier function, *Nutrition*, 16(7–8), 606–611, 2000.

270. Minard, G. and K.A. Kudsk, Nutritional support and infection: does the route matter? *World J. Surg.*, 22(2), 213–219, 1998.

271. Meydani, S.N. and C.A. Dinarello, Influence of dietary fatty acids on cytokine production and its clinical implications, *Nutr. Clin. Pract.*, 8(2), 65–72, 1993.

272. Battistella, F.D. et al., A prospective, randomized trial of intravenous fat emulsion administration in trauma victims requiring total parenteral nutrition, *J. Trauma*, 43(1), 52–58; discussion 58–60, 1997.

273. Minard, G. and L.K. Lysen, Enteral access devices, in *The Science and Practice of Nutrition Support: A Case-Based Core Curriculum.* Gottschlich, M.M., Ed., Dubuque, IA: Kendall/Hunt, 2001.

274. McCormick, J.T. et al., Effect of diagnosis and treatment of sinusitis in critically ill burn victims, *Burns*, 29(1), 79–81, 2003.

275. Tisherman, S.A., P.E. Marik, and J. Ochoa, Promoting enteral feeding 101, *Crit. Care Med.*, 30(7), 1653–1654, 2002.

276. Sefton, E.J. et al., Enteral feeding in patients with major burn injury: the use of nasojejunal feeding after the failure of nasogastric feeding, *Burns*, 28(4), 386–390, 2002.

277. Mentec, H. et al., Upper digestive intolerance during enteral nutrition in critically ill patients: frequency, risk factors, and complications, *Crit. Care Med.*, 29(10), 1955–1961, 2001.

278. Lyons, M. and L.H. Clemens, Energy deficits associated with nasogastric feeding in patients with burns, *J. Burn Care Rehabil.*, 21(4), 372–374; discussion 371, 2000.

279. Gowardman, J. et al., Intermittent enteral nutrition — a comparative study examining the effect on gastric pH and microbial colonization rates, *Anaesth. Intensive Care*, 31(1), 28–33, 2003.

280. Esparza, J. et al., Equal aspiration rates in gastrically and transpylorically fed critically ill patients, *Intensive Care Med.*, 27(4), 660–664, 2001.

281. Heyland, D.K. et al., Effect of postpyloric feeding on gastroesophageal regurgitation and pulmonary microaspiration: results of a randomized controlled trial, *Crit. Care Med.*, 29(8), 1495–1501, 2001.

282. Montecalvo, M.A. et al., Nutritional outcome and pneumonia in critical care patients randomized to gastric versus jejunal tube feedings. The Critical Care Research Team, *Crit. Care Med.*, 20(10), 1377–1387, 1992.

283. Kortbeek, J.B., P.I. Haigh, and C. Doig, Duodenal versus gastric feeding in ventilated blunt trauma patients: a randomized controlled trial, *J. Trauma*, 46(6), 992–996; discussion 996–998, 1999.

284. Kearns, P.J. et al., The incidence of ventilator-associated pneumonia and success in nutrient delivery with gastric versus small intestinal feeding: a randomized clinica trial, *Crit. Care Med.*, 28(6), 1742–1746, 2000.

285. McClave, S.A. et al., North American Summit on Aspiration in the Critically Ill Patient: consensus statement, *J. Parenter. Enteral Nutr.*, 26(6 Suppl.), S80–S85, 2002.

286. Drakulovic, M.B. et al., Supine body position as a risk factor for nosocomial pneumonia in mechanically ventilated patients: a randomised trial, *Lancet*, 354(9193), 1851–1858, 1999.

287. Vincent, J.L. et al., The prevalence of nosocomial infection in intensive care units in Europe. Results of the European Prevalence of Infection in Intensive Care (EPIC) Study. EPIC International Advisory Committee, *JAMA*, 274(8), 639–644, 1995.

288. Gattinoni, L. et al., Effect of prone positioning on the survival of patients with acute respiratory failure, *N. Engl. J. Med.*, 345(8), 568–573, 2001.

289. van der Voort, P.H. and D.F. Zandstra, Enteral feeding in the critically ill: comparison between the supine and prone positions: a prospective crossover study in mechanically ventilated patients, *Crit. Care*, 5(4), 216–220, 2001.

290. Messerole, E. et al., The pragmatics of prone positioning, *Am. J. Respir. Crit. Care Med.*, 165(10), 1359–1363, 2002.

291. Peng, Y.Z., Z.Q. Yuan, and G.X. Xiao, Effects of early enteral feeding on the prevention of enterogenic infection in severely burned patients, *Burns*, 27(2), 145–149, 2001.

292. Gottschlich, M.M. et al., The 2002 Clinical Research Award. An evaluation of the safety of early vs. delayed enteral support and effects on clinical, nutritional, and endocrine outcomes after severe burns, *J. Burn Care Rehabil.*, 23(6), 401–415, 2002.

293. Jenkins, M.E., M.M. Gottschlich, and G.D. Warden, Enteral feeding during operative procedures in thermal injuries, *J. Burn Care Rehabil.*, 15(2), 199–205, 1994.

294. Spain, D.A., When is the seriously ill patient ready to be fed? *J. Parenter. Enteral Nutr.*, 26(6 Suppl.), S62–S65; discussion S65–S68, 2002.

295. Scaife, C.L., J.R. Saffle, and S.E. Morris, Intestinal obstruction secondary to enteral feedings in burn trauma patients, *J. Trauma*, 47(5), 859–863, 1999.

296. McClave, S.A. and W.K. Chang, Complications of enteral access, *Gastrointest. Endosc.*, 58(5), 739–751, 2003.

297. Liljedahl, S.O. et al., Effect of human growth hormone in patients with severe burns, *Acta Chir. Scand.*, 122, 1–14, 1961.

298. Carroll, P.V. and G. Van den Berghe, Safety aspects of pharmacological GH therapy in adults, *Growth Horm. IGF Res.*, 11(3), 166–172, 2001.

299. Demling, R.H., Comparison of the anabolic effects and complications of human growth hormone and the testosterone analog, oxandrolone, after severe burn injury, *Burns*, 25(3), 215–221, 1999.

300. Puolakkainen, P.A. et al., The enhancement in wound healing by transforming growth factor-1 (TGF-a 1) depends on the topical delivery system, *J. Surg. Res.*, 58(3), 321–329, 1995.

301. Tredget, E.E. et al., Transforming growth factor- in thermally injured patients with hypertrophic cars: effects of interferon -2b, *Plast. Reconstr. Surg.*, 102(5), 1317–1328; discussion 1329–1330, 1998.

302. Villet, S., R.L. Chiolero, M.D. Bollmann, J. Revelly, M. Cayeux, J. Delarue, and M.M. Berger, Negative impact of hypocaloric feeding and energy balance on clinical outcome in ICU patients. *Clin. Nutr.*, 24(4), 502–509, 2005.

303. Messiner, R., M. Griffen, R. Crass, Small bowel necrosis related to enteral nutrition after duodenal surgery. *Am. Surg.*, 71(12), 993–995, 2005.

304. Herndon, D.N., R.E. Barrow, M. Stein, Increased mortality with intravenous supplemental feeding in severely burned patients. J. Burn. Care Rehabil., 10(4), 309–313, 1989.

12 Nutrition and Wound Healing in Cancer

Perry Shen and Shayn Martin

CONTENTS

INTRODUCTION

Successful wound healing in the cancer patient can be a formidable task. The effects of malignancy on a patient's nutritional status are multifaceted and can make the achievement of wound healing a challenge. Cancer alters the body's ability to maintain sustenance by manipulating both gastrointestinal caloric intake and subsequent nutritional processing. Malnutrition with varying degrees of weight loss is a common sequela of many solid tumors. Depending on the inciting malignancy, some degree of malnutrition has been identified in 30 to 90% of studied groups.[1] Up to one third of a large population in a multicenter survey demonstrated weight losses greater than 4%.[2] At its greatest magnitude, malnutrition manifests as cachexia, which is characterized by progressive total body muscle and fat wasting. The most severe presentations are identified in the presence of head and neck as well as upper gastrointestinal cancers (i.e., esophagus, stomach, and pancreas). Weight loss in excess of 10% was demonstrated in 14% of patients with colon cancer and between 25 and 40% of those with gastric and pancreatic cancer.[2] Conversely, such severe losses were seen in only 4 to 7% of patients with leukemias, sarcomas, or breast cancer.

Cachexia results from the inappropriate wasting of skeletal muscle and adipose tissue. This is in contrast to simple starvation, which preferentially depletes fat stores, thus sparing lean muscle mass. The mechanisms driving cancer cachexia are multiple and appear to be a complex interaction between the digestive and immune systems. As the mainstay of treatment for many malignancies remains complete surgical resection, the implications of cachexia on wound healing are significant. An understanding of the pathophysiology of cancer cachexia and the effects of malignancy on wound healing will allow treatment regimens to be devised to combat this difficult aspect of oncologic care.

PATHOPHYSIOLOGY OF CANCER CACHEXIA

Cachexia in the setting of malignancy is a complex process with abnormalities identified in caloric intake, metabolism of nutrients, and humoral/inflammatory responses (Figure 12.1). Individual cancers uniquely affect each of those components, resulting in various degrees of the cachectic state.

ALTERED CALORIC AND NUTRITIONAL INTAKE

The ability to consume an adequate quantity of calories and nutrients is commonly decreased in the setting of malignancy. Dietary intake is often inappropriately decreased, even when the malignant condition has increased caloric needs.[3] Anorexia is frequently present, manifesting as a loss of appetite with early satiety. This can be present in as many as one half of newly diagnosed cancer patients. Alterations in the taste and smell of food contribute to this phenomenon.[2] Depression, which is not uncommon among the oncologic population, can greatly decrease a patient's appetite.[1]

A direct effect on the gastrointestinal tract can result in decreased nutritional intake. Cancer of the head and neck or upper gastrointestinal tract can result in dysphagia and odynophagia secondary to mechanical effects. Decreased gastric emptying and intestinal dysfunction lead to decreased bowel motility and subsequent early satiety, nausea, and vomiting. Tumor bulk can impinge upon the upper gastrointestinal tract, resulting in early satiety. Growth of tumor anywhere within the abdomen can compress or directly obstruct the intestinal lumen, resulting in partial or complete bowel obstructions. Also, postoperative changes after bowel surgery can

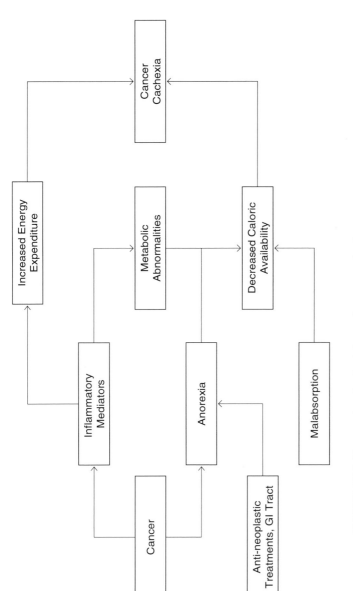

FIGURE 12.1 Presumed pathophysiology of cancer cachexia.

alter gastrointestinal physiology, resulting in abnormal function. Furthermore, intestinal mucosal atrophy or bacterial overgrowth within blind loops may contribute to nutrient malabsorption.[4]

The nonsurgical cancer treatments have also been associated with many conditions that negatively impact dietary intake. Chemotherapeutic agents can cause nausea, vomiting, cramping, and bloating. Mucositis, mucosal erosive lesions, and paralytic ileus have all been observed.[1]

METABOLIC DISORDERS

The normal metabolic function is severely deranged in the cancer patient. The body responds inappropriately to metabolic demands on the host. Normal control systems malfunction, resulting in depletion of muscle and adipose stores. Despite experiencing decreased nutritional intake, the body is unable to downregulate energy expenditure.[5] Instead, the tumor causes an increase in energy expenditure thought to be secondary to an increased adrenergic state and an inflammatory response to the malignancy.[1] Lung and pancreatic cancer have been particularly associated with a hypermetabolic state and, subsequently, demonstrate more severe weight loss.[6]

The metabolism of carbohydrates is altered by malignancy. Anaerobic glycolysis is favored by tumor cells, resulting in the production of lactate. Lactate is inefficiently recycled to glucose by gluconeogenesis in the Cori cycle. A substantial net loss of energy occurs through this wasteful process.[7] Further altered carbohydrate metabolism includes reduced pancreatic insulin secretion as well as glucose intolerance, which is secondary to peripheral insulin resistance.[8]

Abnormal lipid metabolism demonstrates an increased oxidation of fatty acids with subsequent mobilization of peripheral fat. Malignancy stimulates an increased rate of lipolysis in adipose tissue. This is in contrast to normal subjects who are capable of regulating lipid oxidation during starvation.[9] This is believed to be a result of stimulation by a lipid-mobilizing factor that acts directly on adipocytes in a cyclic adenosine monophosphate (cAMP)-dependent manner. Lipoprotein lipase activity is decreased, resulting in diminished uptake of fatty acids from circulating lipoproteins.[7] Ultimately, this results in depletion of total body lipid stores.

Additionally, the metabolism of proteins is abnormal, as demonstrated by increased protein turnover with a reduction in muscle protein synthesis.[1] This protein catabolism escapes normal regulatory control, resulting in protein depletion and subsequent muscle atrophy. The escalation of hepatic acute phase reactants in the setting of malignancy also depletes protein stores.[5] The breakdown of protein is mediated by a proteolytic inducing factor that utilizes an adenosine triphosphate (ATP)-ubiquitin-dependent pathway.[10] This has been observed even in the presence of adequate protein consumption, again owing to the loss of homeostatic control in the oncologic patient.

The increased energy expenditure and metabolic abnormalities in cancer patients are of greater magnitude than would be explained by the tumor itself. This has been determined to be a result of an alteration in the release of multiple inflammatory mediators. Listed in Table 12.1 are the humoral mediators thought to be associated with cancer cachexia as well as their proposed effects.

TABLE 12.1
Inflammatory Mediators Believed to Be Involved in Cancer Cachexia

Mediator	Source	Involvement in Cachexia
TNF α	Macrophages	Suppresses lipoprotein lipase; increases protein breakdown; induces acute-phase protein response; anorexia and weight loss; elevates energy expenditure; pyrexia; increases triglycerides; decreases insulin production; increases insulin resistance
IL-1	Macrophages	Anorexia and weight loss; early satiety; increases protein breakdown; antibodies attenuate some aspects of cachexia in animals
IL-6	Macrophages	Induces acute-phase protein response
	Fibroblasts	Antibodies suppress cachexia in animals
	T-lymphocytes	
IFN γ	T-lymphocytes	Effects similar to TNF
	NK cells	Antibodies reversed cachexia in animals
PIF	Tumor cells	Induces skeletal muscle proteolysis; causes rapid weight loss in animals
LMF	Tumor cells	Induces adipocyte lipolysis; causes weight loss in animals
CNTF	Glial cells of peripheral nervous system	Weight loss; induces protein breakdown; fever
	Skeletal muscle	Induces acute-phase protein response

Note: TNF α: tumor necrosis factor alpha, IL-1: Interleukin 1, IL-6: Interleukin 6, IFN γ: interferon gamma, NK cells: natural killer cells, PIF: proteolysis-inducing factor, LMF: lipid-mobilizing factor, CNTF: ciliary neurotrophic factor.

Neuropeptide Y and leptin are substances thought to be associated with poor appetite in cancer patients. Neuropeptide Y is believed to stimulate appetite and feeding, and its effects are significantly decreased in the presence of malignancy.[11] Leptin is a hormone produced by fat which suppresses appetite and has been observed to be elevated in some disease states.[5] Because leptin levels are influenced by cytokine levels, it has been thought that cachexia may be driven by leptin, although studies to date have been unable to define its role.[12]

Multiple cytokines are thought to contribute to the pathogenesis of cancer cachexia. Tumor necrosis factor alpha (TNF-α) has a broad range of effects, including anorexia and weight loss with protein and fat breakdown. Lipoprotein lipase activity is decreased in the presence of TNF-α.[13] Also, some work suggests increased muscle degradation possibly via an ubiquitin-dependent proteolytic pathway.[14] Further effects include alterations in carbohydrate metabolism with insulin resistance, decreased insulin levels, and increased cortisol and glucagon levels.[5] TNF also affects energy expenditure by inducing an increased inflammatory response with fevers and elevated acute phase protein synthesis.[15] While the effects of TNF are well documented, the cachectic response to cancer has not been reversed with administration of TNF antibodies.[16]

The cytokine interleukin 6 (IL-6) has also been implicated by its induction of the inflammatory response with increased production of acute phase proteins.[17] Patients with non-small cell lung cancer and weight loss were found to have elevated IL-6 levels over those without weight loss.[18] In animal models, there has been some suppression of cachexia with administration of IL-6 antibodies.[19] Despite this, there has been a poor association with degree of weight loss and IL-6 levels.[20]

Ciliary neurotrophic factor (CNTF) is related to IL-6 and has similar mechanisms contributing to cachexia. Weight loss with protein breakdown has been observed with CNTF administration in rodents.[21] As with IL-6, CNTF induces an acute phase response resulting in fevers and overall increased expenditure.[22] The cytokine IL-1 has effects similar to CNTF, producing anorexia, weight loss, and protein depletion.[5] Some success has been achieved with blockade of IL-1 with antibodies, demonstrating some improvement in the cachectic state.[23]

As described above, cancer patients exhibit factors that contribute to depletion of protein and lipid stores. A skeletal muscle proteolysis-inducing factor (PIF) has been identified in patients demonstrating severe weight loss as characterized by greater than 10%.[10,24] Studies indicate that PIF is produced by the tumor and that it acts preferentially on skeletal muscle to decrease lean body mass.[25,26] Lipid catabolism is driven by a lipid mobilizing factor (LMF) that induces lipolysis through a cAMP-driven mechanism.[27] LMF has been identified in patients with cancer cachexia but was absent in those with simple starvation.[27] These two substances demonstrate compelling evidence as to their contribution to the cachectic state.

TREATMENT OF CANCER CACHEXIA

The most effective management of cancer cachexia rests in successful treatment of the malignancy. As this is not always immediately possible, other methods have been attempted to combat the cachectic process. Pharmacologic interventions include appetite stimulants and agents that act as inflammatory mediators. Steroids are commonly used agents for appetite stimulation. Studies have shown that prednisolone and dexamethasone significantly improve appetite, although long-term weight loss is unaffected.[28,29] The progestational agents have demonstrated some success in stimulating appetite and slowing weight loss. Megestrol acetate at various doses increased appetite and, although the rate of weight loss was slowed, lean body mass was not increased.[30–33]

Modulation of the inflammatory response to cancer is a novel technique that attempts to alter the aberrant control mechanisms that lead to cachexia. Despite extensive effort, identifying effective modulators has been a difficult task due to the complexity and redundancy of the body's immune system. There has been some success with nonsteroidal anti-inflammatory agents in attenuating the wasting process. Ibuprofen has been observed to improve protein metabolism, likely due to reductions in IL-6, cortisol, and acute phase reactant levels.[34,35] A blunting of the acute phase response has also been associated with a decrease in energy expenditure.[36] Prospective data in the setting of pancreatic cancer demonstrated that ibuprofen may be capable of weight stabilization.[37] There are also data that suggest that the nonsteroidal anti-inflammatory indomethacin may prolong survival in patients with metastatic disease.[38]

WOUND HEALING

Wound healing in the cancer patient may be compromised, as the malignant condition can complicate many aspects of the healing process. In normal subjects, the process of healing follows a well-studied and delineated pattern consisting of three stages — inflammatory, proliferative, and remodeling. Briefly, the inflammatory stage begins at the time of wound closure and lasts approximately 4 d. Immediate vasoconstriction occurs, and platelet aggregation with thrombus formation is evident.[39] Exposed collagen bundles interact with platelets and blood products to initiate the coagulation cascade with the assistance of release thromboplastin.[40] Platelets involved in the clot release growth factor, including platelet-derived growth factor (PDGF), transforming growth factor β(TGF-β), insulin growth factor-1 (IGF-1), and epidermal growth factor (EGF), which function to attract neutrophils, monocytes, fibroblasts, and smooth muscle cells.[41] Vasodilation shortly follows to augment the influx of blood cells and proteins into the wound.[39] Macrophages and neutrophils then debride the wound and reduce the quantity of bacteria through the process of phagocytosis and enzymatic breakdown. Monocytes also stimulate angiogenesis and the initial fibroblast production of collagen.[40]

The proliferative stage that follows is dominated by collagen synthesis and neovascularization. This stage lasts for approximately 3 weeks during which time the wound becomes stronger. Local tissue hypoxia stimulates the ingrowths of new blood vessels, increasing the oxygen levels within the wound.[40] Fibroblasts proliferate and migrate as they are stimulated by PDGF, EGF, and basic fibroblast growth factor (bFGF).[42] Fibroblasts produce collagen that slowly becomes cross-linked and thus, significantly increases wound strength. Myofibroblasts migrate into the wound matrix, and the wound begins to contract.[40] Capillary ingrowth and collagen deposition result in granulation tissue, which provides a surface for epithelialization that provides skin covering over the wound.[39] IGF-1, bFGF, TGF-β, PDGF, and keratinocyte growth factor released by fibroblasts stimulate the formation of the connective tissue matrix. At the completion of the proliferative stage, the wound appears healed and has obtained approximately 30% of its prewounding strength.

The final stage is remodeling, during which time collagen becomes remodeled and cross-linking is completed. This may last for as long as 2 yr, following which the wound ultimately achieves approximately 80 to 85% of the strength of normal skin.[43] Each of the steps in wound healing can be complicated in the setting of active malignancy. The disease and the use of radiation and chemotherapy each uniquely obstruct the normal healing process.

EFFECTS OF RADIATION THERAPY

Radiation therapy disrupts the healing of wounds in multiple ways. The initial inflammatory response to injury is retarded, thus slowing the initial phases of healing.[44] Neovascularization is decreased, resulting in tissue hypoxia and subsequent poor connective tissue healing and collagen synthesis.[39] Hypoxia also results from degeneration of existing vessels with basement membrane disruption and increased vascular permeability.[5] Fibroblasts fail to proliferate, and their number becomes depleted. The combination of the above events ultimately leads to tissue fibrosis.

Various factors, including total dose, administration schedule, target tissue, and timing of therapy with respect to surgery contribute to the effect on wound healing. Radiation administration in the preoperative period of time can complicate healing unless the dose is quite low. In animals, a 300 rads preoperative dose had no identifiable effect on healing compared to a dose of over 1000 rads, which significantly slowed healing.[40] The timing before an operation is an important factor as well. Wounds produced within 12 weeks of preoperative radiation demonstrate some evidence of delayed healing, with decreased tensile strength that worsens as the temporal proximity decreases.[45] A group of 849 rectal cancer patients who received radiation during a 5 to 7 d period of time before resection experienced a significantly higher wound infection rate when compared to surgery alone.[46] Despite this, certain tissue is more resilient to radiation therapy. Recently, a group of patients with head and neck sarcoma were found to have fewer healing complications after radiation therapy than a group with extremity sarcoma receiving comparable treatment.[47] Though radiation in the preoperative setting can make subsequent healing difficult, it is generally felt to be safe when administered at least 6 to 8 weeks before resection.

Postoperative radiation effects on healing are also highly dependent on timing. If radiation is given after the completion of the proliferative stage of healing, there will be no clinically significant impact on overall wound healing. After colon resection, radiation to the colon within 24 h resulted in significantly decreased wound strength at 5 and 15 d after surgery.[48] In one study, radiation therapy after the proliferative stage of healing was felt to be complete resulted in only a 3% incidence of wound complications versus 22% in patients receiving radiation within 1 week. Therefore, radiation administration after 1 week of healing avoided most clinically relevant wound problems.

EFFECTS OF CHEMOTHERAPY

Chemotherapy can adversely affect the healing process in many of the same ways as radiation. Treatments can reduce the inflammatory response, decrease fibroblast proliferation, and impede angiogenesis, thus slowing healing and increasing the risk of infection.[49] The various types of chemotherapeutics have been studied in human and animal models, revealing an effect on healing depending on the mechanism of action.

ANTHRACYCLINE ANTITUMOR ANTIBIOTICS

The antitumor antibiotics prevent DNA and RNA synthesis and, thus, affect cellular division and protein synthesis. Doxorubicin is a well-studied anthracycline that is believed to impede wound healing by downregulating the production of growth factors. Doxorubicin has been found to significantly impair wound breaking strength in several studies. Studies in mice receiving doxorubicin up to 42 d before and 21 d after operation indicated that wound healing is negatively affected.[50–52] Though when treatment was delayed to 28 d, postoperative wound breaking strength was not significantly decreased.[53] In humans, preoperative doxorubicin administered up to 14 to 21 d before mastectomy was associated with wound complications in 71% of patients compared to 10% after surgery alone.[54] These effects are felt to be secondary to a reduction in collagen synthesis.[50] However, other studies have used preoperative cytotoxic chemotherapy prior to mastectomy with no significant wound complications, so these results must be interpreted with caution.[55a]

ALKYLATING AGENTS

Alkylating agents produce breaks in DNA molecules, and at high enough doses, they reduce fibroblast proliferation. At low doses, cyclophosphamide, an alkylating agent, has been found to significantly impact wound healing.[39] In animal models, the strength of healing wounds was affected, though, when given at high doses (165 to 500 mg/kg) anywhere from 3 d prior to 7 d after operation.[55] When cyclophosphamide was administered at moderate doses (200 mg/kg), wound bursting strength was decreased when the timing of dosage was 1 to 4 d after wounding, while if given 1 to 4 days before surgery, wound strength was not significantly different.[55] Despite this data in animals, studies in humans showed no impact on wound healing, regardless of timing and medication dosage.[56,57] Regardless, it seems that the effect of alkylating agents on wound healing depends mostly on timing of dosage with respect to resection.[58]

VINCA ALKALOIDS

Vinca alkaloids, an example of which is vincristine, bind to cytoplasmic motility structures and, therefore, block DNA transfer during cell replication. When administered to mice on the day of wounding, vincristine was associated with a decrease in wound healing strength which resolved by 1 week postoperatively.[58] A series in children with nephroblastoma receiving preoperative vincristine also demonstrated no significant effects on wound healing.[59]

FOLIC ACID ANALOGS

Methotrexate is a folic acid analog that decreases DNA synthesis by inhibiting dihydrofolate reductase. Animals treated with methotrexate demonstrated evidence of early weakening of wound strength, which resolved over time.[39] Studies in humans with head and neck cancer demonstrated no effect on wound healing with the administration of methotrexate.[39]

CISPLATIN

Cisplatin inhibits DNA synthesis by cross-linking strands of DNA. Wounds tested in cisplatin-treated mice were weaker in the early phases of healing, although this resolved by day 16.[60] In a study of head and neck cancers in humans, preoperative cisplatin with radiation was felt to inhibit wound healing, requiring 25% longer hospitalization when compared to surgery with radiation alone.[61]

In general, chemotherapy and surgical intervention can be safely used together to provide a multimodality approach to the management of malignancy. The timing of chemotherapy in relation to surgery is the most important factor. For the most part, preoperative chemotherapy has little effect on subsequent wound healing. Some agents such as doxorubicin may require longer delays before surgery to avoid complications. In the postoperative period, chemotherapy can significantly impair healing and should be avoided until the proliferative stage of healing is felt to be completed. This usually means that chemotherapy can be safely started at about 4 to 6 weeks after resection.

GROWTH FACTORS IN WOUND HEALING

The difficulty with wound healing encountered in cancer patients has stimulated much work in determining ways of maximizing the healing process. Exogenous growth factors have been found to improve wound healing in both animal models and, to a limited degree, in the clinical realm.

TGF-β is a growth factor produced by bone, kidney, macrophages, platelets, and lymphocytes.[62] It is important in the process of cellular replication and has been shown to improve wound healing in animals. When applied topically to rat and guinea pig wounds, tensile strength was increased at 5 and 7 d, respectively.[63,64] The impairing effects of doxorubicin on wound healing were reversed by the topical administration of TGF-β in rats treated at the time of wounding.[65] When surface beam irradiation was administered in a rat model, TGF-β had no effect on wound healing, although it was effective in the setting of total body radiation.[66] This was felt to be due to the lack of fibroblasts in the surface-beam irradiated animals. Clinical evaluation of TGF-β in wound healing is limited.

EGF is produced by platelets and has its effect on epithelial cells by stimulating proliferation and migration. The initial work with EGF was determined to be ineffective when administered in single doses. Subsequently, it was found that the sustained administration of EGF was beneficial in wound healing. When skin incisions in rats were treated with EGF-impregnated subcutaneous sponges, wound DNA and hydroxyproline levels were significantly increased.[67] In another study, the tensile strength of rat wounds treated with topical EGF was three times that of control wounds.[68] In humans, a randomized prospective study revealed enhanced wound healing of partial-thickness skin wounds when a EGF and Silvadene mixture was applied.[68] This effect was also seen in a group of chronic nonhealing wounds that healed only after the administration of EGF.[69]

PDGF is a chemotactic for inflammatory cells, fibroblasts, and smooth muscle cells that is also produced by platelets.[70] Skin incisions in rats treated with topical PDGF demonstrated improved wound-breaking strength over controls.[71] This is in contrast to PDGF-treated gastric wounds that showed no significant response.[72] There was also no benefit observed in doxorubicin-treated animals when PDGF was administered.[51] Prospective data in humans have been promising, with PDGF decreasing wound volume in chronic pressure sores after 28 d of treatment.[73] In another study, wounds that demonstrated no response after an average of 198 weeks of therapy healed after 10.6 weeks of PDGF administration.[74] This benefit was also seen when PDGF was administered to a group of chronic wounds for 8 weeks. In this group, 81% of treated wounds achieved complete epithelialization versus only 15% in the control group.[74]

bFGF has its greatest effect on fibroblasts, chondrocytes, and endothelial cells.[39] Rats with full-thickness incisional wounds demonstrated improved tensile strength after topical treatment with bFGF.[75] This benefit was also seen in the presence of diabetes, obesity, and steroid treatment.[76] Despite this benefit in animals, there is limited human data to support its use clinically.

NUTRITION SUPPORT IN CANCER PATIENTS

The metabolic effects of cancer and its detrimental relationship to whole body integrity have been well described. In addition, the application of chemotherapy and radiation therapy can have deleterious effects on wound healing in those patients who undergo surgical intervention for their malignancy. In spite of these findings, defining the optimal mode of perioperative nutritional support and determining which patients will benefit most from such supplementation remain controversial. Refinements in the technical aspects of many of the most challenging surgical procedures and the perioperative anesthetic management have led to reductions in the perioperative morbidity and mortality.[77,78] Improvements in the physician's ability to identify the nutritionally depleted surgical patient at risk for postoperative complications has also improved.[79] Current trends in surgical oncology have led to more aggressive surgical procedures in treating not only primary cancers but also those with metastatic or recurrent disease. Therefore, the role of perioperative nutritional support has the potential to play a vital role in improving outcome for these patients. Multiple studies have been performed to evaluate the route of delivery, the composition of the formula, and, most recently, the supplemental additives designed to stimulate immune function.[80] This portion of the chapter will review the nutritional assessment of the cancer patient with regards to objective criteria, clinical parameters, and the metabolic consequences of operative stress. This will be followed by a review of the role of parenteral and enteral nutrition in the clinical management of the cancer patient and what new advances are on the horizon.

NUTRITIONAL ASSESSMENT OF THE CANCER PATIENT

The nutritional status of the cancer patient is determined by a careful history (including diet history) and physical examination, followed by additional confirmatory tests. Anthropometric measures of nutritional status (e.g., weight, midarm muscle circumference, triceps fat fold) are performed. Biochemical tests, such as serum albumin, prealbumin, and transferrin, may give some indication of real-time nutritional status. Peripheral blood lymphocyte count and assessment of delayed hypersensitivity using skin testing to common antigens have been used as indicators of immunocompetence. Taking objective measurements of body compartments with tools, such as body impedance analysis or dual-photon absorptiometry, can also be done.[7]

Probably the most direct method to assess for malnutrition is to determine the percentage of unintentional weight loss that the patient has suffered as a result of his or her disease. Because disproportionately large degrees of protein catabolism accompany acute inflammatory illnesses and cancer wasting, an unintentional weight loss of 10% or more of premorbid weight due to disease translates into a contraction of 15 to 20% of the critical protein-containing compartment of the body. This degree of loss has been shown to cause impaired physiologic functions and increased morbidity and mortality.[81] Clinical trials have repeatedly demonstrated that patients who exceed this threshold benefit from aggressive nutritional support.[82,83]

Though several techniques and methods have been mentioned in the nutritional assessment of the cancer patient, none of these is perfect. The measurement of triceps skin fold is dependent on accurate measurements and varies with the type of caliper used.[84] Albumin levels can be seriously affected by any abnormality altering body fluid retention and distribution, such as the surgical procedure itself.[85] Transferrin may be a more accurate indicator of malnutrition than albumin, because it has a shorter half-life, but it is not only affected by body water changes in the seriously ill, it is also altered by body iron status.[86] Even body weight can be misleading as a nutritional parameter. In patients with gastrointestinal/hepatobiliary malignancies who have cirrhosis and ascites, the weight of the ascites masks the loss of lean body mass. Studies using sophisticated means of assessing total body protein have demonstrated that nearly all patients who are categorized into Childs–Pugh class B or class C have lost more than 20% of total body protein; half of patients with Childs–Pugh classification of A fall into the same category.[87]

Unfortunately, most indices used are poor indicators of response to therapy in patients with malignancy, although they remain good response indices in uncomplicated simple starvation. Thus, while serum albumin may be a good outcome predictor, it can be difficult to improve serum albumin in patients with malignancy with nutritional support only.[85]

Two other measurements of nutritional status that have been used in clinical practice are the creatinine–height index and the prognostic nutritional index (PNI). The creatinine–height index, which is the amount of urinary creatinine excreted in 24 h corrected for the patient's height, is an accurate reflection of muscle mass, because a constant percentage (approximately 2%) of muscle creatine is converted to creatinine each day. Although this index is useful, incomplete urine collections, excessive meat ingestion, corticosteroid therapy, and abnormal or unstable renal function can alter apparent or actual creatinine excretion independent of muscle mass. Gender-specific tables exist for normative values, and a patient whose index is 80% or less of the normative value can be considered to have a moderate to severe degree of malnutrition (Table 12.2).

TABLE 12.2
Normative Values for Creatinine Excretion Based on Height

Men[a]		Women[b]	
Height (cm)	Ideal Creatinine (mg)	Height (cm)	Ideal Creatinine (mg)
157.5	1288	147.3	830
160.0	1325	149.9	851
162.6	1359	152.4	875
165.1	1386	154.9	900
167.6	1426	157.9	925
170.2	1467	160.0	949
172.7	1513	162.6	977
175.3	1555	165.1	1006
177.8	1596	167.6	1044
180.3	1642	170.2	1076
182.9	1691	172.7	1109
185.4	1739	175.3	1141
188.0	1785	177.8	1174
190.5	1831	180.3	1206
193.0	1891	182.9	1240

[a] Creatinine coefficient (men) = 23 mg/kg of ideal body weight.
[a] Creatinine coefficient (women) = 18 mg/kg of ideal body weight.
Note: Creatinine–height index = actual 24 h urinary creatinine excretion divided by the normative value for height and sex.

Source: From *Gastrointestinal Oncology: Principles and Practice. Gastrointestinal Cancer: Nutritional Support*, Lippincott Williams & Wilkins, 2002, p.131. With permission.

The PNI is a nutritional index that represents a weighted regression of nutritional and physiologic measures. The original model was developed from 161 nonemergency surgical patients referred to a nutritional support service. The patients underwent extensive nutritional evaluation and were then evaluated after a major surgical procedure. Five values showed significant differences between complicated and uncomplicated patients: triceps skinfold, albumin, transferrin, total lymphocyte count, and delayed hypersensitivity, but only albumin, transferrin, triceps skinfold, and delayed hypersensitivity had substantial predictive outcome. The PNI was then tested and confirmed prospectively in 100 patients.[88] Surprisingly, weight loss is not a component of this index. It has been shown to be a valid predictor of postoperative complications and mortality among inpatient cancer patients who are about to undergo surgery.[83] Though the PNI is actually a reflection of both nutritional status and severity of illness, a value greater than 40% suggests moderate to severe malnutrition.[7]

A recent study[89] compared physician bedside clinical evaluation with more sophisticated methods of assessment of the degree of malnutrition. In an effort to determine reproducibility and validity of clinical assessment of nutritional status, the authors studied 59 patients in a general surgical ward. After clinical assessment, including history of weight loss, patients were divided into one of three groups: normal nutritional status, mild malnutrition, and severe malnutrition. These categories were then compared with results of multiple laboratory tests. There was good interobserver agreement of clinical status, with 81% complete agreement on 48 patients, on whom subsequent comparisons were made with biochemical indexes.

In addition, there was good correlation between the clinical evaluation and the biochemical assessment, with appropriate differences being statistically significant between normal and severe malnutrition in all cases, and in the majority of patients between mild and severe malnutrition. A high degree of correlation between measured variables was also evident. When an examination of the outcome of these patients was undertaken, the incidence of postoperative infection was highly correlated ($P < 0.005$) with the clinical evaluation, as was the use of antibiotics. This high degree of correlation between simple clinical evaluation and more sophisticated techniques of body composition led the authors to conclude that a carefully performed history and physical by a clinician are sufficient for nutritional assessment. The ability of the clinician to predict a significant degree of malnutrition by a simple physical and medical history was demonstrated to be equivalent to that of the most sophisticated methods currently available for confirmation of malnutrition.[89]

CLINICAL CONSEQUENCES OF MALNUTRITION IN THE POSTOPERATIVE PERIOD

The stress of surgical intervention combined with the dysfunctional metabolism in the cancer patient potentially increases the risk of postoperative complications. The role of malnutrition in this setting plays an important role. It is vitally important to determine the degree of malnutrition and then understand what effect that degree of malnutrition has on clinical outcome. The equally imperative corollary is whether or not reversal of this malnourished state can decrease perioperative morbidity and mortality.

The effect of malnutrition in the cancer patient undergoing surgery has been evaluated in several papers. Conti et al.[90] described 48 patients undergoing esophagogastrectomy for carcinoma of the distal esophagus and cardia. The average weight loss of those having no postoperative complications was 13.5%, whereas those having fatal complications had a preoperative weight loss of 20%.

The significance of such studies is difficult to interpret. Many are associated with compounding factors. A study by DeWys et al.[2] demonstrated a significant difference in survival based on prior weight loss and performance status in colorectal and gastric cancer, but not in pancreas cancer. It would appear that weight loss is a prognostic variable for survival in the majority of gastrointestinal malignancies.

In another study of patients with colorectal cancer,[91] serum albumin and total lymphocyte count were examined. Postoperative complications were increased if either value, alone or in combination, was abnormal. Postoperative mortality was increased only when both values were abnormal. Hickman[92] found that patients with colorectal cancer who had low preoperative serum albumin concentration had a greater postoperative complication rate and greater mortality, and preoperative body weight loss demonstrated similar predictive capacity for poor outcome. In the majority of situations, serum albumin appeared to be a strong predictor of outcome, although not necessarily a direct indicator of malnutrition.

Belghiti et al.[93] examined 75 patients with squamous cell carcinoma of the esophagus and found that 50% had abnormal nutritional or immunological indices. Patients with normal nutritional evaluation had a resectability rate of 71%, whereas those with abnormal values were only resectable in 29% of cases. Similar observations were made according to antecedent weight loss, with 38% of those with greater than 11% weight loss being resectable, compared to 76% of those with no weight loss. Postoperative leak rates were statistically greater in the malnourished.

Other studies have examined the complications of operation in cancer patients. Bozzeti et al.[94] examined the nutritional status of 162 cancer patients undergoing elective clean or clean contaminated operation. Preoperatively, the percent weight loss, arm muscle circumference, triceps skinfold thickness, creatinine–height index, total serum protein, serum albumin, total iron-binding capacity, cholinesterase, peripheral lymphocytes, complement C3–C4, and skin tests were all evaluated.

Postoperative sepsis occurred in 40 patients (25%), with diminished mean values for total serum protein, serum albumin, total iron-binding capacity, and cholinesterase, compared to values for 114 patients with no complications. Multivariate analysis demonstrated only total serum protein and total iron-binding capacity to be independent variables. However, many of these patients had only minimal preoperative abnormalities for some indices, e.g., mean percent usual body weight was $95 \pm 8\%$.

PERIOPERATIVE PARENTERAL NUTRITION

The effect of surgical intervention in the malnourished cancer patients can have devastating consequences. Several prospective randomized studies have been performed to examine whether the initiation of parenteral nutrition in the perioperative period can reduce postoperative morbidity and mortality. Listed in Table 12.3 are the major prospective randomized trials on this topic. One of the first randomized trials to address this question was reported in 1977 by Holter and Fischer.[95] The study group, 30 patients with upper gastrointestinal malignancy who had lost > 4.5 kg in the 3 month period before surgery, received 80 gm protein and 2000 kcal/d intravenously, starting 72 h before surgery and continuing for 10 d afterwards. The control group, 26 patients with a similar weight loss, did not receive nutritional support. Mortality was the same in the two groups, but major postoperative complications (prolonged ileus, intestinal obstruction, fistula formation, wound dehiscence, anastomotic leakage) occurred more frequently in the control group. Intravenous nutrition reduced (but not significantly) the rate of major complications from 19 to 13%. This study has been criticized for its small number of patients and the inability of 72 h of preoperative nutritional support to alter nutritional state significantly.

Moghissi et al.[96] also carried out a randomized study in patients with esophageal cancer undergoing thoracotomy. Fifteen patients were entered, and ten were randomized to receive approximately 35 kcal/kg and 0.2 gm nitrogen/kg daily for 5 to 7 d before and 6 to 7 d after surgery. Five patients in the control group were given

TABLE 12.3

Prospective Randomized Trials of Perioperative Total Parenteral Nutrition (TPN) in Cancer Patients

Author	Year	Number	Tumor Type	Timing of TPN	Complication Rate	Perioperative Mortality
Williams[154]	1976	74	Gastroesophageal	Preoperative	No difference	No difference
Holter[95]	1977	56	Gastrointestinal	Preoperative and postoperative	No difference	No difference
Moghissi[96]	1977	15	Esophageal	Preoperative and postoperative	No difference	NR
Heatley[97]	1979	74	Gastroesophageal	Preoperative	No difference	No difference
Mullen[155]	1980	145	Gastrointestinal	Preoperative	DECREASED	DECREASED
Simms[156]	1980	20	Gastroesophageal	Preoperative and Postoperative	NR	No difference
Thompson[157]	1981	21	Gastrointestinal	Preoperative and Postoperative	No difference	NR
Lim[158]	1981	24	Esophageal	Preoperative	No difference	No difference
Sako[159]	1981	68	Head and neck	Preoperative and Postoperative	NR	No difference
Muller[160]	1982	125	Gastrointestinal	Preoperative	DECREASED	DECREASED
Yamada[161]	1983	34	Gastric	Postoperative	No difference	No difference
Askanazi[162]	1986	35	Bladder	Postoperative	No difference	No difference
Muller[160]	1986	110	Gastroesophageal	Preoperative	DECREASED	No difference
Bellanton[163]	1988	100	Gastrointestinal	Preoperative	No difference	No difference
Woolfson[164]	1989	122	Head and neck, gastroesophagea, bladder	Postoperative	No difference	No difference
Buzby (VA group)[101]	1991	395*	gastrointestinal, lung	Preoperative and postoperative	No difference	No difference
Sandstrom[165]	1993	300	Gastrointestinal, bladder	Postoperative	No difference	No difference
Brennan[102]	1994	117	Pancreas	Postoperative	INCREASED	No difference
Fan[103]	1994	124	Hepatocellular	Preoperative and postoperative	DECREASED	No difference

* 66% of the patients had malignant disease.
Note: NR: not reported

only dextrose–saline (6 kcal/kg) over the same period. Patients in both groups had similar weight loss before operation (1.8 to 5.9 kg). Increased morbidity — impaired wound healing — was documented in four of the five patients in the control group. Because of the small number of patients, statistical significance was not obtained.

The first study to demonstrate significant beneficial effects was performed by Heatley et al., who randomized 74 patients with stomach or esophageal cancer to preoperative total parenteral nutrition (TPN) plus an oral diet versus an oral diet alone for 7 to 10 d.[97] All patients with esophageal anastomoses were given postoperative TPN, regardless of randomization. The overall complication rate, mortality rate, and hospital length of stay were not different between the groups. Subset analysis revealed a significantly lower percentage of wound infections in the treated group; and the difference was magnified if a second subset of patients with low serum albumin (< 3.5 gm/dl) were included.

Mullen et al.[98] compared the effect of 10 d of preoperative TPN ($n = 50$) with that of a standard oral hospital diet ($n = 95$) in patients undergoing surgery for intra-abdominal malignancy. The groups were matched for nutritional status and assessed by serum albumin < 3.5 gm/dl, negative responses to skin antigens, and weight loss > 5 kg in the preceding 12 months. Although this study demonstrated a significant decrease in major complications and mortality in the group receiving TPN, the intake of those receiving oral nutrition was not controlled. In a similar study, Muller et al. randomized 160 upper GI and colorectal cancer patients to 10 d of preoperative TPN plus oral diet versus oral diet alone.[99] This clinical trial reported a significant reduction in the major complication rate (intra-abdominal abscess, peritonitis, anastomotic leakage, ileus) and mortality in the treatment group. There are significant concerns with this trial. When the surgeons in this study began stapling their anastomoses, anastomotic leakage — which was the major cause of the mortality and morbidity — was substantially reduced, whether or not patients received nutritional supplementation.

These studies have been criticized because of small numbers of patients, lack of randomization, use of unsuitable control groups, differences in nutritional status before surgery, and inadequate quantity or duration of nutrition. Detsky et al.[100] carried out a meta-analysis of trials of perioperative nutritional support and, despite the limitations of many of the studies, found that nutritional supplementation reduced the morbidity rate by 21% and the mortality rate by 32% after major surgery, although it was not possible to identify clearly which particular patients would benefit. Major iatrogenic complications associated with TPN were documented in 7% of patients.

Because of problems in the methodology and design of previous randomized clinical trials evaluating the impact of perioperative TPN in the reduction of postoperative morbidity and mortality, Buzby et al.[101] performed a critical review of previous randomized trials and determined that the defects in these studies fell into four major categories: defects in statistical design (inadequate sample size, inappropriate procedures for randomization); inappropriate patient selection (presence of malnutrition not an eligibility requirement for study participation); inappropriate treatment regimens (inadequate TPN regimen in treated patients, use of forced enteral feeding in control subjects); inadequate definition of endpoint criteria (lack of objective criteria defining presence of complications).

These considerations led to the development of the Veterans Affairs Total Parenteral Nutrition Cooperative Group study.[82] This was a prospective, multicenter study that followed 395 patients undergoing thoracic or abdominal surgery who were randomized to 7 to 15 d of preoperative and 3 d of postoperative TPN versus no intravenous nutritional support. All patients were given an oral diet if clinically indicated (mean daily caloric intake in the TPN group was 2944 kcal and in the control group was 1280 kcal). Sixty-six percent of the patients were cancer patients. The overall complication rate and mortality were not different between the groups, suggesting no benefit to routine perioperative support. In addition, the incidence of infectious complications and the length of hospital stay were greater in the TPN group. However, subgroup analysis revealed that if patients were severely malnourished (as defined by the Nutrition Risk Index or the Subjective Global Assessment),[89] they had a significantly lower noninfectious complication rate without an increase in the infectious complications. Noninfectious complications included major complications, such as anastomotic leakage, bronchopleural fistula, and organ dysfunction.

Two prospective randomized studies have examined the role of perioperative TPN in pancreatic cancer and hepatocellular carcinoma with differing conclusions. Brennan et al.[102] randomized 117 patients with pancreatic cancer undergoing major pancreatic resection to receive postoperative parenteral nutrition (mean 12 d) or standard intravenous fluids. The majority of patients demonstrated mild malnutrition based on weight loss and serum albumin. Major complications that could potentially be influenced by the addition of TPN (fistula, abscess, obstruction, anastomotic leakage, reoperation) were significantly higher in the group that received parenteral nutrition. There were no differences in postoperative mortality or length of hospital stay between the two groups. Fan et al.[103] studied 124 patients with hepatocellular carcinoma who underwent major hepatic resection randomized to 7 d of preoperative and 7 d of postoperative TPN versus intravenous fluids and an oral diet. A significant reduction in the postoperative complication rate was demonstrated primarily due to a reduction in the subset of infectious complications. Again, there were no significant differences in the mortality or hospital length of stay.

In assessing the clinical implications of these various studies, it appears that routine perioperative TPN is not associated with a significant benefit in the surgical cancer patient, regardless of the type of malignancy or the magnitude of the operation. The use of TPN can be associated with an increased risk of infectious complications. However, subset analyses seem to indicate that if after conducting a nutritional assessment of the patient, whether by clinical or objective measures, a severe level of malnutrition is determined, then these patients may benefit from perioperative TPN, as the risks of nutritionally related complications outweigh the risks of TPN-related complications.

PERIOPERATIVE ENTERAL NUTRITION

Several prospective randomized studies have also examined the role of enteral feeding in the perioperative period in cancer patients, and these are listed in Table 12.4. The proposed advantages of enteral nutrition over parenteral include the following:

- Maintenance of gut mucosal mass
- Maintenance of brush border enzyme activity
- Support of gut immune function
- Preservation of gut mucosal barrier function
- Maintenance of a balanced luminal microflora environment

TABLE 12.4
Prospective Randomized Trials of Perioperative Enteral Feeding in Cancer Patients

Author	Year	Number	Tumor Type	Timing of Enteral Nutrition	Control	Complication Rate	Perioperative Mortality
Shukla[104]	1984	110	Gastrointestina, oral, breast	Preoperative	IVF	DECREASED	DECREASED
Smith[106]	1985	50	Gastrointestinal	Postoperative	IVF	No difference	No difference
Spirtos[105]	1988	60	Gynecologic	Postoperative	IVF	No difference	No difference
Meijerink[107]	1992	151	Gastric, colorectal	Preoperative	TPN and IVF	NR	No difference
Baigrie[108]	1996	97	Gastroesophageal	Postoperative	TPN	No difference	No difference
Beier-Holgerson[109]	1996	60[a]	Abdominal	Postoperative	IVF	DECREASED	No difference
Shirabe[110]	1997	26	Hepatic	Postoperative	TPN	No difference	No difference
Bozzetti[111]	2001	317	Gastrointestinal	Postoperative	TPN	DECREASED	No difference

[a] Approximately two thirds of patients had a diagnosis of cancer; 66% of the patients had malignant disease.
Note: NR: not reported.

A randomized study by Shukla et al.[104] compared preoperative enteral feeding versus regular oral diet/postoperative crystalloid solutions in 110 patients with gastrointestinal, oral, and breast cancers. The enterally fed group had decreased postoperative wound infections, less mortality, and shorter length of stay. Unfortunately, no formal statistical analysis was performed on the results.

Spirtos et al.[105] randomized 60 patients with gynecologic cancer to early postoperative enteral feeding versus standard intravenous crystalloid solutions. Approximately 25% of the patients were considered malnourished. More calories and nutrition were received by the fed group, but there were not significant differences in the overall or infectious complication rate, mortality, or length of hospital stay.

Smith et al.[106] randomized 50 patients with gastrointestinal cancers to postoperative enteral feeding via feeding jejunostomy versus standard intravenous fluids. Complications defined as "related to the surgical procedure" were not different between the groups. Length of stay was significantly prolonged in the jejunostomy group, and overall mortality was similar. Catheter-related complications were high, and one death was directly attributable to the feedings.

Meijerink et al.[107] randomized 151 gastric and colorectal cancer patients to 10 d of preoperative enteral nutrition versus 10 d of preoperative TPN versus no nutritional intervention. All patients were described as "depleted," but no specific parameters for this designation were reported. The overall complication rate and length of hospital stay were not reported, but there was a significant reduction in the number of intra-abdominal abscesses and septic events in the group fed enterally compared with the unfed controls. There were no differences in the postoperative mortality for any of the groups. There were no differences in any of the clinical outcomes between the enterally fed and TPN group, respectively. Subset analysis of patients with weight loss greater than 10% again demonstrated a reduction of intra-abdominal abscesses in the enterally fed and TPN groups compared with the control patients.

Baigrie et al.[108] compared postoperative enteral feeding with a feeding jejunostomy vs. TPN in 97 patients undergoing esophagectomy or gastrectomy. Catheter-related complications between the two groups were similar, but 45% of patients in the TPN group suffered major complications. However, there were no statistically significant differences in clinical outcomes reported between the two groups.

Beier-Holgersen et al.[109] randomized 60 patients undergoing "major abdominal" operations to postoperative enteral feeding compared to a placebo solution (unfed control). Approximately two thirds of the operations were for cancer, and only a few of the patients were malnourished. Specific data about the preoperative nutritional status of the patients were not reported in the study. A significant reduction in the overall complication rate and infectious complications was demonstrated in the enteral feeding group. No significant differences in mortality and length of stay were found.

Shirabe et al.[110] randomized 26 patients undergoing hepatic resection for malignancy into two groups: early postoperative enteral feeding and TPN. The enteral feeding group demonstrated a significantly greater immune response in the postoperative period, and there was a nonsignificant trend toward decreased infectious complications in the enteral feeding group.

Bozzeti et al.[111] reported a large randomized multicenter clinical trial of 317 patients with gastrointestinal cancer who were considered malnourished, but were candidates for elective surgery. The treatment group received postoperative enteral nutrition, and the control group received parenteral nutrition with a primary endpoint of postoperative complications. There was a statistically significant difference in complication rate of 34% versus 49% for the enteral feeding and parenteral feeding groups, respectively ($p = 0.005$). The hospital stay was 13.4 d in the enteral nutrition group and 15.0 d for the parenteral nutrition group ($p = 0.009$). Fourteen patients crossed over to the parenteral nutrition group due to intolerance of enteral feeds.

Though there are fewer studies comparing perioperative enteral feeding to TPN or intravenous fluids in patients with malignant disease, the results seem to mirror the conclusions of the previous studies examining parenteral nutrition. The routine use of enteral feeding in the perioperative period is not indicated, but in those patients who exhibit signs, symptoms, and biochemical evidence of severe malnutrition, enteral feeding in the preoperative and postoperative period may help to decrease postoperative complications. Because of the reasons mentioned at the beginning of this section, it is to be preferred over TPN in those patients who can tolerate it. The optimal delivery method and enteral feeding schedule have yet to be determined.

NUTRITIONAL SUPPORT AND CHEMOTHERAPY

Prospective cohort analyses suggest that malnutrition is a risk factor for diminished responsiveness to chemotherapy, increased toxicity of the drugs, poorer quality of life, and shorter survival.[112] However, early clinical trials (see Table 12.5) that examined the efficacy of nutritional support in chemotherapy were largely negative and resulted in a meta-analysis that concluded that routine nutritional support in this setting was not indicated.[113] Subsequent intervention trials, which have stratified the patients by nutritional status, have generally shown that gains in nutritional status can be realized in malnourished patients undergoing chemotherapy, although a reduction in toxicity still has not been reproducibly demonstrated.[114,115] If such patients subsequently proceed to surgery, the nutritional support appears to improve their perioperative course.[115]

Cancer patients who receive chemotherapy may develop severe and prolonged mucositis and enterocolitis, which precludes using the GI tract for nutritional support. Under these circumstances, TPN should be provided to malnourished patients until the enteritis resolves and oral feeding can be resumed. In addition, under circumstances in which chemotherapy may be contraindicated due to severe malnutrition, parenteral nutrition may be beneficial in optimizing nutritional status and allowing the initiation of a chemotherapeutic regimen. As in the perioperative setting, when enteral nutrition is feasible, it should be the preferred method of nutritional support.

NUTRITIONAL SUPPORT AND RADIATION THERAPY

The radiation-induced nutritional disorders depend on the tumor localization, the region irradiated, the dose and length of radiotherapy, the fractionation, the volume irradiated, and the combination with other therapeutic modalities.[116] The acute

TABLE 12.5
Results of Prospective Randomized Controlled Trials Evaluating Nutritional Therapy (NT) in Patients Receiving Chemotherapy

Author	Tumor Type	Patients		Survival		Tumor Response (%)		Treatment Toxicity		Infection Rate (%)	
		NT	Control	NT	Control	NT	Control	Heme	GI	NT	Control
				Parenteral Nutrition							
Nixon et al.[128]	Colorectal	20	25	79	308 (mean)	15	12	Worse	No difference	5	4
Samuels et al.[166]	Testicular	16	14	72%	77% (2.5 yr)	63	79	Better	No difference	17	4
Shamberger et al.[167]	Sarcoma	14	18	13%	44% (4 yr)	14	50	No difference	No difference	42	33
Valdivieso et al.[168]	Small-cell lung	30	35	11 months	12 month (median)	43	66	No difference	Worse	27	18
Clamon et al.[169]	Small-cell lung	57	62	51%	57% (1 yr)	48	43	Better	NA	35	5
Issell et al.[170]	Squamous-cell lung	13	13	NA	NA	31	8	Better	Better	NA	NA
Jordan et al.[171]	Adenocarcinoma lung	19	24	22 weeks	40 week (median)	12	30	Worse	No difference	32	8

Enteral Nutrition

Study	Tumor								
Elkort et al.[172]	Breast	24	23	84%	87% (1 yr)	No difference		No difference	No difference
Evans et al.[173]	Non-small cell	30	36	8 months	6 months (median)	28	15	NA	NA
	Colorectal	21	33	9 months	24 months (median)	10	16	NA	No difference
Tandon et al.[174]	GI	31	39	94%	85%	35	21	NA	Better
Bounous et al.[175]	Metastatic	9	12	NA	NA	56	64	No difference	No difference

Note: NA = not available.

Source: From *Cancer: Principles and Practice of Oncology*, 5th ed., Lippincott-Raven, 1997, p.2849. With permission.

radiation-induced reactions are usually of limited duration and, for this reason, tend to interfere with the nutritional status to a lesser extent than the permanent chronic consequences of irradiation. Weight loss and malnutrition tend to develop particularly in patients in whom segments of the gastrointestinal tract are subjected to irradiation.

The use of aggressive nutritional support in patients undergoing radiation therapy has been most extensively studied in individuals who have aero digestive cancers, because such patients tend to have mechanical difficulties with deglutition, they have a high prevalence of substantial malnutrition,[117] and radiation therapy is a commonly used modality of treatment in this cancer population. Table 12.6 lists the results of prospective randomized trials examining the role of nutritional support in cancer patients treated with radiation therapy. These trials do not demonstrate any consistent significant benefit in terms of survival or treatment toxicity. In patients with head and neck cancers, nutritional support has also been shown to significantly improve objective indicators of the quality of life,[118] which may be enough to justify its use for these types of patients.

RECOMMENDATIONS FOR NUTRITIONAL SUPPORT IN CANCER PATIENTS

A thorough review of the literature of nutritional support in cancer patients has only served to demonstrate the inconsistency and methodologic flaws of various well-intentioned clinical trials. Most of the data for these studies come from the use of parenteral and enteral nutrition in the perioperative period. However, the increasing role of multimodality therapy also brings chemotherapy and radiation therapy into the equation. The following recommendations come from an attempt to combine the conclusions from the aforementioned reports with a realistic commonsense desire to provide the cancer patient with the best chance for a successful intervention, whatever the modality.

For cancer patients undergoing elective major oncologic surgery, perioperative nutritional support is indicated in the following situations:

1. When no oral intake is anticipated for 7 to 10 d postoperatively, enteral feedings should be initiated 2 to 3 d after the operation. This can be accomplished through a nasoduodenal feeding tube or a feeding jejunostomy placed at the time of operation. If the risk of aspiration is low, and there are no surgical anastomotic concerns, a nasogastric or surgical gastrostomy tube can be used as well. If the gut cannot be used, then parenteral feedings should be initiated postoperatively.

2. If after 7 d the patient cannot take oral nutrition when it was originally thought he or she would be able to, then parenteral nutrition should be initiated at that time. A nasogastric or nasoduodenal feeding tube can then be inserted and enteral feedings started at the same time. It usually takes 3 to 4 d to reach caloric goals, and the TPN can then be decreased as the enteral feedings are increased.

TABLE 12.6
Results of Prospective Randomized Controlled Trials Evaluating Nutritional Therapy (NT) in Patients Treated with Radiation Therapy

| Author | Tumor Type | Patients | | Survival | | Treatment Toxicity | |
		NT	Control	NT	Control	Heme	GI
		Parenteral Nutrition					
Solassol et al.[176]	Ovarian	42	39	9 months	8 months[a]	NA	Better
Kinsella et al.[177]	Pelvic	17	15	47%	47%	NA	NA
Ghavimi et al.[178]	Childhood	14	14	27%	29%	Worse	Worse
Donaldson et al.[179]	Childhood	12	13	8%	8%[b]	NA	Worse
		Enteral Nutrition					
Douglass et al.[180]	GI	13	17	62%	76%	No difference	NA
Brown et al.[181]	Pelvic	30	17	NA	NA	Better	No difference
Bounous et al.[182]	Abdomen/pelvic	9	9	NA	NA	Better	Better
Daly et al.[183]	Head and neck	22	18	NA	NA	NA	Worse
Moloney et al.[184]	Various	42	42	36%	38%	NA	NA

[a] Median.
[b] Posttherapy.
Note: NA = Not available.

Source: From Cancer: Principles and Practice of Oncology, 5th ed., Lippincott-Raven, 1997, p.2849. With permission.

3. Patients with severe preoperative malnutrition (preoperative weight loss greater than 10% and serum albumin level less than 3.5 g/dl) should receive 7 to 10 d of preoperative nutritional support. The preferred method is enteral feedings as described in number 2. TPN can be administered until enteral feedings are at goal rate. If the gut cannot be used, then parenteral nutrition should be given for the entire period.

Cancer patients undergoing chemotherapy or radiation therapy who are severely malnourished should receive pretreatment nutritional support for 7 to 15 d, and this should continue during therapy until the patient's clinical and biochemical parameters improve. Patients with enteritis or stomatitis from chemotherapy or radiation therapy should receive TPN. For those individuals with aero digestive malignancies unable to tolerate oral intake, a feeding gastrostomy should be placed. Traditionally, these patients underwent placement of a percutaneous endoscopic gastrostomy tube for administration of enteral feedings during chemoradiation therapy. However, in a recent review of the literature,[119] at least 19 cases of metastatic head and neck carcinoma were found at the site of percutaneous endoscopic gastrostomies that were inserted by the "pull" method for the placement of gastrostomy tubes. It is theorized that this technique may induce metastasis by direct implantation of tumor cells because of contact between the gastrostomy tube and tumor cells. Laparoscopic gastrostomy tube placement has been shown to be a safe, effective, and minimally invasive method of enteral access in these patients.[120] Percutaneous radiologic gastrostomy under fluoroscopic guidance is another alternative in this setting. However, there are some reports in the literature[121–123] that suggest a higher incidence of tube-related complications when compared to surgically or endoscopically placed gastrostomies.

NUTRIENT EXCESS AND TUMOR GROWTH

A major concern with the use of aggressive nutritional supplementation in the malnourished cancer patient is the potential to stimulate tumor growth. The animal tumor model has been studied regarding this issue, with investigators measuring tumor volume, weight, mitotic activity, DNA/RNA concentration, and protein synthesis rates to determine the presence of tumor growth during nutritional supplementation. Several reports have demonstrated tumor growth to be significantly increased by nutritional support, and in some cases, the rate of cancer stimulation was greater than that of the host tissues.[124–126] However, these studies have been criticized for using transplanted tumors with rapid doubling times and large tumor–host weight ratios.

Human studies of tumor growth stimulation by nutrition are scarce, though one report by Jin et al.[115] suggests there may be some increase in DNA synthesis during nutritional repletion in malnourished cancer patients. One of the problems is lack of a reliable and accurate method to assess tumor growth stimulation caused by nutritional supplementation. In malignant cells, growth is effected by protein synthesis, and this has been used as a determinant of cellular proliferation.[127] Mullen et al.[98] measured tumor protein synthesis rates in a nonrandomized study and reported that in patients with gastrointestinal cancer, there was no difference in rates between groups receiving adequate parenteral ($n = 13$) or inadequate oral ($n = 12$) nutrition. Nixon et al.[128] found neither clinical nor biochemical evidence of tumor growth in patients with metastatic colorectal carcinoma when patients were fed intravenously ($n = 55$) or orally ($n = 61$). These studies suggest that nutritional support does not stimulate tumor growth, although the methods of growth assessment used were considered relatively crude.

A more recent study by Bozzeti et al.[129] measured tumor cell growth in 19 malnourished patients with gastric cancer who received either 10 d of preoperative TPN or no nutritional support. Tumor cell proliferation was evaluated by measuring variations in S-phase cell fraction using 3H-thymidine labeling index (TLI). The overall TLI value between the two groups was not significantly different, though 50% of patients in the TPN group exhibited some tumor cell proliferation. A review of this topic by Cozzaglio et al.[130] concluded there is no clinically significant effect of TPN on tumor growth in humans. However, the available studies in the literature are limited by the small number of patients, lack of a sure and reproducible method to analyze tumor growth, and trial design flaws.

The potential for tumor growth stimulation by nutritional supplementation may increase tumor susceptibility to cycle-specific chemotherapeutic agents by placing more cancer cells in the vulnerable DNA synthesis phase of the cell cycle. Reynolds et al.[131] investigated the effect of methotrexate on tumor growth in rats. Animals were placed on a protein-free diet or standard oral nutritional regimen and then given methotrexate. A better response to therapy was observed in the rats given an oral diet compared to the group on a protein-free diet. A similarly enhanced response to chemotherapy was found in rats fed on continuous parenteral or intrajejunal feeding for 10 d before chemotherapy.[132] Another study combined nutritional support with doxorubicin (cell-cycle-specific agent) and cyclophosphamide (cell-cycle-nonspecific agent) in a rat model with subcutaneously implanted AC33 breast cancer, and found that in animals receiving pulsed TPN, the antitumor effect of doxorubicin, but not cyclophosphamide, was enhanced.[133] The effect of parenteral nutrition on AC33 breast tumor cell kinetics has revealed that 2 h of TPN was sufficient to increase the number of cells in the S-phase with a corresponding decrease in the ratios of G0/G1 and G2/M cancer cell populations.[134] These results must be interpreted with caution before extrapolating them to the effects of TPN on human chemotherapeutic regimens. The tumors in these animal models were rapidly growing with doubling times of 2 to 3 d and resulted in the death of the animals within 6 weeks.[124]

It is true, however, that the sensitivity of human breast cancers to chemotherapy is also dependent on the number of cells in the S-phase of the cell cycle. Remvikos et al.[135] demonstrated that patients with tumors having greater than 10% of the cells in S-phase had an increased response to chemotherapy. Park et al.[136] was one of the first to study the effect of nutrient support on the response of cancer cells to chemotherapy. It was demonstrated that a 3 d pulse of oral arginine supplementation could stimulate human breast cancer protein synthesis and expression of activation antigens *in vivo*. A prospective randomized, double-blind placebo controlled trial was performed in patients receiving neoadjuvant chemotherapy for breast cancer.[185] Ninety-six patients were randomized to receive 3 d of the amino acid arginine versus placebo prior to chemotherapy (doxorubicin, cyclophosphamide, vincristine, prednisolone). There was no significant difference in overall clinical response rate between the arginine group (77%) and the placebo group (71%). Further study is required before this approach can be considered a standard for clinical practice.

FUTURE DIRECTIONS: IMMUNONUTRITION

The use of nutritional supplements in excess of what is necessary to meet basal metabolic requirements in order to provide additional clinical benefit to the individual is called targeted nutrient therapy.[7] These substances may act more as a pharmaceutical agent with specific physiologic actions rather than just meet nutritional needs. The following section will discuss the potential benefit of the addition of omega-3 fatty acids, glutamine, arginine, and RNA during nutritional support of malnourished cancer patients.

Conventional enteral and parenteral nutritional formulations use a vegetable oil rich in omega-6 polyunsaturated fatty acids as a source of fat. In the targeted nutrient therapy setting, these standard fatty acids are replaced with one or both of the two major omega-3 polyunsaturated fatty acids, eicosapentaenoic acid and docosahexaenoic acid, with the hope these nutrients will help to attenuate or reverse the effects of cancer cachexia. This substitution of fatty acids not only changes the fatty acid composition of immune cell membranes, it also alters the immune response.[137] Studies have shown that supplemental n-3 fatty acids appear to downregulate the systemic reaction to inflammatory regulators in healthy volunteers, but in malnourished cancer patients or those stressed by major surgery, levels of mediators such as TNF-α are increased, and lymphocyte responsiveness is enhanced.[137-141] It appears the immunomodulation of n-3 fatty acids is affected by the overall health status of the individual taking the supplementation. Other substances thought to have an effect on the immune system beyond that of merely nutrient value include arginine, RNA, and glutamine. Many studies in tumor-bearing or otherwise stressed animal models have demonstrated that nutritional supplementation with arginine, RNA, or glutamine can improve cell-mediated immune responses and, in some instances, enhance survival.[142-144]

Various studies, including a meta-analysis, have examined the clinical benefit of multimodality supplements, including n-3 fatty acids, RNA, arginine, and glutamine for patients with gastrointestinal cancer undergoing surgery.[145-149] When immunologic and biochemical parameters were examined, the administration of ˈese multimodality immunomodulatory formulas produced significant decreases in levels of mediators of systemic inflammation, simultaneous increases in cell-ˈated immunity, and, in some cases, an enhancement of net protein bal-ˈ,150-152 In most of these trials, these changes translated into a significant in perioperative infections[145-148] and length of hospital stay[145,146,148] when ˈo both standard enteral and parenteral nutrition.

exception was a study performed by Heslin et al.,[153] who performed ˈandomized study comparing early enteral feeding versus intravenous crystalloid solutions in 195 patients undergoing resection of upper gastrointestinal cancers. The enteral feedings were supplemented with an immune-enhancing formulation of arginine, RNA, and omega-3 fatty acids. Patients in the study had a mean preoperative weight loss of only 5% and possessed normal mean serum albumin levels. Though the treatment group received significantly more protein, carbohydrate, lipids, and immune-enhancing nutrients than did the control group, there were no significant differences in complication rate, perioperative mortality, or length of hospital stay. This study confirms the concept that aggressive nutritional support, even with immunonutrients, does not benefit adequately nourished patients.

Though there appears to be substantial evidence to indicate the clinical benefit of multimodality immunomodulatory formulas in malnourished cancer patients undergoing surgery, there is still controversy regarding its widespread application, and it is not uniformly recommended.[80] Further research may be helpful in further defining those groups of patients who would truly benefit from nutritional supplementation and determining the ultimate efficacy of immunonutrient-supplemented enteral feedings.

REFERENCES

1. Nitenberg, G. and Raynard, B., Nutritional support of the cancer patient: issues and dilemmas, *Crit. Rev. Oncol. Hematol.*, 34, 137–168, 2000.
2. Dewys, W.D., Begg, C., Lavin, P.T., Band, P.R., Bennett, J.M., Bertino, J.R., Cohen, M.H., Douglass, H.O., Jr., Engstrom, P.F., Ezdinli, E.Z., Horton, J., Johnson, G.J., Moertel, C.G., Oken, M.M., Perlia, C., Rosenbaum, C., Silverstein, M.N., Skeel, R.T., Sponzo, R.W., and Tormey, D.C. Prognostic effect of weight loss prior to chemotherapy in cancer patients. Eastern Cooperative Oncology Group, *Am. J. Med.*, 69, 491–497, 1980.
3. Bosaeus, I., Daneryd, P., Svanberg, E., and Lundholm, K., Dietary intake and resting energy expenditure in relation to weight loss in unselected cancer patients, *Int. J. Cancer*, 93, 380–383, 2001.
4. Tisdale, M.J., Cancer anorexia and cachexia, *Nutrition*, 17, 438–442, 2001.
5. Barber, M.D., Ross, J.A., Fearon, K.C., Disordered metabolic response with cancer and its management, *World J. Surg.*, 24, 681–689, 2000.
6. Fredrix, E.W., Soeters, P.B., Wouters, E.F., Deerenberg, I.M., von Meyenfeldt, M.F., and Saris, W.H., Effect of different tumor types on resting energy expenditure, *Cancer Res.*, 51, 6138–6141, 1991.
7. Mason, J.B. and Choi, S.W., Gastrointestinal cancer: nutritional support, in *Gastrointestinal Oncology: Principles and Practice*, Kelsen D.P. et al., Eds., Lippincott Williams & Wilkins, Philadelphia, 2002, chap. 9.
8. Rofe, A.M., Bourgeois, C.S., Coyle, P., Taylor, A., and Abdi, E.A., Altered insulin response to glucose in weight-losing cancer patients, *Anticancer Res.*, 14, 647–650, 1994.
9. Shaw, J.H. and Wolfe, R.R., Fatty acid and glycerol kinetics in septic patients and in patients with gastrointestinal cancer. The response to glucose infusion and parenteral feeding, *Ann. Surg.*, 205, 368–376, 1987.
10. Todorov, P., Cariuk, P., McDevitt, T., Coles, B., Fearon, K., and Tisdale, M., Characterization of a cancer cachectic factor, *Nature*, 379, 739–742, 1996.

11. Chance, W.T., Balasubramaniam, A., Thompson, H., Mohapatra, B., Ramo, J., and Fischer, J.E., Assessment of feeding response of tumor-bearing rats to hypothalamic injection and infusion of neuropeptide Y, *Peptides*, 17, 797–801, 1996.

12. Mantzoros, C.S., The role of leptin in human obesity and disease: a review of current evidence, *Ann. Intern. Med.*, 130, 671–680, 1999.

13. Fried, S.K. and Zechner, R., Cachectin/tumor necrosis factor decreases human adipose tissue lipoprotein lipase MRNA levels, synthesis, and activity, *J. Lipid Res.*, 30, 1917–1923, 1989.

14. Garcia-Martinez, C., Lopez-Soriano, F.J., and Argiles, J.M., Acute treatment with tumour necrosis factor- induces changes in protein metabolism in rat skeletal muscle, *Mol. Cell Biochem.*, 125, 11–18, 1993.

15. Starnes, H.F., Jr., Warren, R.S., Jeevanandam, M., Gabrilove, J.L., Larchian, W., Oettgen, H.F., and Brennan, M.F., Tumor necrosis factor and the acute metabolic response to tissue injury in man, *J. Clin. Invest.*, 82, 1321–1325, 1988.

16. Smith, B.K. and Kluger, M.J., Anti-TNF- antibodies normalized body temperature and enhanced food intake in tumor-bearing rats, *Am. J. Physiol.*, 265, R615–R619, 1993.

17. Castell, J.V., Gomez-Lechon, M.J., David, M., Fabra, R., Trullenque, R., and Heinrich, P.C., Acute-phase response of human hepatocytes: regulation of acute-phase protein synthesis by interleukin-6, *Hepatology*, 12, 1179–1186, 1990.

18. Scott, H.R., McMillan, D.C., Crilly, A., McArdle, C.S., and Milroy, R., The relationship between weight loss and interleukin 6 in non-small-cell lung cancer, *Br. J. Cancer*, 73, 1560–1562, 1996.

19. Strassmann, G., Fong, M., Kenney, J.S., and Jacob, C.O., Evidence for the involvement of interleukin 6 in experimental cancer cachexia, *J. Clin. Invest.*, 89, 1681–1684, 1992.

20. Soda, K., Kawakami, M., Kashii, A., and Miyata, M., Manifestations of cancer cachexia induced by colon 26 adenocarcinoma are not fully ascribable to interleukin-6, *Int. J. Cancer*, 62, 332–336, 1995.

21. Henderson, J.T., Seniuk, N.A., Richardson, P.M., Gauldie, J., and Roder, J.C., Systemic administration of ciliary neurotrophic factor induces cachexia in rodents, *J. Clin. Invest.*, 93, 2632–2638, 1994.

22. Espat, N.J., Auffenberg, T., Rosenberg, J.J., Rogy, M., Martin, D., Fang, C.H., Hasselgren, P.O., Copeland, E.M., and Moldawer, L.L., Ciliary neurotrophic factor is catabolic and shares with IL-6 the capacity to induce an acute phase response, *Am. J. Physiol.*, 271, R185–R190, 1996.

23. Oldenburg, H.S., Rogy, M.A., Lazarus, D.D., Van Zee, K.J., Keeler, B.P., Chizzonite, R.A., Lowry, S.F., and Moldawer, L.L., Cachexia and the acute-phase protein response in inflammation are regulated by interleukin-6, *Eur. J. Immunol.*, 23, 1889–1894, 1993.

24. Belizario, J.E., Katz, M., Chenker, E., and Raw, I., Bioactivity of skeletal muscle proteolysis-inducing factors in the plasma proteins from cancer patients with weight loss, *Br. J. Cancer*, 63, 705–710, 1991.

25. Khan, S. and Tisdale, M.J., Catabolism of adipose tissue by a tumour-produced lipid-mobilising factor, *Int. J. Cancer*, 80, 444–447, 1999.

Lorite, M.J., Thompson, M.G., Drake, J.L., Carling, G., and Tisdale, M.J., Mechanism muscle protein degradation induced by a cancer cachectic factor, *Br. J. Cancer*, 850–856, 1998.

S.A. and Tisdale, M.J., Production of lipolytic and proteolytic factors by a tumor-producing cachexia in the host, *Cancer Res.*, 47, 5919–5923, 1987.

28. Willox, J.C., Corr, J., Shaw, J., Richardson, M., Calman, K.C., and Drennan, M., Prednisolone as an appetite stimulant in patients with cancer, *Br. Med. J. (Clin. Res. Ed.)*, 288, 27, 1984.

29. Moertel, C.G., Schutt, A.J., Reitemeier, R.J., and Hahn, R.G., Corticosteroid therapy of preterminal gastrointestinal cancer, *Cancer*, 33, 1607–1609, 1974.

30. Loprinzi, C.L., Ellison, N.M., Schaid, D.J., Krook, J.E., Athmann, L.M., Dose, A.M., Mailliard, J.A., Johnson, P.S., Ebbert, L.P., and Geeraerts, L.H., Controlled trial of megestrol acetate for the treatment of cancer anorexia and cachexia, *J. Natl. Cancer Inst.*, 82, 1127–1132, 1990.

31. Bruera, E., Macmillan, K., Kuehn, N., Hanson, J., and MacDonald, R.N., A controlled trial of megestrol acetate on appetite, caloric intake, nutritional status, and other symptoms in patients with advanced cancer, *Cancer*, 66, 1279–1282, 1990.

32. Feliu, J., Gonzalez-Baron, M., Berrocal, A., Artal, A., Ordonez, A., Garrido, P., Zamora, P., Garcia de Paredes, M.L., and Montero, J.M., Usefulness of megestrol acetate in cancer cachexia and anorexia. A placebo-controlled study, *Am. J. Clin. Oncol.*, 15, 436–440, 1992.

33. McMillan, D.C., Preston, T., Watson, W.S., Simpson, J.M., Fearon, K.C., Shenkin, A., Burns, H.J., and McArdle, C.S., Relationship between weight loss, reduction of body cell mass and inflammatory response in patients with cancer, *Br. J. Surg.*, 81, 1011–1014, 1994.

34. McMillan, D.C., Leen, E., Smith, J., Sturgeon, C., Preston, T., Cooke, T.G., and McArdle, C.S., Effect of extended ibuprofen administration on the acute phase protein response in colorectal cancer patients, *Eur. J. Surg. Oncol.*, 21, 531–534, 1995.

35. Preston, T., Fearon, K.C., McMillan, D.C., Winstanley, F.P., Slater, C., Shenkin, A., and Carter, D.C., Effect of ibuprofen on the acute-phase response and protein metabolism in patients with cancer and weight loss, *Br. J. Surg.*, 82, 229–234, 1995.

36. Wigmore, S.J., Falconer, J.S., Plester, C.E., Ross, J.A., Maingay, J.P., Carter, D.C., and Fearon, K.C., Ibuprofen reduces energy expenditure and acute-phase protein production compared with placebo in pancreatic cancer patients, *Br. J. Cancer*, 72, 185–188, 1995.

37. McMillan, D.C., Wigmore, S.J., Fearon, K.C., O'Gorman, P., Wright, C.E., and McArdle, C.S., A prospective randomized study of megestrol acetate and ibuprofen in gastrointestinal cancer patients with weight loss, *Br. J. Cancer*, 79, 495–500, 1999.

38. Lundholm, K., Gelin, J., Hyltander, A., Lonnroth, C., Sandstrom, R., Svaninger, G., Korner, U., Gulich, M., Karrefors, I., Norli, B., Anti-inflammatory treatment may prolong survival in undernourished patients with metastatic solid tumors, *Cancer Res.*, 54, 5602–5606, 1994.

39. Cornell, K. and Waters, D.J., Impaired wound healing in the cancer patient: effects of cytotoxic therapy and pharmacologic modulation by growth factors, *Vet. Clin. North Am. Small Anim. Pract.*, 25, 111–131, 1995.

40. Springfield, D.S., Surgical wound healing, *Cancer Treat. Res.*, 67, 81–98, 1993.

41. Bennett, N.T. and Schultz, G.S., Growth factors and wound healing: biochemical properties of growth factors and their receptors, *Am. J. Surg.*, 165, 728–737, 1993.

42. Wahl, S.M., Wong, H., and McCartney-Francis, N., Role of growth factors in inflammation and repair, *J. Cell Biochem.*, 40, 193–199, 1989.

43. Peacock, E.E., Jr., Collagenolysis: the other side of the equation, *World J. Surg.*, 4, 297–302, 1980.

44. Vegesna, V., Withers, H.R., Holly, F.E., and McBride, W.H., The effect of local and systemic irradiation on impairment of wound healing in mice, *Radiat. Res.*, 135, 431–433, 1993.

45. Arbeit, J.M., Hilaris, B.S., and Brennan, M.F., Wound complications in the multimo-dality treatment of extremity and superficial truncal sarcomas, *J. Clin. Oncol.*, 5, 480–488, 1987.

46. Stockholm Rectal Cancer Study Group, Preoperative short-term radiation therapy in operable rectal carcinoma. A prospective randomized trial, *Cancer*, 66, 49–55, 1990.

47. O'Sullivan, B., Gullane, P., Irish, J., Neligan, P., Gentili, F., Mahoney, J., Sellmann, S., Catton, C., Waldron, J., Brown, D., Witterick, I., Freeman, J., and Bell, R., Preoperative radiotherapy for adult head and neck soft tissue sarcoma: assessment of wound complication rates and cancer outcome in a prospective series, *World J. Surg.*, 27, 875–883, 2003.

48. Murphy, K., Frith, C., Lang, N., et al., Effect of radiotherapy on healing of colonic anastomoses, *Surgery Forum*, 31, 222, 1980.

49. Karppinen, V. and Myllarniemi, H., Vascular reactions in the healing laparotomy wound under cytostatic treatment, *Acta Chir. Scand.*, 136, 675–680, 1970.

50. Devereux, D.F., Thibault, L., Boretos, J., and Brennan, M.F., The quantitative and qualitative impairment of wound healing by adriamycin, *Cancer*, 43, 932–938, 1979.

51. Lawrence, W.T., Norton, J.A., Harvey, A.K., Gorschboth, C.M., Talbot, T.L., and Grotendorst, G.R., Doxorubicin-induced impairment of wound healing in rats, *J. Natl. Cancer Inst.*, 76, 119–126, 1986.

52. Lawrence, W.T., Talbot, T.L., and Norton, J.A., Preoperative or postoperative doxo-rubicin hydrochloride (adriamycin): which is better for wound healing? *Surgery*, 100, 9–13, 1986.

53. Lawrence, W.T., Norton, J.A., Sporn, M.B., Gorschboth, C., and Grotendorst, G.R., The reversal of an adriamycin induced healing impairment with chemoattractants and growth factors, *Ann. Surg.*, 203, 142–147, 1986.

54. Bland, K.I., Palin, W.E., von Fraunhofer, J.A., Morris, R.R., Adcock, R.A., and Tobin, G.R., Experimental and clinical observations of the effects of cytotoxic chemother-apeutic drugs on wound healing, *Ann. Surg.*, 199, 782–790, 1984.

55. Cohen, S.C., Gabelnick, H.L., Johnson, R.K., and Goldin, A., Effects of cyclophos-phamide and adriamycin on the healing of surgical wounds in mice, *Cancer*, 36, 1277–1281, 1975.

55a. Perloff, M. and Lesnick, G.J., Chemotherapy before and after mastectomy in stage III breast cancer, *Arch. Surg.* Jul; 117(7), 879–881, 1982.

56. Cohen, S.C., Gabelnick, H.L., Johnson, R.K., and Goldin, A., Effects of antineoplastic agents on wound healing in mice, *Surgery*, 78, 238–244, 1975.

57. Finney, R., Adjuvant chemotherapy in the radical treatment of carcinoma of the breast — a clinical trial, *Am. J. Roentgenol. Radium. Ther. Nucl. Med.*, 111, 137–141, 1971.

58. Nissen-Meyer, R., Kjellgren, K., Malmio, K., Mansson, B., and Norin, T., Surgical adjuvant chemotherapy: results with one short course with cyclophosphamide after mastectomy for breast cancer, *Cancer*, 41, 2088–2098, 1978.

59. Bracken, R.B., Sutow, W.W., Jaffe, N., Ayala, A., and Guarda, L., Preoperative chemotherapy for Wilms' tumor. *Urology*, 19, 55–60, 1982.

60. Stiernberg, C.M., Williams, R.M., and Hokanson, J.A., Influence of cisplatin on wound healing — an experimental model, *Otolaryngol. Head Neck Surg.*, 95, 210–212, 1986.

Schaefer, S.D., Middleton, R., Reisch, J., and Frenkel, E.P., Cis-Platinum induction chemotherapy in the multi-modality initial treatment of advanced stage IV carcinoma of the head and neck, *Cancer*, 51, 2168–2174, 1983.

th, M.H., Peptide growth factors and wound healing, *Clin. Plast. Surg.*, 17, 1990.

63. Mustoe, T.A., Pierce, G.F., Thomason, A., Gramates, P., Sporn, M.B., and Deuel, T.F., Accelerated healing of incisional wounds in rats induced by transforming growth factor-β, *Science*, 237, 1333–1336, 1987.

64. Ksander, G.A., Ogawa, Y., Chu, G.H., McMullin, H., Rosenblatt, J.S., and McPherson, J.M., Exogenous transforming growth factor-β 2 enhances connective tissue formation and wound strength in guinea pig dermal wounds healing by secondary intent, *Ann. Surg.*, 211, 288–294, 1990.

65. Curtsinger, L.J., Pietsch, J.D., Brown, G.L., von Fraunhofer, A., Ackerman, D., Polk, H.C., Jr., and Schultz, G.S., Reversal of adriamycin-impaired wound healing by transforming growth factor-β, *Surg. Gynecol. Obstet.*, 168, 517–522, 1989.

66. Cromack, D.T., Porras-Reyes, B., Purdy, J.A., Pierce, G.F., and Mustoe, T.A., Acceleration of tissue repair by transforming growth factor 1: identification of *in vivo* mechanism of action with radiotherapy-induced specific healing deficits, *Surgery*, 113, 36–42, 1993.

67. Buckley, A., Davidson, J.M., Kamerath, C.D., and Woodward, S.C., Epidermal growth factor increases granulation tissue formation dose dependently, *J. Surg. Res.*, 43, 322–328, 1987.

68. Brown, G.L., Nanney, L.B., Griffen, J., Cramer, A.B., Yancey, J.M., Curtsinger, L.J., III, Holtzin, L., Schultz, G.S., Jurkiewicz, M.J., and Lynch, J.B., Enhancement of wound healing by topical treatment with epidermal growth factor, *N. Engl. J. Med.*, 321, 76–79, 1989.

69. Brown, G.L., Curtsinger, L., Jurkiewicz, M.J., Nahai, F., and Schultz, G., Stimulation of healing of chronic wounds by epidermal growth factor, *Plast. Reconstr. Surg.*, 88, 189–194, 1991.

70. Deuel, T.F., Senior, R.M., Huang, J.S., and Griffin, G.L., Chemotaxis of monocytes and neutrophils to platelet-derived growth factor, *J. Clin. Invest.*, 69, 1046–1049, 1982.

71. Pierce, G.F., Mustoe, T.A., Lingelbach, J., Masakowski, V.R., Griffin, G.L., Senior, R.M., and Deuel, T.F., Platelet-derived growth factor and transforming growth factor-β enhance tissue repair activities by unique mechanisms, *J. Cell. Biol.*, 109, 429–440, 1989.

72. Mustoe, T.A., Landes, A., Cromack, D.T., Mistry, D., Griffin, A., Deuel, T.F., and Pierce, G.F., Differential acceleration of healing of surgical incisions in the rabbit gastrointestinal tract by platelet-derived growth factor and transforming growth factor, type , *Surgery*, 108, 324–329, 1990.

73. Robson, M.C., Phillips, L.G., Thomason, A., Robson, L.E., and Pierce, G.F., Platelet-derived growth factor BB for the treatment of chronic pressure ulcers, *Lancet*, 339, 23–25, 1992.

74. Knighton, D.R., Ciresi, K.F., Fiegel, V.D., Austin, L.L., and Butler, E.L., Classification and treatment of chronic nonhealing wounds. Successful treatment with autologous platelet-derived wound healing factors (PDWHF), *Ann. Surg.*, 204, 322–330, 1986.

75. McGee, G.S., Davidson, J.M., Buckley, A., Sommer, A., Woodward, S.C., Aquino, A.M., Barbour, R., and Demetriou, A.A., Recombinant basic fibroblast growth factor accelerates wound healing, *J. Surg. Res.*, 45, 145–153, 1988.

76. Klingbeil, C.K., Cesar, L.B., and Fiddes, J.C., Basic fibroblast growth factor accelerates tissue repair in models of impaired wound healing, *Prog. Clin. Biol. Res.*, 365, 443–458, 1991.

77. Lieberman, M.D., Kilburn, H., Lindsey, M., and Brennan, M.F., Relation of perioperative deaths to hospital volume among patients undergoing pancreatic resection for malignancy, *Ann. Surg.*, 222, 638–645, 1995.

78. Yeo, C.J., Cameron, J.L., Sohn, T.A., Lillemoe, K.D., Pitt, H.A., Talamini, M.A., Hruban, R.H., Ord, S.E., Sauter, P.K., Coleman, J., Zahurak, M.L., Grochow, L.B., and Abrams, R.A., Six hundred fifty consecutive pancreaticoduodenectomies in the 1990s: pathology, complications, and outcomes, *Ann. Surg.*, 226, 248–257, 1997.

79. Smale, B.F., Mullen, J.L., Buzby, G.P., and Rosato, E.F., The efficacy of nutritional assessment and support in cancer surgery, *Cancer*, 47, 2375–2381, 1981.

80. Heslin, M.J. and Brennan, M.F., Advances in perioperative nutrition: cancer, *World J. Surg.*, 24, 1477–1485, 2000.

81. Hill, G.L., Jonathan E. Rhoads Lecture. Body composition research: implications for the practice of clinical nutrition, *J. Parenter. Enteral Nutr.*, 16, 197–218, 1992.

82. The Veterans Affairs Total Parenteral Nutrition Cooperative Study Group, Perioperative total parenteral nutrition in surgical patients, *N. Engl. J. Med.*, 325, 525–532, 1991.

83. Bastow, M.D., Rawlings, J., and Allison, S.P., Benefits of supplementary tube feeding after fractured neck of femur: a randomised controlled trial, *Br. Med. J. (Clin. Res. Ed.)*, 287, 1589–1592, 1983.

84. Burgert, S.L. and Anderson, C.F., A comparison of triceps skinfold values as measured by the plastic McGaw caliper and the Lange caliper, *Am. J. Clin. Nutr.*, 32, 1531–1533, 1979.

85. McCauley, R.L. and Brennan, M.F., Serum albumin levels in cancer patients receiving total parenteral nutrition, *Ann. Surg.*, 197, 305–309, 1983.

86. Eriksson, B. and Douglass, H.O., Jr., Intravenous hyperalimentation. An adjunct to treatment of malignant disease of upper gastrointestinal tract, *JAMA*, 243, 2049–2052, 1980.

87. Prijatmoko, D., Strauss, B.J., Lambert, J.R., Sievert, W., Stroud, D.B., Wahlqvist, M.L., Katz, B., Colman, J., Jones, P., and Korman, M.G., Early detection of protein depletion in alcoholic cirrhosis: role of body composition analysis, *Gastroenterology*, 105, 1839–1845, 1993.

88. Buzby, G.P., Mullen, J.L., Matthews, D.C., Hobbs, C.L., and Rosato, E.F., Prognostic nutritional index in gastrointestinal surgery, *Am. J. Surg.*, 139, 160–167, 1980.

89. Baker, J.P., Detsky, A.S., Wesson, D.E., Wolman, S.L., Stewart, S., Whitewell, J., Langer, B., and Jeejeebhoy, K.N., Nutritional assessment: a comparison of clinical judgement and objective measurements, *N. Engl. J. Med.*, 306, 969–972, 1982.

90. Conti, S., West, J.P., and Fitzpatrick, H.F., Mortality and morbidity after esophago-gastrectomy for cancer of the esophagus and cardia, *Am. Surg.*, 43, 92–96, 1977.

91. Winters, J.O. and Leider, Z.L., The value of instant nutritional assessment in predicting postoperative complications and death in gastrointestinal surgical patients, *Am. Surg.*, 49, 533–535, 1983.

92. Hickman, D.M., Miller, R.A., Rombeau, J.L., Twomey, P.L., and Frey, C.F., Serum albumin and body weight as predictors of postoperative course in colorectal cancer, *J. Parenter. Enteral Nutr.*, 4, 314–316, 1980.

93. Belghiti, J., Langonnet, F., Bourstyn, E., and Fekete, F., Surgical implications of malnutrition and immunodeficiency in patients with carcinoma of the oesophagus, *Br. J. Surg.*, 70, 339–341, 1983.

94. Bozzetti, F., Migliavacca, S., Gallus, G., Radaelli, G., Scotti, A., Bonalumi, M.G., Ammatuna, M., Sequeira, C., and Terno, G., "Nutritional" markers as prognostic indicators of postoperative sepsis in cancer patients, *J. Parenter. Enteral Nutr.*, 9, 464–470, 1985.

95. Holter, A.R. and Fischer, J.E., The effects of perioperative hyperalimentation on complications in patients with carcinoma and weight loss, *J. Surg. Res.*, 23, 31–34, 1977.

96. Moghissi, K., Hornshaw, J., Teasdale, P.R., and Dawes, E.A., Parenteral nutrition in carcinoma of the oesophagus treated by surgery: nitrogen balance and clinical studies, *Br. J. Surg.*, 64, 125–128, 1977.

97. Heatley, R.V., Williams, R.H., and Lewis, M.H., Pre-operative intravenous feeding — a controlled trial, *Postgrad. Med. J.*, 55, 541–545, 1979.

98. Mullen, J.L., Buzby, G.P., Gertner, M.H., Stein, T.P., Hargrove, W.C., Oram-Smith, J., and Rosato, E.F., Protein synthesis dynamics in human gastrointestinal malignancies, *Surgery*, 87, 331–338, 1980.

99. Muller, J.M., Brenner, U., Dienst, C., and Pichlmaier, H., Preoperative parenteral feeding in patients with gastrointestinal carcinoma, *Lancet*, 1, 68–71, 1982.

100. Detsky, A.S., Baker, J.P., O'Rourke, K., and Goel, V., Perioperative parenteral nutrition: a meta-analysis, *Ann. Intern. Med.*, 107, 195–203, 1987.

101. Buzby, G.P., Williford, W.O., Peterson, O.L., Crosby, L.O., Page, C.P., Reinhardt, G.F., and Mullen, J.L., A randomized clinical trial of total parenteral nutrition in malnourished surgical patients: the rationale and impact of previous clinical trials and pilot study on protocol design, *Am. J. Clin. Nutr.*, 47, 357–365, 1988.

102. Brennan, M.F., Pisters, P.W., Posner, M., Quesada, O., and Shike, M., A prospective randomized trial of total parenteral nutrition after major pancreatic resection for malignancy, *Ann. Surg.*, 220, 436–441, 1994.

103. Fan, S.T., Lo, C.M., Lai, E.C., Chu, K.M., Liu, C.L., and Wong, J., Perioperative nutritional support in patients undergoing hepatectomy for hepatocellular carcinoma, *N. Engl. J. Med.*, 331, 1547–1552, 1994.

104. Shukla, H.S., Rao, R.R., Banu, N., Gupta, R.M., and Yadav, R.C., Enteral hyperalimentation in malnourished surgical patients, *Indian J. Med. Res.*, 80, 339–346, 1984.

105. Spirtos, N.M. and Ballon, S.C., Needle catheter jejunostomy: a controlled, prospective, randomized trial in patients with gynecologic malignancy, *Am. J. Obstet. Gynecol.*, 158, 1285–1290, 1988.

106. Smith, R.C., Hartemink, R.J., Hollinshead, J.W., and Gillett, D.J., Fine bore jejunostomy feeding following major abdominal surgery: a controlled randomized clinical trial, *Br. J. Surg.*, 72, 458–461, 1985.

107. Meijerink, W.J., von Meyenfeldt, M.F., Rouflart, M.M., and Soeters, P.B., Efficacy of perioperative nutritional support, *Lancet*, 340, 187–188, 1992.

108. Baigrie, R.J., Devitt, P.G., and Watkin, D.S., Enteral versus parenteral nutrition after oesophagogastric surgery: a prospective randomized comparison, *Aust. N.Z. J. Surg.*, 66, 668–670, 1996.

109. Beier-Holgersen, R. and Boesby, S., Influence of postoperative enteral nutrition on postsurgical infections, *Gut*, 39, 833–835, 1996.

110. Shirabe, K., Matsumata, T., Shimada, M., Takenaka, K., Kawahara, N., Yamamoto, K., Nishizaki, T., and Sugimachi, K., A comparison of parenteral hyperalimentation and early enteral feeding regarding systemic immunity after major hepatic resection — the results of a randomized prospective study, *Hepatogastroenterology*, 44, 205–209, 1997.

111. Bozzetti, F., Braga, M., Gianotti, L., Gavazzi, C., and Mariani, L., Postoperative enteral versus parenteral nutrition in malnourished patients with gastrointestinal cancer: a randomised multicentre trial, *Lancet*, 358, 1487–1492, 2001.

112. Andreyev, H.J., Norman, A.R., Oates, J., and Cunningham, D., Why do patients with weight loss have a worse outcome when undergoing chemotherapy for gastrointestinal malignancies? *Eur. J. Cancer*, 34, 503–509, 1998.

113. McGeer, A.J., Detsky, A.S., and O'Rourke, K., Parenteral nutrition in cancer patients undergoing chemotherapy: a meta-analysis, *Nutrition*, 6, 233–240, 1990.

114. De Cicco, M., Panarello, G., Fantin, D., Veronesi, A., Pinto, A., Zagonel, V., Monfardini, S., and Testa, V., Parenteral nutrition in cancer patients receiving chemotherapy: effects on toxicity and nutritional status, *J. Parenter. Enteral Nutr.*, 17, 513–518, 1993.

115. Jin, D., Phillips, M., and Byles, J.E., Effects of parenteral nutrition support and chemotherapy on the phasic composition of tumor cells in gastrointestinal cancer, *J. Parenter. Enteral Nutr.*, 23, 237–241, 1999.

116. Thiel, H.J., Fietkau, R., and Sauer, R., Malnutrition and the role of nutritional support for radiation therapy patients, *Recent Results Cancer Res.*, 108, 205–226, 1988.

117. Mick, R., Vokes, E.E., Weichselbaum, R.R., and Panje, W.R., Prognostic factors in advanced head and neck cancer patients undergoing multimodality therapy, *Otolaryngol. Head Neck Surg.*, 105, 62–73, 1991.

118. Senft, M., Fietkau, R., Iro, H., Sailer, D., and Sauer, R., The influence of supportive nutritional therapy via percutaneous endoscopically guided gastrostomy on the quality of life of cancer patients, *Support. Care Cancer*, 1, 272–275, 1993.

119. Sinclair, J.J., Scolapio, J.S., Stark, M.E., and Hinder, R.A., Metastasis of head and neck carcinoma to the site of percutaneous endoscopic gastrostomy: case report and literature review, *J. Parenter. Enteral Nutr.*, 25, 282–285, 2001.

120. Maccabee, D. and Sheppard, B.C., Prevention of percutaneous endoscopic gastrostomy stoma metastases in patients with active oropharyngeal malignancy, *Surg. Endosc.*, 17, 1678, 2003.

121. Cosentini, E.P., Sautner, T., Gnant, M., Winkelbauer, F., Teleky, B., and Jakesz, R., Outcomes of surgical, percutaneous endoscopic, and percutaneous radiologic gastrostomies, *Arch. Surg.*, 133, 1076–1083, 1998.

122. Hoffer, E.K., Cosgrove, J.M., Levin, D.Q., Herskowitz, M.M., and Sclafani, S.J., Radiologic gastrojejunostomy and percutaneous endoscopic gastrostomy: a prospective, randomized comparison, *J. Vasc. Interv. Radiol.*, 10, 413–420, 1999.

123. Neeff, M., Crowder, V.L., McIvor, N.P., Chaplin, J.M., and Morton, R.P., Comparison of the use of endoscopic and radiologic gastrostomy in a single head and neck cancer unit, *Aust. N.Z. J. Surg.*, 73, 590–593, 2003.

124. Steiger, E., Oram-Smith, J., Miller, E., Kuo, L., and Vars, H.M., Effects of nutrition on tumor growth and tolerance to chemotherapy, *J. Surg. Res.*, 18, 455–466, 1975.

125. Daly, J.M., Copeland, E.M., III, Dudrick, S.J., and Delaney, J.M., Nutritional repletion of malnourished tumour-bearing and nontumour bearing rats: effects on body weight, liver, muscle and tumour, *J. Surg. Res.*, 28, 507–518, 1980.

126. Cameron, I.L. and Pavlat, W.A., Stimulation of growth of a transplantable hepatoma in rats by parenteral nutrition, *J. Natl. Cancer Inst.*, 56, 597–602, 1976.

127. McNurlan, M.A. and Clemens, M.J., Inhibition of cell proliferation by interferons. Relative contributions of changes in protein synthesis and breakdown to growth control of human lymphoblastoid cells, *Biochem. J.*, 237, 871–876, 1986.

128. Nixon, D.W., Moffitt, S., Lawson, D.H., Ansley, J., Lynn, M.J., Kutner, M.H., Heymsfield, S.B., Wesley, M., Chawla, R., and Rudman, D., Total parenteral nutrition as an adjunct to chemotherapy of metastatic colorectal cancer, *Cancer Treat. Rep.*, 65 Suppl. 5, 121–128, 1981.

129. Bozzetti, F., Gavazzi, C., Cozzaglio, L., Costa, A., Spinelli, P., and Viola, G., Total parenteral nutrition and tumor growth in malnourished patients with gastric cancer, *Tumori*, 85, 163–166, 1999.

130. Cozzaglio, L. and Bozzetti, F., Does parenteral nutrition increase tumor growth? A review, *Tumori*, 80, 169–174, 1994.

131. Reynolds, H.M., Jr., Daly, J.M., Rowlands, B.J., Dudrick, S.J., and Copeland, E.M., III, Effects of nutritional repletion on host and tumor response to chemotherapy, *Cancer*, 45, 3069–3074, 1980.

132. Daly, J.M., Reynolds, H.M., Jr., Copeland, E.M., III, and Dudrick, S.J., Effects of enteral and parenteral nutrition on tumor response to chemotherapy in experimental animals, *J. Surg. Oncol.*, 16, 79–86, 1981.

133. Torosian, M.H., Mullen, J.L., Miller, E.E., Wagner, K.M., Stein, T.P., and Buzby, G.P., Adjuvant, pulse total parenteral nutrition and tumor response to cycle-specific and cycle-nonspecific chemotherapy, *Surgery*, 94, 291–299, 1983.

134. Torosian, M.H., Tsou, K.C., Daly, J.M., Mullen, J.L., Stein, T.P., Miller, E.E., and Buzby, G.P., Alteration of tumor cell kinetics by pulse total parenteral nutrition. Potential therapeutic implications, *Cancer*, 53, 1409–1415, 1984.

135. Remvikos, Y., Beuzeboc, P., Zajdela, A., Voillemot, N., Magdelenat, H., and Pouillart, P., Correlation of pretreatment proliferative activity of breast cancer with the response to cytotoxic chemotherapy, *J. Natl. Cancer Inst.*, 81, 1383–1387, 1989.

136. Park, K.G., Heys, S.D., Blessing, K., Kelly, P., McNurlan, M.A., Eremin, O., and Garlick, P.J., Stimulation of human breast cancers by dietary L-arginine, *Clin. Sci. (London)*, 82, 413–417, 1992.

137. Endres, S., Ghorbani, R., Kelley, V.E., Georgilis, K., Lonnemann, G., van der Meer, J.W., Cannon, J.G., Rogers, T.S., Klempner, M.S., and Weber, P.C., The effect of dietary supplementation with n-3 polyunsaturated fatty acids on the synthesis of interleukin-1 and tumor necrosis factor by mononuclear cells, *N. Engl. J. Med.*, 320, 265–271, 1989.

138. Wigmore, S.J., Fearon, K.C., Maingay, J.P., and Ross, J.A., Down-regulation of the acute-phase response in patients with pancreatic cancer cachexia receiving oral eicosapentaenoic acid is mediated via suppression of interleukin-6, *Clin. Sci. (London)*, 92, 215–221, 1997.

139. Endres, S., Meydani, S.N., Ghorbani, R., Schindler, R., and Dinarello, C.A., Dietary supplementation with n-3 fatty acids suppresses interleukin-2 production and mononuclear cell proliferation, *J. Leukoc. Biol.*, 54, 599–603, 1993.

140. Gogos, C.A., Ginopoulos, P., Salsa, B., Apostolidou, E., Zoumbos, N.C., and Kalfarentzos, F., Dietary omega-3 polyunsaturated fatty acids plus vitamin E restore immunodeficiency and prolong survival for severely ill patients with generalized malignancy: a randomized control trial, *Cancer*, 82, 395–402, 1998.

141. Furukawa, K., Tashiro, T., Yamamori, H., Takagi, K., Morishima, Y., Sugiura, T., Otsubo, Y., Hayashi, N., Itabashi, T., Sano, W., Toyoda, Y., Nitta, H., and Nakajima, N., Effects of soybean oil emulsion and eicosapentaenoic acid on stress response and immune function after a severely stressful operation, *Ann. Surg.*, 229, 255–261, 1999.

142. Saito, H., Trocki, O., Wang, S.L., Gonce, S.J., Joffe, S.N., and Alexander, J.W., Metabolic and immune effects of dietary arginine supplementation after burn, *Arch. Surg.*, 122, 784–789, 1987.

143. Fanslow, W.C., Kulkarni, A.D., Van Buren, C.T., and Rudolph, F.B., Effect of nucleotide restriction and supplementation on resistance to experimental murine candidiasis, *J. Parenter. Enteral Nutr.*, 12, 49–52, 1988.

144. Fox, A.D., Kripke, S.A., De Paula, J., Berman, J.M., Settle, R.G., and Rombeau, J.L., Effect of a glutamine-supplemented enteral diet on methotrexate-induced enterocolitis, *J. Parenter. Enteral Nutr.*, 12, 325–331, 1988.

145. Gianotti, L., Braga, M., Vignali, A., Balzano, G., Zerbi, A., Bisagni, P., and Di, C.V., Effect of route of delivery and formulation of postoperative nutritional support in patients undergoing major operations for malignant neoplasms, *Arch. Surg.*, 132, 1222–1229, 1997.

146. Braga, M., Gianotti, L., Radaelli, G., Vignali, A., Mari, G., Gentilini, O., and Di, C.V., Perioperative immunonutrition in patients undergoing cancer surgery: results of a randomized double-blind phase 3 trial, *Arch. Surg.*, 134, 428–433, 1999.

147. Senkal, M., Zumtobel, V., Bauer, K.H., Marpe, B., Wolfram, G., Frei, A., Eickhoff, U., and Kemen, M., Outcome and cost-effectiveness of perioperative enteral immunonutrition in patients undergoing elective upper gastrointestinal tract surgery: a prospective randomized study, *Arch. Surg.*, 134, 1309–1316, 1999.

148. Daly, J.M., Weintraub, F.N., Shou, J., Rosato, E.F., and Lucia, M., Enteral nutrition during multimodality therapy in upper gastrointestinal cancer patients, *Ann. Surg.*, 221, 327–338, 1995.

149. Heys, S.D., Walker, L.G., Smith, I., and Eremin, O., Enteral nutritional supplementation with key nutrients in patients with critical illness and cancer: a meta-analysis of randomized controlled clinical trials, *Ann. Surg.*, 229, 467–477, 1999.

150. Braga, M., Gianotti, L., Cestari, A., Vignali, A., Pellegatta, F., Dolci, A., and Di, C.V., Gut function and immune and inflammatory responses in patients perioperatively fed with supplemented enteral formulas, *Arch. Surg.*, 131, 1257–1264, 1996.

151. Gianotti, L., Braga, M., Fortis, C., Soldini, L., Vignali, A., Colombo, S., Radaelli, G., and Di, C.V., A prospective, randomized clinical trial on perioperative feeding with an arginine-, omega-3 fatty acid-, and RNA-enriched enteral diet: effect on host response and nutritional status, *J. Parenter. Enteral Nutr.*, 23, 314–320, 1999.

152. Hochwald, S.N., Harrison, L.E., Heslin, M.J., Burt, M.E., and Brennan, M.F., Early postoperative enteral feeding improves whole body protein kinetics in upper gastrointestinal cancer patients, *Am. J. Surg.*, 174, 325–330, 1997.

153. Heslin, M.J., Latkany, L., Leung, D., Brooks, A.D., Hochwald, S.N., Pisters, P.W., Shike, M., and Brennan, M.F., A prospective, randomized trial of early enteral feeding after resection of upper gastrointestinal malignancy, *Ann. Surg.*, 226, 567–577, 1997.

154. Williams, R.H., Heatley, R.V., and Lewis, M.H., Proceedings: a randomized controlled trial of preoperative intravenous nutrition in patients with stomach cancer, *Br. J. Surg.*, 63, 667, 1976.

155. Mullen, J.L., Buzby, G.P., Matthews, D.C., Smale, B.F., and Rosato, E.F., Reduction of operative morbidity and mortality by combined preoperative and postoperative nutritional support, *Ann. Surg.*, 192, 604–613, 1980.

156. Simms, J.M., Oliver, E., and Smith, J.A., A study of total parenteral nutrition (TPN) in major gastric and esophageal resection for neoplasia, *J. Parenter. Enteral Nutr.*, 4, 422, 1980.

157. Thompson, B.R., Julian, T.B., and Stremple, J.F., Perioperative total parenteral nutrition in patients with gastrointestinal cancer, *J. Surg. Res.*, 30, 497–500, 1981.

158. Lim, S.T., Choa, R.G., Lam, K.H., Wong, J., and Ong, G.B., Total parenteral nutrition versus gastrostomy in the preoperative preparation of patients with carcinoma of the oesophagus, *Br. J. Surg.*, 68, 69–72, 1981.

159. Sako, K., Lore, J.M., Kaufman, S., Razack, M.S., Bakamjian, V., and Reese, P., Parenteral hyperalimentation in surgical patients with head and neck cancer: a randomized study, *J. Surg. Oncol.*, 16, 391–402, 1981.

160. Muller, J.M., Keller, H.W., Brenner, U., Walter, M., and Holzmuller, W., Indications and effects of preoperative parenteral nutrition, *World J. Surg.*, 10, 53–63, 1986.

161. Yamada, N., Koyama, H., Hioki, K., Yamada, T., and Yamamoto, M., Effect of postoperative total parenteral nutrition (TPN) as an adjunct to gastrectomy for advanced gastric carcinoma, *Br. J. Surg.*, 70, 267–274, 1983.

162. Askanazi, J., Hensle, T.W., Starker, P.M., Lockhart, S.H., LaSala, P.A., Olsson, C., and Kinney, J.M., Effect of immediate postoperative nutritional support on length of hospitalization, *Ann. Surg.*, 203, 236–239, 1986.

163. Bellantone, R., Doglietto, G.B., Bossola, M., Pacelli, F., Negro, F., Sofo, L., and Crucitti, F., Preoperative parenteral nutrition in the high risk surgical patient, *J. Parenter. Enteral Nutr.*, 12, 195–197, 1988.

164. Woolfson, A.M. and Smith, J.A., Elective nutritional support after major surgery: a randomized trial, *Clin. Nutr.*, 8, 15, 1989.

165. Sandstrom, R., Drott, C., Hyltander, A., Arfvidsson, B., Schersten, T., Wickstrom, I., and Lundholm, K., The effect of postoperative intravenous feeding (TPN) on outcome following major surgery evaluated in a randomized study, *Ann. Surg.*, 217, 185–195, 1993.

166. Samuels, M.L., Selig, D.E., Ogden, S., Grant, C., and Brown, B., IV Hyperalimentation and chemotherapy for stage III testicular cancer: a randomized study, *Cancer Treat. Rep.*, 65, 615–627, 1981.

167. Shamberger, R.C., Brennan, M.F., Goodgame, J.T., Jr., Lowry, S.F., Maher, M.M., Wesley, R.A., and Pizzo, P.A., A prospective, randomized study of adjuvant parenteral nutrition in the treatment of sarcomas: results of metabolic and survival studies, *Surgery*, 96, 1–13, 1984.

168. Valdivieso, M., Frankmann, C., Murphy, W.K., Benjamin, R.S., Barkley, H.T., Jr., McMurtrey, M.J., Jeffries, D.G., Welch, S.R., and Bodey, G.P., Long-term effects of intravenous hyperalimentation administered during intensive chemotherapy for small cell bronchogenic carcinoma, *Cancer*, 59, 362–369, 1987.

169. Clamon, G.H., Feld, R., Evans, W.K., Weiner, R.S., Moran, E.M., Blum, R.H., Kramer, B.S., Makuch, R.W., Hoffman, F.A., and Dewys, W.D., Effect of adjuvant central IV hyperalimentation on the survival and response to treatment of patients with small cell lung cancer: a randomized trial, *Cancer Treat. Rep.*, 69, 167–177, 1985.

170. Issell, B.F., Valdivieso, M., Zaren, H.A., Dudrick, S.J., Freireich, E.J., Copeland, E.W., and Bodey, G.P., Protection against chemotherapy toxicity by IV hyperalimentation, *Cancer Treat. Rep.*, 62, 1139–1143, 1978.

171. Jordan, W.M., Valdivieso, M., Frankmann, C., Gillespie, M., Issell, B.F., Bodey, G.P., and Freireich, E.J., Treatment of advanced adenocarcinoma of the lung with Ftorafur, doxorubicin, cyclophosphamide, and cisplatin (FACP) and intensive IV hyperalimentation, *Cancer Treat. Rep.*, 65, 197–205, 1981.

172. Elkort, R.J., Baker, F.L., Vitale, J.J., and Cordano, A., Long-term nutritional support as an adjunct to chemotherapy for breast cancer, *J. Parenter. Enteral Nutr.*, 5, 385–390, 1981.

173. Evans, W.K., Nixon, D.W., Daly, J.M., Ellenberg, S.S., Gardner, L., Wolfe, E., Shepherd, F.A., Feld, R., Gralla, R., and Fine, S., A randomized study of oral nutritional support versus ad lib nutritional intake during chemotherapy for advanced colorectal and non-small-cell lung cancer, *J. Clin. Oncol.*, 5, 113–124, 1987.

174. Tandon, S.P., Gupta, S.C., Sinha, S.N., and Naithani, Y.P., Nutritional support as an adjunct therapy of advanced cancer patients, *Indian J. Med. Res.*, 80, 180–188, 1984.

175. Bounous, G., Gentile, J.M., and Hugon, J., Elemental diet in the management of the intestinal lesion produced by 5-fluorouracil in man, *Can. J. Surg.*, 14, 312–324, 1971.

176. Solassol, C., Joyeux, J., and Dubois, J.B., Total parenteral nutrition (TPN) with complete nutritive mixtures: an artificial gut in cancer patients, *Nutr. Cancer*, 1, 13, 1979.

177. Kinsella, T.J., Malcolm, A.W., Bothe, A., Jr., Valerio, D., and Blackburn, G.L., Prospective study of nutritional support during pelvic irradiation, *Int. J. Radiat. Oncol. Biol. Phys.*, 7, 543–548, 1981.

178. Ghavimi, F., Shils, M.E., Scott, B.F., Brown, M., and Tamaroff, M., Comparison of morbidity in children requiring abdominal radiation and chemotherapy, with and without total parenteral nutrition, *J. Pediatr.*, 101, 530–537, 1982.

179. Donaldson, S.S., Wesley, M.N., Ghavimi, F., Shils, M.E., Suskind, R.M., and Dewys, W.D., A prospective randomized clinical trial of total parenteral nutrition in children with cancer, *Med. Pediatr. Oncol.*, 10, 129–139, 1982.

180. Douglass, H.O., Jr., Milliron, S., Nava, H., Eriksson, B., Thomas, P., Novick, A., and Holyoke, E.D., Elemental diet as an adjuvant for patients with locally advanced gastrointestinal cancer receiving radiation therapy: a prospectively randomized study, *J. Parenter. Enteral Nutr.*, 2, 682–686, 1978.

181. Brown, M.S., Buchanan, R.B., and Karran, S.J., Clinical observations on the effects of elemental diet supplementation during irradiation, *Clin. Radiol.*, 31, 19–20, 1980.

182. Bounous, G., Le Bel, E., Shuster, J., Gold, P., Tahan, W.T., and Bastin, E., Dietary protection during radiation therapy, *Strahlentherapie*, 149, 476–483, 1975.

183. Daly, J.M., Hearne, B., Dunaj, J., LePorte, B., Vikram, B., Strong, E., Green, M., Muggio, F., Groshen, S., and DeCosse, J.J., Nutritional rehabilitation in patients with advanced head and neck cancer receiving radiation therapy, *Am. J. Surg.*, 148, 514–520, 1984.

184. Moloney, M., Moriarty, M., and Daly, L., Controlled studies of nutritional intake in patients with malignant disease undergoing treatment, *Hum. Nutr. Appl. Nutr.*, 37, 30–35, 1983.

185. Heys, S.D., et al., Potentiation of the response to chemotherapy in patients with breast cancer by dietary supplementation with L-arginine: results of a randomised controlled trial, *Int. J. Oncol.*, 12(1), 221–225, 1998.

13 Nutrition and Wound Healing at the Age Extremes

Hannah G. Piper, Tom Jaksic, and Patrick J. Javid

CONTENTS

INTRODUCTION

Wound healing is a remarkable process that involves multiple stages executed in a timely fashion to reestablish an effective barrier to the outside world. It is fascinating that most wounds will heal even under physiologically challenging conditions. In general, wounded adults have adequate nutritional reserve to mount an appropriate inflammatory response, allowing healing to occur without local or systemic complications. However, for patients who are either very young or very old, this same healing process poses unique problems and considerations. For patients at the age extremes, underlying nutritional status can have a significant impact on the ability to heal efficiently. Both neonates and the elderly have reduced nutritional stores that can impede recovery from injury. An understanding of the metabolism of the very young and the very old is necessary to provide adequate nutritional support to optimize wound healing.

NUTRITIONAL NEEDS OF THE INFANT

BODY COMPOSITION AND ENERGY REQUIREMENTS

The body composition of the young child contrasts with the adult in several ways that significantly affect nutritional requirements. Listed in Table 13.1 are the macro-nutrient stores of the neonate, child, and healthy young adult as a percentage of total body weight.[1,2,3] Carbohydrate stores are limited in all age groups and provide only a short-term supply of glucose when utilized. Despite this fact, neonates have a high demand for glucose and have shown elevated rates of glucose turnover when compared to the adult.[4] Short periods of fasting can predispose the newborn to hypoglycemia. Thus, when infants are burdened with critical illness, they must turn to the breakdown of protein stores in order to generate glucose through the process of gluconeogenesis. Lipid reserves are also reduced in the neonate and gradually increase with age. The lowest proportion of lipid stores is found in premature infants, as the majority of polyunsaturated fatty acids accumulate in the third trimester.[5] The most dramatic difference between young adults and pediatric patients is in the relative quantity of stored protein. Protein reserves are nearly doubled in the adult as compared to the neonate. Hence, infants cannot afford to lose significant amounts of protein during the course of protracted critical illness or injury.

Neonates and children also have much higher baseline energy requirements. Studies have demonstrated that the resting energy expenditure for neonates is two to three times that of adults when standardized for body weight.[6–8] Clearly, the child's need for rapid growth and development is a large component of this increase in energy requirement. Moreover, the relatively large body surface area of the young child may increase heat loss and thereby contribute to elevations in energy expenditure.

The basic requirements for protein and energy in the healthy neonate and child based on recommendations by the National Academy of Sciences are listed in Table 13.2.[9] It should be noted that the recommended dietary protein provision for the neonate

---

TABLE 13.1
The Body Composition of Neonates, Children, and Adults as a Percentage of Total Body Weight

Age	Percent Protein	Percent Fat	Percent Carbohydrate
Neonates	11	14	0.4
Children (age 10 yr)	15	17	0.4
Adults	18	19	0.4

Source: From Jaksic, T., *Surg. Clin. N. Am.*, 82, 381, 2002. With permission.

TABLE 13.2
Estimated Requirements for Energy and Protein in Healthy Humans of Different Age Groups

Age	Protein (g/kg/d)	Energy (kcal/kg/d)
Neonates	2.2	120
Children (age 10 yr)	1.0	70
Adults	0.8	35

is almost three times that of the healthy adult. In premature infants, a minimum protein allotment of 2.8 g/kg/d is required to maintain *in utero* growth rates.[10] Together, the increased metabolic demand and limited nutrient reserves of the infant mandate early nutritional support in times of traumatic injury and critical illness.

Micronutrients are also important for normal growth and development. Vitamins and trace elements are needed for vital enzymatic reactions, and if not available in the child's regular diet, they should be supplemented to meet the recommended daily reference intake (Table 13.3). However, because these micronutrients are not consumed by the biochemical reactions for which they are required, providing excessive amounts in times of physiologic stress is not necessary and, in fact, may lead to toxicity.

THE NUTRITIONAL MANAGEMENT OF THE CRITICALLY ILL CHILD

Children undergo profound yet predictable changes in metabolism with the onset and continuation of critical illness. The turnover rates of all nutrients increase substantially, and net protein breakdown is greatly accelerated. Despite a modest increase in protein synthesis, net protein balance (the difference between protein synthesis and protein degradation) is considerably negative. Muscle protein is broken down, and amino acids are sent to the liver for conversion into acutely needed inflammatory mediators and acute phase reactants. The remaining amino acids are used to manufacture glucose through the process of gluconeogenesis to supply a diverse array of tissues. Although these changes represent excellent short-term adaptations in the child, the metabolic stress response can become injurious if left unrestrained, as it depletes body protein stores, dampens growth, and may contribute to multiple organ failure.

Protein Metabolism

At baseline, infants are known to have higher rates of protein turnover than adults, and even greater rates of protein turnover have been measured in premature and low birth weight infants.[11] Extremely low birth weight infants receiving no dietary protein can lose in excess of 1.2 g/kg/d of endogenous protein.[12] Although the healthy adult can subsist with a neutral protein balance, infants must maintain a positive protein balance to attain adequate growth and development.

TABLE 13.3
Recommended Micronutrient Dietary Reference Intakes for Children

Age	Calcium (mg/d)	Magnesium (mg/d)	Phosphorus (mg/d)	Vitamin A (μg/d)	Vitamin C (mg/d)	Vitamin D (μg/d)	Vitamin E (mg/d)	Vitamin K (μg/d)	Vitamin B$_{12}$ (μg/d)	Zinc (mg/d)	Iron (mg/d)	Thiamine (mg/d)
0 to 6 months	210	30	100	400	40	5	4	2	0.4	3	0.27	0.2
7 to 12 months	270	75	275	500	50	5	5	2.5	0.5	3	11	0.3
1 to 3 yr	500	80	460	300	15	5	6	30	0.9	3	7	0.5
4 to 8 yr	800	130	500	400	25	5	7	55	1.2	4	10	0.6
9 to 13 yr	1300	240	1250	600	45	5	11	60	1.8	7	8	0.9
14 to 18 yr	1300	410 (m) 360 (f)	1250	900 (m) 700 (f)	75 (m) 65 (f)	5	15	75	2.4	11 (m) 9 (f)	11 (m) 15 (f)	1.2 (m) 1.0 (f)

Source: Adapted from Standing Committee on the Scientific Evaluation of Dietary Reference Intakes, *Dietary Reference Intakes*, National Academy Press, Washington, D.C., 1998. With permission.

In the metabolically stressed patient, protein turnover is doubled when compared to healthy subjects.[13–15] This process redistributes amino acids from skeletal muscle to the liver, wound, and tissues taking part in the inflammatory response. The mediators of the inflammatory response, acutely needed enzymes, serum proteins, and glucose, are thereby synthesized from degraded body protein stores. The well-established increase in hepatically derived acute phase proteins (including C-reactive protein, fibrinogen, transferrin, and -1-acid glycoprotein), along with the concomitant decrease in transport proteins (albumin and retinol binding protein) is evidence of this protein redistribution.

As substrate turnover is increased during the pediatric stress response, rates of both whole body protein degradation and whole body protein synthesis are accelerated. However, protein breakdown predominates, leading to a hypercatabolic state with ensuing net negative protein and nitrogen balance.[16] Protein loss is evident in elevated levels of excreted urinary nitrogen during critical illness. Evidence of severe protein loss includes skeletal muscle wasting, weight loss, delayed wound healing, and immune dysfunction.[17]

The increase in protein breakdown associated with the metabolic stress response takes place for two fundamental reasons. First, the body needs to reroute its amino acid utilization from structural proteins to those required for the inflammatory response and wound healing. In addition, the body appears to have an increased need for glucose production during times of metabolic stress, and rates of gluconeogenesis are accelerated during illness and injury.[18–20] Accelerated glucose production is necessary, because glucose is a versatile energy source used by tissues involved in the inflammatory response. It has been shown, for example, that glucose utilization by leukocytes is significantly increased in settings of inflammation.[21] Unfortunately, the nutritional provision of additional dietary glucose to critically ill patients does not suppress the body's need for increased glucose production, and therefore, net protein breakdown to fuel glucose production continues to predominate.[19,22,23]

Although increased muscle protein catabolism is a successful short-term adaptation during critical illness, it is limited and ultimately harmful to the pediatric patient who has reduced protein stores and elevated protein demands at baseline. Without elimination of the inciting stress, the progressive breakdown of diaphragmatic, cardiac, and skeletal muscle can lead to respiratory compromise, fatal arrhythmia, and loss of lean body mass. Moreover, a prolonged negative protein balance may have a significant impact on the child's growth and development. Healthy, nonstressed neonates require a positive protein balance of nearly 2 g/kg/d.[24,25] In contrast, critically ill, premature neonates requiring mechanical ventilation have a protein balance of −1 g/kg/d.[26,27] Critically ill neonates who require extracorporeal membrane oxygenation (ECMO) have exceedingly high rates of protein loss with a net protein balance of −2.3 g/kg/d.[13]

The protein catabolic response is concerning, because it is well known to correlate with morbidity and mortality in the surgical patient. Fortunately, amino acid supplementation in critically ill children tends to promote increased nitrogen retention and positive protein balance.[23,28] The mechanism appears to be an increase in protein synthesis, although the rate of protein degradation remains constant.[29,30] The

TABLE 13.4
Recommended Protein Requirements for
Critically Ill Infants and Children

Age (yr)	Estimated Protein Requirement (g/kg/d)
0 to 2	2.0 to 3.0
2 to 13	1.5 to 2.0
13 to 18	1.5

Source: From Jaksic, T., *Surg. Clin. N. Am.*, 82, 383, 2002.
With permission.

provision of dietary protein sufficient to optimize protein synthesis, facilitate wound healing and the inflammatory process, and preserve skeletal muscle mass is the single most important nutritional intervention in critically ill children. Importantly, the quantity of protein needed to enhance protein accrual is greater in critically ill than in healthy children. Listed in Table 13.4 are the recommended quantities of dietary protein for critically ill children. During extreme physiologic stress, including children with extensive burn injury or neonates on ECMO, additional protein supplementation may be necessary to meet metabolic demands. Toxicity from excessive protein administration has been reported, particularly in children with impaired renal and hepatic function. The provision of protein at levels greater than 3.5 g/kg/d is rarely indicated and is often associated with azotemia. Studies using protein provisions of 6 g/kg/d have demonstrated significant morbidity, including azotemia, pyrexia, strabismus, and lower IQ scores.[31,32]

Carbohydrate Metabolism

Glucose production and availability are a priority in the pediatric metabolic stress response. Glucose is the primary energy source for the brain, erythrocyte, and renal medulla and is also used extensively in the inflammatory response. In the past, nutritional support for critically ill patients included large amounts of glucose in an attempt to reduce endogenous glucose production. Unfortunately, excess glucose increases CO_2 production, engenders fatty liver, and does not attenuate endogenous glucose turnover.[33] Thus, a surplus of carbohydrate may increase the ventilatory burden in the critically ill patient. Recent data from studies of critically ill neonates has also shown that excessive carbohydrates may be paradoxically associated with an increased rate of protein breakdown.[34]

When designing a nutritional regimen for the critically ill child, excessive carbohydrate calories are generally avoided, and a mixed diet, including both glucose and lipid substrates, is utilized to meet the patient's caloric requirements. When the postoperative neonate is fed a high glucose diet, the corresponding respiratory quotient (RQ) is approximately 1.0, and may be higher than 1.0 in select patients, implying net lipogenesis.[35] A mixed dietary regimen of glucose and lipid (2 to 4 g/kg/d) lowers the effective RQ in neonates to 0.8.[36] This approach will provide the child with full nutritional supplementation while alleviating the increased ventilatory burden and risks of hyperglycemia.

Lipid Metabolism

Along with protein and carbohydrate metabolism, lipid turnover is generally increased in the systemic response to critical illness, major surgery, and trauma in the pediatric patient.[37] The increased lipid metabolism is thought to be proportional to the overall degree of illness. The process of lipid turnover involves both the synthesis of triglycerides from free fatty acids and glycerol as well as triglyceride breakdown. Approximately 30 to 40% of free fatty acids are oxidized for energy, and RQ values may decline during illness, reflecting an increased utilization of fat as an energy source.[38] This suggests that fatty acids are a prime source of energy in metabolically stressed pediatric patients. In addition to the rich energy supply from lipid substrate, the glycerol moiety released from triglycerides may be converted to pyruvate and used to manufacture glucose. However, like protein catabolism, it has been shown that extra dietary glucose provisions do not decrease fatty acid turnover in times of illness.

The increased demand for lipid utilization in critical illness coupled with the limited lipid stores in the neonate places the metabolically stressed child at high risk for the development of essential fatty acid deficiency.[39,40] Preterm infants develop biochemical evidence of essential fatty acid deficiency as soon as 2 d after the initiation of a fat-free diet.[41] In the human, the polyunsaturated fatty acids, linoleic acid and linolenic acid, are considered essential fatty acids, because the body cannot manufacture them by desaturating other fatty acids. Linoleic acid is used by the body to synthesize arachidonic acid, an important intermediate in prostaglandin synthesis. The prostaglandin family includes the leukotrienes and thromboxanes, which serve as mediators in such wide-ranging processes as vascular permeability, smooth muscle reactivity, and platelet aggregation. If the body lacks dietary linoleic acid, the formation of arachidonic acid (a tetraene, with four double bonds) cannot take place, and eicosatrienoic acid (a triene, with three double bonds) accumulates in its place. Clinically, a fatty acid profile can be performed on human serum, and an elevated triene to tetraene ratio greater than 0.4 is characteristic of biochemical essential fatty acid deficiency. This condition may present in the child as dermatitis, alopecia, thrombocytopenia, increased susceptibility to infection, and overall failure to thrive. To avoid essential fatty acid deficiency in neonates, the allotment of linoleic and linolenic acid is recommended at concentrations of 4.5 and 0.5% of total calories, respectively.[42]

Parenterally delivered lipid solutions administered in a mixed fuel nutritional regimen limit the need for excessive glucose provision. Lipid emulsions provide a higher quantity of energy per gram than glucose (9 kcal/g versus 4 kcal/g), thereby reducing the overall rate of CO_2 production, the RQ value, and the incidence of hepatic steatosis.[43] Further, the adequate provision of lipids eliminates the risk of essential fatty acid deficiency. In general, lipid and carbohydrate feeding appear to be equally efficacious in ameliorating net protein catabolism in surgical neonates.[36]

When starting a patient on intravenous lipid administration, there are several risks to consider. These include hypertriglyeridemia, a possible increased risk of infection, and decreased alveolar oxygen diffusion capacity.[44–46] Most pediatric institutions initiate lipid provisions at 0.5 to 1.0 g/kg/d and increase delivery over a period of days to a goal of 2 to 4 g/kg/d. During this time, triglyceride levels are monitored closely. Lipid administration is generally restricted to between 30 and 40% of total caloric intake in ill children in an effort to prevent immune dysfunction, although this practice has not been validated in a formal clinical trial.

Energy Metabolism

The pediatric metabolic response is characterized by dramatic increases in the systemic turnover of protein, carbohydrate, and lipid substrates. In the adult patient, these changes have been associated with an elevated resting energy expenditure.[47] Clearly, the increase in substrate turnover requires the input of energy and therefore increases the basal energy expenditure for the critically ill patient. However, whether total energy requirements are actually increased in critically ill babies is an expanding area of pediatric clinical research. The question is important, because caloric provisions have significant consequences on the child's overall recovery.

In general, in the pediatric patient, any increase in resting energy expenditure during illness or after an operation is variable, and far less than originally hypothesized. In children with severe burn injuries, the resting energy expenditure during the initial flow phase of injury is increased by 50% but returns to normal during convalescence.[48] Multiple studies have shown that newborns who undergo major surgery have a variable increase in energy expenditure of 3 to 20% that returns to baseline within 24 h of the operation.[38,49,50] At 5 d postoperatively, there is no discernible difference in energy expenditure rates between stable, extubated surgical neonates and normal infants.[51] The energy expenditure of critically ill neonates on ECMO is nearly identical to age- and diet-matched nonstressed controls.[52] In addition, effective analgesia may prevent any increase in the neonate's energy expenditure. patent ductus arteriosis (PDA) ligation in the neonate causes no change in energy expenditure when fentanyl analgesia is used.[53] In this same group of patients, whole body protein turnover and breakdown were significantly reduced postoperatively when compared to preoperative values.[50]

The data suggest that critically ill and postoperative infants have only a small and transient increase in energy expenditure. The unique energy requirements of the critically ill pediatric patient are thought to involve changes in the overall growth of the child. It is known that growth in the child is halted or delayed during periods of physiologic stress. In addition, levels of physical activity are low secondary to sedative agents and the nature of intensive care treatment. Thus it is possible that any increase in the energy requirement from accelerated substrate turnover is alleviated by a decrease in energy utilization for purposes of growth and development. In general, energy and caloric requirements for the critically ill child are the same as those for the nonstressed child of similar age (Table 13.5). The practice of providing high calorie diets to critically ill children may result in overfeeding and its untoward consequences.[54]

TABLE 13.5
Estimated Energy Requirements for
Critically Ill Neonates, Children, and
Nonobese Adolescents

Age (yr)	Estimated Energy Requirement (kcal/kg/d)
0 to 4	100
4 to 6	90
6 to 8	80
8 to 10	70
10 to 12	60
12 to 18	50

Source: From Jaksic, T., *Surg. Clin. N. Am.*, 82, 384, 2002. With permission.

When constructing an appropriate nutritional regimen for the sick child, the recommended dietary caloric intake for age-matched healthy children represents a reasonable starting point for caloric provisions. This quantity of caloric allotment should afford adequate weight gain while optimizing positive protein balance. For example, postoperative parenterally fed neonates given adequate amino acid intake require a total of only 85 to 90 kcal/kg/d of energy to achieve sufficient protein accretion rates during the first 3 d postoperatively.[29] Children fed enterally require 10% more calories due to obligate intestinal malabsorption. Increased caloric allotments may be necessary in children with labored breathing, such as those with bronchopulmonary dysplasia or congenital diaphragmatic hernia.[55] Caloric provision for the pediatric patient during convalescence should be guided by the attainment of adequate growth parameters.

Of note, energy expenditure measurements in critically ill children have demonstrated high individual variability in numerous studies. Therefore the actual measurement of resting energy expenditure, using indirect calorimetry or stable isotopic techniques, is recommended when prolonged nutritional support is required. Serial measurements of energy expenditure may be necessary to determine the individual child's pattern throughout illness and into convalescence. Predictive equations for energy expenditure used in conjunction with factors to account for physiologic stress have proven inaccurate and should not be relied upon when determining caloric provisions.[56,57]

NUTRITION IN THE ELDERLY PATIENT

The population of elderly adults in North America is increasing at a remarkable rate. Currently 1 of every 8 adults is over the age of 65, and the oldest elderly (greater than 85 yr) represent the fastest-growing segment of our population. By the year 2050, it is estimated that more than 20% of the population will be over the age of

65.[58] The health care worker must therefore be familiar with the nutritional changes that coincide with old age. Similar to the pediatric patient, the elderly patient has specific and unique metabolic demands that impact nutrient requirements. Knowledge of the metabolic differences compared to younger adults is paramount to implementing adequate nutritional provisions for the ill elderly patient.

ENERGY REQUIREMENTS IN THE ELDERLY PATIENT

As adults age, there is a known progressive decrease in total energy expenditure. This is due to both a decline in basal metabolic rate and physical activity energy expenditure together accounting for a decrease per decade of approximately 165 kcal/d for men and 103 kcal/d for women.[59] This change in energy expenditure impacts the energy needs of the elderly patient, and thus the recommended dietary allowance (RDA) for caloric intake in this population is lower than that in the younger adult population. Elderly patients need approximately 1200 to 1600 kcal/d compared to younger adults who need 1900 to 2300 kcal/d.[60] Similar to the pediatric patient, overfeeding carries significant risk, including net generation of CO_2, thereby compounding baseline respiratory difficulties common in this population and leading to an increased risk of hepatic steatosis.

There are several factors contributing to the age-dependent decrease in energy expenditure. The reduction in basal metabolic rate is primarily due to a generalized loss of skeletal muscle mass, known as sarcopenia, associated with the aging process. Invasive studies have demonstrated that sarcopenia involves a reduction in type II skeletal muscle fibers, although type I fibers are usually preserved.[61] Although there is no strict quantitative definition of sarcopenia, data from one large survey using dual-energy x-ray absorptiometry in 883 elderly patients found that between 13 and 24% of patients under the age of 70 had a muscle mass two or more standard deviations below the mean for young healthy patients compared to 50% of those patients over the age of 80.[62] The pathophysiology resulting in sarcopenia and the full functional implications for the elderly patient are not completely understood. However, there seems to be a positive feedback phenomenon. The more pronounced the sarcopenia, the more difficult daily tasks become until eventually these tasks are abandoned. The only known effective treatment for sarcopenia is progressive resistance training. Interestingly, the ability of muscle fibers to adapt to applied resistance is not lost with age;[63] however, as the tasks of daily living are curtailed, there is less resistance training and worsening sarcopenia. It is important to assess progressive loss of muscle mass when determining an elderly patient's energy requirements.

A second important factor contributing to decreased total energy expenditure is the reduction in physical activity that coincides with aging. Physical activity is the most variable component of daily energy expenditure. In sedentary elderly adults, it can account for as little as 15% of total energy expenditure; however, it can account for up to 50% of expenditure in highly active elderly adults.[64] While the data are not conclusive, it appears that even within subgroups of elderly patients who remain physically active, an overall reduction in energy requirements still takes place. When quantifying the amount of energy used for physical activity, often used is a physical activity level (PAL) ratio that can be multiplied by the resting metabolic rate to obtain total daily energy expenditure.[65] A study by Starling et al. using doubly labeled water calorimetry determined that women between the ages of 56 and 90 had an average PAL of 1.6, and men of the same age range had an average PAL of 1.73.[65] Clearly, there is individual variability; therefore, to most accurately evaluate the energy expenditure in a given elderly patient, resting energy expenditure should be determined by using calorimetry.

Finally, chronic disease also contributes to the decline in total energy expenditure in the elderly. Occasionally, an increase in basal metabolic rate can occur in the setting of chronic disease (for example, in disease processes that induce an inflammatory state); however, there usually remains an overall decrease in total energy expenditure due to the accompanying decrease in physical activity.[66] Patients with Alzheimer's disease, on average, expend 14% less energy daily than healthy controls those with congestive heart failure expend 20 to 26% less energy and for those with Parkinson's disease, energy expenditure is up to 56% lower per day.[65]

Although the decline in energy expenditure in elderly adults is multifactorial and differs depending on the individual, in most cases there is a progressive reduction in total energy expenditure. The practitioner must therefore pay careful attention to the changes in energy metabolism when devising the nutritional regimen for the ill elderly patient.

Macronutrient and Micronutrient Needs in Elderly Adults

Compared to the infant, the elderly patient starts with a larger proportion of body protein per kilogram of body weight. In addition, given the differences in growth rates between the infant and the older adult, the elderly patient does not need the high quantities of protein required by the young child. However, while rates of whole body protein breakdown remain stable in the elderly population, the overall rate of protein synthesis is reduced. This contributes to a decreased rate of total protein turnover, which may contribute to the age-related decline in resting energy expenditure. The attenuation of protein synthesis is seen most prominently in the setting of critical illness or injury, when the elderly patient needs to increase the rate of whole body protein synthesis.[67] Elderly patients may have difficulty stimulating an increase in the synthesis of acute phase reactants and immune globulins needed during acute illness.[68,69] This can result in a dampened immune response and even problems with enteral absorption if there is significant hypoalbuminemia leading to intestinal edema.[70] There is some evidence to suggest that providing semielemental protein is beneficial in these situations, resulting in improved visceral organ protein stores.[71–73]

Given the changes in protein metabolism, there is debate over the adequate daily protein provision for the healthy elderly patient. While some authors believe the standard adult RDA for protein (0.8 g/kg/d) should suffice, others advocate an increased rate of protein intake of 1.0 g/kg/d to overcome the reduction in the rate of protein synthesis. It is clear, given the age-related changes in protein metabolism, that elderly adults have a low tolerance for the dramatic increase in protein catabolism seen with critical illness or injury. Thus in the critically ill elderly patient, efforts should be made to optimize protein balance, and an increased allotment of protein is often recommended (up to 1.5 g/kg/d), especially in situations in which active collagen synthesis will be taking place.[74]

In addition to energy and protein metabolism, changes in micronutrient availability and absorption must also be considered in the elderly patient. For example, atrophic gastritis becomes more common with advancing age and is a cause of malabsorption.[75] Given the associated hypochlorhydria and ensuing increase in gastric pH, elderly adults are at risk for deficient binding of vitamin B_{12}, poor absorption of iron, folate, and calcium, and small bowel bacterial overgrowth.[76,77] In severe cases, vitamin B_{12} supplementation may be warranted while monitoring serial levels of B_{12}. Levels of vitamin D may also be significantly reduced in elderly adults. This is thought to be secondary to an age-dependent reduction in skin synthesis of vitamin D and renal hydroxylation required for conversion of vitamin D into an active metabolite, as well as decreased intake.[78] In fact, researchers who conducted a cross-sectional assessment of dietary intake among 1740 healthy adults aged 51 to 85 found that more than 60% of those surveyed reported dietary intake deficient in vitamin D, vitamin E, folate, and calcium.[78] The current micronutrient dietary reference intakes (RDIs) for adults are listed in Table 13.6.

Finally, it is well established that with age, adults gradually increase their basal levels of cholecystekinin (CCK), a hormone that promotes satiety in addition to its effects on gallbladder motility.[58] Thus it is possible that the elderly subject feels full after ingesting smaller nutritional allotments and has a decreased appetite when compared to the younger adult.[79] This could potentially make it more difficult to ingest the necessary macro- and micronutrients on a daily basis.

Energy Metabolism and Critical Illness

While recent data demonstrate that the neonate develops only a subtle and brief elevation in energy expenditure with the onset and duration of critical illness, the elderly patient, in contrast, experiences a dramatic increase in energy needs with severe illness. In this way, the elderly subject acts in similar fashion to the younger adult. Although a baby can divert energy needed for growth to fuel the process of illness-induced metabolic turnover, elderly adults must increase their resting energy expenditure in order to power the increase in nutrient turnover associated with illness or injury. It is estimated that uncomplicated intra-abdominal surgery increases metabolic rate by 10%, uncomplicated injuries increase metabolism by 20%, peritonitis by 20 to 40%, and third-degree burns by at least 50%.[80] Thus, increased dietary caloric provisions may be required in elderly adults to meet the increased systemic metabolic demands. However, given the baseline reduction in resting energy expenditure found in elderly patients, the practitioner should be careful of overfeeding, especially when the patient is being nourished with total parenteral nutrition (TPN) or tube feeds. In contrast, when the elderly patient is eating independently, the practitioner more often encounters the problem of undernutrition. During illness, cytokines such as interleukin-1, interleukin-6, and tumor necrosis factor (TNF) are released, leading to a catabolic state accompanied by a decrease in appetite.[81] If this is associated with underlying problems with sense of smell and taste, difficulty

TABLE 13.6
Recommended Micronutrient Dietary Reference Intakes for Adults

Age	Calcium (mg/d)	Magnesium (mg/d)	Phosphorus (mg/d)	Vitamin A (µg/d)	Vitamin C (mg/d)	Vitamin D (µg/d)	Vitamin E (mg/d)	Vitamin K (µg/d)	Vitamin B$_{12}$ (µg/d)	Zinc (mg/d)	Iron (mg/d)	Thiamine (mg/d)
19 – 30 yr	1300	400 (m) / 310 (f)	700	900 (m) / 700 (f)	90 (m) / 75 (f)	5	15	120 (m) / 90 (f)	2.4	9.4 (m) / 6.8 (f)	8 (m) / 18 (f)	1.2 (m) / 1.1 (f)
31 – 50 yr	1000	420 (m) / 320 (f)	700	900 (m) / 700 (f)	90 (m) / 75 (f)	5	15	120 (m) / 90 (f)	2.4	9.4 (m) / 6.8 (f)	8 (m) / 18 (f)	1.2 (m) / 1.1 (f)
51 – 70 yr	1200	420 (m) / 320 (f)	700	900 (m) / 700 (f)	90 (m) / 75 (f)	10	15	120 (m) / 90 (f)	2.4	9.4 (m) / 6.8 (f)	8	1.2 (m) / 1.1 (f)
> 70 yr	1200	420 (m) / 320 (f)	700	900 (m) / 700 (f)	90 (m) / 75 (f)	15	15	120 (m) / 90 (f)	2.4	9.4 (m) / 6.8 (f)	8	1.2 (m) / 1.1 (f)

Source: Adapted from Standing Committee on the Scientific Evaluation of Dietary Reference Intakes, *Dietary Reference Intakes*, National Academy Press, Washington, D.C., 1998. With permission.

swallowing, dry mouth, dental problems, depression, or dementia, the patient will often take in far fewer calories than are necessary during a time of illness.[75]

Malnutrition in the Elderly Adult

Malnutrition in the elderly adult is a significant problem worldwide. Survey estimates indicate that 4 to 31% of free living older adults living independently have clinical malnutrition,[82] and this number may approach 60% in institutionalized or nursing home patients.[83,84] These numbers are not surprising when one considers the daily living conditions of the elderly adult: approximately 30% of older adults live alone, 25% require assistance with activities of daily living, and many suffer from poor dentition, decreased smell and taste sensitivity, as well as psychosocial factors such as depression.[75] In addition, common disease processes found in the elderly population can mandate fluid restriction or result in gastrointestinal malabsorption, further limiting nutritional intake in these patients.[75] The majority of elderly adults consume insufficient quantities of vitamin D, vitamin E, folate, calcium, dairy products, grains, fruits, and vegetables.[78]

Thus when an elderly patient presents with a surgical disease process, the patient is often found to have associated deficiencies in macro- or micronutrients. The clinical implications of malnutrition in this population are significant. Hospitalized elderly adults with concomitant malnutrition have increased lengths of hospital stay and increased risk of morbidity and mortality during admission and within the first 90 d of discharge.[84] There are several clinical signs that can be used to assess for malnutrition in elderly patients and, if present, could warrant dietary supplementation to optimize recovery. Signs to watch for include cheilosis and angular stomatitis, dehydration, glossitis, poorly healing wounds or ulcers, loss of subcutaneous fat, and loss of muscular mass. In addition, a decreased level of plasma zinc, a low lymphocyte count, and low albumin are all markers of malnutrition[81] (Table 13.7).

The role of supplemental nutrition for elderly patients both during hospitalization and in the pre-hospital period is a current focus of clinical nutritional research. In general, both macronutrient and micronutrient supplementation has proven beneficial for elderly patients. For example, in elderly outpatients, dietary supplementation

TABLE 13.7
Risk Factors for Malnutrition in the Elderly Patient

Clinical Sign	Well Nourished	Undernourished
Weight loss	N/A	> 5% in past month
		> 10% in past 3 months
BMI	18.5 to 24.9	< 8.5
Serum albumin	4.5 to 3.5 g/dl	< 3.5 g/dl
Serum zinc	11 to 33 μmol/l	< 11 μmol/l
Lymphocyte count	5000 to 1500/ml	< 1500/ml
		< 900/ml (severe)

with calcium and vitamin D can reduce the risk of long bone fractures,[85,86] and protein supplementation appears to reduce postoperative rehabilitation time in elderly patients with hip fractures.[87] The administration of protein–calorie supplements to hospitalized elderly patients has been shown to increase rates of weight gain and significantly reduce mortality in the most undernourished subgroup.[88]

The timing and route of nutritional supplementation is still somewhat controversial. Enteral nutrition is generally favored and can be given in various forms, including thickened beverages, shakes, or tube feeds. However, when considering elderly patients, one needs to be realistic in determining how capable the patient is of consuming the proposed diet as well as the potential risks and discomforts of a feeding tube. In addition, enteral feeds are frequently interrupted due to diagnostic and therapeutic procedures requiring that the patient be fasted. Achieving adequate caloric delivery can therefore be problematic.[89] Regardless, some patients will benefit from short courses of supplemental tube feeds, but the use of chronic tube feeds in hospitalized or nursing home patients is not clearly beneficial.[90] Although there are significant risks associated with TPN, it is an option for those malnourished patients who cannot tolerate enteral intake. In a study by Mullen et al., malnourished patients who were given at least 7 d of preoperative TPN were less likely to develop postoperative complications.[91] Finally, in a multicenter Veteran's Administration cooperative study, 395 preoperative patients with malnutrition by clinical screening were randomized to receive preoperative parenteral nutrition or the standard hospital diet. This study found that severely malnourished subjects in the preoperative TPN arm of the study had a decreased incidence of postoperative complications when compared to patients who did not receive TPN as well as a control group of well-nourished patients.[92] These studies suggest that the nutritional state of the elderly patient has a direct influence on clinical outcome, and that severe malnutrition can be reversed with aggressive preoperative nutritional supplementation.

WOUND HEALING AND NUTRITIONAL SUPPORT IN THE PEDIATRIC PATIENT

Wound healing in the infant is thought to follow the same basic physiologic principles as in the adult patient. In general, pediatric wound healing adheres to distinct stages and requires the coordination of multiple anatomic and physiologic systems. In many ways, children have a greater capacity for wound healing given the fact that they often have fewer and less serious medical comorbidities.

However, wound healing in the pediatric patient is also characterized by the immaturity of the multiple systems involved in the healing process.[93] For example, the neonate has an underdeveloped immune system at birth that gradually acquires full immunocompetence with antigenic exposure over time. The newborn child, and in particular the premature infant, relies upon passive immunity early in life. Thus the infant may have difficulty mobilizing the immune and inflammatory mediators required for the initial coordination of the wound healing process. The young child may also have difficulty overcoming bacterial and secondary infections that frequently complicate healing, not only because of an immature immune system but also because the skin is a less protective barrier during the early stages of life.[94]

The infant has a skin structure that is relatively weak but increases in strength over time.[95] For example, the neonate's skin has weaker intercellular attachments than that of older children and adults. Thus, minimal injury or friction to the skin surface can result in separation of the epidermis from the dermis. In addition to being thin, infant skin is also characterized by fewer hair follicles and sebaceous glands.[95] These changes in infant skin are confined primarily to the epidermis, while the dermis is well developed even in the extremely premature neonate. When considering protecting a hospitalized infant's skin from breakdown, it is also important to consider the differences in weight distribution among young infants, children, and adults. Infants need the most protection on the occiput that bears the majority of weight while in the supine position. The sacrum becomes the point of maximal weight bearing as we age.[96]

The skin of the neonate, and in particular premature neonates less than 33 weeks gestation, may not be an effective barrier to permeable fluids and the external environment.[97] Although it is unclear whether this contributes to an increased degree of skin injury when traumatized, it can make the young child more susceptible to wound formation. It is also known that the infant has a relatively large skin surface-to-body-volume ratio, thereby increasing the risk of wound formation.[95] While there has been much discussion in the pediatric and fetal literature about the phenomenon of scarless wound closure in the fetus, there is clear scar formation in the third gestation of pregnancy and thereafter.[98] Pediatric patients may be more prone to forming keloids and hypertrophic scars than adults due to abundant collagen formation.[99]

Nutrition plays a significant role in the wound healing process in the infant. It is well established that amino acid substrate is required for several stages in wound healing, including clot formation, fibroblast proliferation, neovascularization, wound remodeling, and immunologic-mediated phagocytosis.[100,101] Proteins also have a significant role in wound healing, contributing to both structure and essential enzyme synthesis. In addition, collagen synthesis may be delayed by hypoproteinemia.[102] Given the limited protein reserves of the neonate and the associated net increase in protein loss with critical illness and traumatic injury, protein becomes a vital macronutrient. Adequate carbohydrate calories are also essential for infants with wounds because of their limited glycogen reserve. Efficient delivery can be monitored by daily weight gain (15 to 20 g/kg/d for newborns and 12 g/kg/d for 1 to 2 year olds). However, caution must be used, because excessive carbohydrates can overwhelm the neonatal bowel and result in osmotic diarrhea.[103]

Certain subsets of pediatric patients will need close surveillance of nutritional provision during times of wound healing. For example, the child with short bowel syndrome represents a unique anatomic and physiologic challenge to growth and nutrient absorption. A working definition for short bowel syndrome in the pediatric age group is a requirement for parenteral nutrition for at least 3 months due to inadequate intestinal absorptive capacity. These children usually have undergone a massive intestinal resection at an early age, and many are missing the terminal ileum, which is vital to normal nutrient absorption. Children with short bowel syndrome often have difficulty attaining adequate levels of the fat-soluble vitamins (A, D, E, K), vitamin B_{12}, folate, iron, and zinc. Many of these micronutrients play important roles in the wound healing process, and thus patients with short bowel syndrome may be at increased risk for poor or delayed wound healing.

In much the same way, children with respiratory difficulty have a unique relationship between nutritional intake and wound healing. This subset of pediatric patients includes premature infants with bronchopulmonary dysplasia and babies born with congenital diaphragmatic hernia (CDH). The increased work of breathing associated with these conditions may result in an elevation of the resting energy expenditure. In contrast to the pediatric metabolic response to critical illness, in which the baby generally does not increase his energy requirements, these conditions provide a physical basis for an increase in energy needs. Therefore these children may require a greater allotment of caloric intake to maintain normal growth and wound healing parameters.

Given the unique nature of the young infant's metabolism and its limited body macronutrient stores, healing of large wounds must be followed closely in the clinical setting. Difficulties with adequate wound healing, such as poor granulation, fistula formation, or recurrent infection, should raise the possibility of insufficient nutritional intake. In this setting, a formal dietary evaluation should be performed, including assessment of micronutrient serum levels (vitamins A, B_{12}, D, E, iron, zinc, and folate). Pediatric patients who are refractory to basic nutritional supplementation will benefit from objective determination of resting energy expenditure. This can be performed with indirect calorimetry or validated stable isotopic techniques.

WOUND HEALING AND NUTRITIONAL SUPPORT IN THE ELDERLY PATIENT

Wound healing can pose a significant problem in elderly patients. In order to heal a wound in an efficient manner, the body needs to mount an effective inflammatory response, mobilize the appropriate resources for angiogenesis, ground substance production and collagen deposition, and eventually remodel the collagen and contract the scar.[104] Elderly patients are at a disadvantage compared to younger adults, because they have lower rates of protein synthesis, are often mildly immunosuppressed, and frequently suffer from micro- and macronutrient deficiencies. Elderly patients are also more likely to have comorbid conditions that interfere with healing wounds. Diabetes, which occurs in over 10% of patients over the age of 60,[102] has serious consequences for wound healing. Not only does hyperglycemia increase the risk of infection and interfere with fibroblast and leukocyte function, but the absence of or insensitivity to insulin has also been shown to impair healing.[105] Peripheral vascular disease and cardiovascular compromise are both common problems in elderly patients and can significantly affect oxygen delivery to the site of injury, prolonging the time required for healing and predisposing to chronic ulceration and skin breakdown.[106] In addition, both chronic renal and hepatic disease are associated with wound healing delays due to problems with managing fluid volume and clotting factor production as well as amino acid metabolism.[106] However, surprisingly, even with numerous factors that could potentially negatively impact upon healing, most simple wounds heal without significant delay.

Although the healing of acute surgical or traumatic wounds is usually not problematic for elderly patients, chronic wounds and, specifically, decubitus pressure ulcers, are particularly concerning. Pressure ulcers are associated with poor nutritional status, with malnourished patients being twice as likely to develop these wounds compared to well-nourished elderly patients.[107] It is estimated that as many as 65% of malnourished elderly people in chronic care facilities have pressure ulcers.[108] Even adequately nourished patients are at risk for developing these wounds. Up to 10% of hospitalized geriatric patients will develop decubitus ulcers during their hospital stay.[106] In addition to ensuring that patients are rotated frequently and physical pressure is eliminated as much as possible, ensuring maximal blood flow, a full nutritional assessment is necessary in the setting of decubitus ulcers and, in fact, is prudent in the elderly population whenever wound healing is problematic.[109]

One of the most important factors for proper wound healing is the ability to channel adequate energy to the wound. The body tends to place a high priority on wound healing, but if there is an infection or abscess elsewhere, requiring additional energy, wound healing can be delayed.[100] The most energy-consuming aspect of wound healing is collagen synthesis and deposition. The estimated caloric requirement is 0.9 kcal/g of collagen. Small wounds do not usually pose a significant metabolic burden, but large wounds can.[88] Generally, an appropriate balance of protein, carbohydrates, and lipids is essential for proper nutrition and the best chances of uneventful wound healing. Deficiencies in protein can lead to problems with skin cell proliferation, tissue reorganization, and collagen synthesis; inadequate intake of carbohydrates can impair fibroblast proliferation;[110] and too few lipids can result in problems with cell membrane and intracellular matrix synthesis, as well as dampened inflammatory reactions.[111,112] There has also been extensive research into the roles of specific single nutrients in the healing process in the hopes that providing supplementation of these components will enhance healing. These nutrients include single amino acids, vitamins, and trace elements.

Two amino acids of special interest are arginine and glutamine. Arginine, although not considered an essential amino acid under normal conditions, when given as a supplement in experimental conditions has been shown to improve collagen deposition and strength.[104] One of the metabolic pathways for arginine includes conversion to ornithine, which is a proline precursor and therefore may directly stimulate collagen production.[113] Arginine is also thought to reduce protein breakdown during catabolic conditions, mainly by stimulating the release of insulin, glucagon, and growth hormone. Glutamine is another potentially useful amino acid for wound healing. It is the most abundant amino acid in the body and is used by many inflammatory cells for fuel as well as for nucleotide synthesis needed for cellular replication.[114] However, despite encouraging findings for both arginine and glutamine, there is little evidence to support routine supplementation in the elderly, and neither amino acid has had a significant effect on preventing pressure ulcers in susceptible patients.[115]

The vitamins of most benefit in wound healing are vitamins C and A. Vitamin C is historically known to be a crucial cofactor for proper collagen cross-linking,[116] and although deficiencies are rare in elderly patients, it is important to provide supplementation if inadequate intake is anticipated. The recommended daily dietary allowance is 60 mg, except for women over the age of 51, who should get 62 mg/d. Vitamin A is also important for wound healing and is particularly effective as a supplement in patients who are being treated with steroids, radiotherapy, or who have diabetes. At supplemental doses of 25,000 U/d in this patient population, healing may be accelerated secondary to an increased inflammatory response and increased collagen synthesis.[80]

Although sometimes forgotten, the trace element zinc has an important role in wound healing because of its role in DNA and protein synthesis. After injury, there is a redistribution of zinc with increased uptake in the wound, liver, and spleen, resulting in a relative decrease in plasma and skin levels.[117] When deficient (levels less than 100 µg/100 ml), wound strength and epithelialization can be affected.[74] Although there is no proven benefit to supplementing patients who are not deficient, if the serum level is low it should be brought to adequate levels. The recommended daily dose for elderly patients is 15 mg.[88] Hospitalized patients are particularly at risk for low serum zinc levels due to decreased oral intake and increased zinc losses through diarrhea or malabsorption.[118] There is also some benefit to using topical zinc ointments, because zinc is absorbed percutaneously and enhances cell division within the epidermal layer. In addition, the topical zinc formulations have mild antibacterial properties.[101]

It is important to remember that a nutritional evaluation for an elderly patient who is critically ill or injured requires ongoing assessment. Elderly adults, similarly to infants and children, are at risk of becoming malnourished while in the hospital because they are not always able to adequately nourish themselves. Although elderly patients do have some nutritional reserve, they can become deficient in both macro- and micronutrients during times of illness due to ongoing catabolism. The sooner nutritive deficiencies are detected and corrected, the more the patient will benefit and the better the chance of uncomplicated wound healing.

FUTURE DIRECTIONS

The dramatic increase in protein breakdown during critical illness coupled with the known association between protein loss and patient mortality and morbidity has stimulated a wide array of research efforts. The measurement of whole body nitrogen balance through urine and stool was once the only way to investigate changes in protein metabolism, but now validated nonradioactive stable isotope tracer techniques exist to measure the precise rates of protein turnover, breakdown, and synthesis.[119]

However, the modulation of protein metabolism in critically ill patients has proved difficult. Dietary supplementation of amino acids increases protein synthesis but appears to have no effect on protein breakdown rates. Thus investigators have recently focused on the use of alternative anabolic agents to decrease protein catabolism. To achieve this goal, researchers have used various pharmacologic tools, including growth hormone, insulin-derived growth factor I (IGF-I), and testosterone with varying degrees of success.[120–122] One of the most promising agents, however, may be the anabolic hormone insulin.

Multiple studies have used insulin to reduce protein breakdown in healthy volunteers and adult burn patients.[123–125] In children with extensive burns, intravenous insulin has been shown to increase lean body mass and mitigate peripheral muscle catabolism.[126] A recent prospective, randomized trial of over 1500 adult postoperative patients in the intensive care unit demonstrated significant reductions in mortality and morbidity with the use of intravenous insulin.[127] Preliminary stable isotopic studies demonstrate that an intravenous insulin infusion may reduce protein breakdown by 32% in critically ill neonates on ECMO.[128] The use of insulin and other hormonal modalities to modulate the protein metabolic response to systemic illness will continue to be an active area of clinical investigation in critically ill adults and children. It is likely that interventions that promote net protein accretion will augment the wound healing process, as additional protein substrate will be available for the various mechanisms involved in wound healing.

REFERENCES

1. Forbes, G.B. and Bruining, G.J., Urinary creatinine excretion and lean body mass, *Am. J. Clin. Nutr.*, 29, 1359–1366, 1976.
2. Foman, S.J., Haschke, F., Zeigler, E.E. et al., Body composition of reference children from birth to age 10 years, *Am. J. Clin. Nutr.*, 35, 1169–1175, 1982.
3. Munro, H.N., Nutrition and muscle protein metabolism, *Fed. Proc.*, 37, 2281–2282, 1978.
4. Long, C.L., Spencer, J.L., Kinney, J.M. et al., Carbohydrate metabolism in normal man and effect of glucose infusion, *J. Appl. Phys.*, 31, 102–109, 1971.
5. Herrera, E. and Amusquivar, E., Lipid metabolism in the fetus and the newborn, *Diabet./Metab. Res. Rev.*, 16, 202–210, 2000.
6. Reichman, B., Chessex, P., Vercellen, G. et al., Dietary composition and macronutrient storage in preterm infants, *Pediatrics*, 72, 322–328, 1983.
7. Schulze, K.F., Stefanski, M., Masterson, J. et al., Energy expenditure, energy balance and composition of weight gain in low birth weight infants fed diets of different protein and energy content, *J. Pediatr.*, 110, 753–759, 1987.
8. Whyte, R.K., Haslam, R., Vlainic, C. et al. Energy balance and nitrogen balance in growing low birthweight infants fed human milk or formula, *Pediatr. Res.*, 18, 891–898, 1983.
9. Food and Nutrition Board, *Recommended Dietary Allowances*, 10th ed., National Academy of Science — National Research Council, Washington, D.C., 1989.
10. Kashyap, S., Schulze, K.F., Forsyth, M. et al., Growth, nutrient retention, and metabolic response in low birth weight infants fed varying intakes of protein and energy, *J. Pediatr.*, 113, 713–721, 1988.
11. Denne, S.C., Karn, C.A., Ahlrichs, J.A. et al., Proteolysis and phenylalanine hydroxylation in response to parenteral nutrition in extremely premature and normal newborns, *J. Clin. Invest.*, 97, 746–754, 1996.
12. Hay, W.W., Lucas, A., Heird, W.C. et al., Workshop summary: nutrition of the extremely low birth weight infant, *Pediatrics*, 104, 1360–1368, 1999.
13. Keshen, T., Miller, R.G., Jahoor, F. et al., Stable isotopic quantitation of protein metabolism and energy expenditure in neonates on and post extracorporeal life support, *J. Pediatr. Surg.*, 32, 958–963, 1997.
14. Jaksic, T., Wagner, D.A., Burke, J.F. et al., Proline metabolism in adult male burned patients and healthy control subjects, *Am. J. Clin. Nutr.*, 54, 408–413, 1991.

15. Cogo, P.E., Carnielli, V.P., Rosso, F. et al., Protein turnover, lipolysis, and endogenous hormonal secretion in critically ill children, *Crit. Care Med.*, 30, 65–70, 2002.

16. Coss-Bu, J.A., Klish, W.J., Walding, D. et al., Energy metabolism, nitrogen balance, and substrate utilization in critically ill children, *Am. J. Clin. Nutr.*, 74, 664–669, 2001.

17. Bilmazes, C., Klein, C.L., Rorbaugh, D.K. et al., Muscle protein catabolism after injury in man, as measured by urinary excretion of 3-methyl-histidine, *Clin. Sci.*, 52, 527–533, 1977.

18. Pierro, A., Metabolism and nutritional support in the surgical neonate, *J. Pediatr. Surg.*, 37, 811–822, 2002.

19. Long, C.L., Kinney, J.M., and Geiger, J.W., Non-suppressability of gluconeogenesis by glucose in septic patients, *Metabolism*, 25, 193–201, 1976.

20. Keshen, T., Miller, R., Jahoor, F. et al., Glucose production and gluconeogenesis are negatively related to body weight in mechanically ventilated, very low birthweight neonatos, *Pediatr. Res.*, 31, 132–138, 1997.

21. Meszaros, K., Bojta, J., Bautista, A.P. et al., Glucose utilization by Kupffer cells, endothelial cells, and granulocytes in endotoxemic rat liver, *Am. J. Phys.*, 267, G7–G12, 1994.

22. Denne, S.C., Karn, C.A., Wang, J. et al., Effect of intravenous glucose and lipid on proteolysis and glucose production in normal newborns, *Am. J. Phys.*, 269, E361–E366, 1995.

23. Mitton, S.G. and Garlick, P.J., Changes in protein turnover after the introduction of parenteral nutrition in premature infants: comparison of breast milk and egg protein-based amino acid solutions, *Pediatr. Res.*, 32, 447–454, 1992.

24. Pencharz, P., Beesley, J., Sauer, P. et al., Total-body protein turnover in parenterally fed neonates: effects of energy source studied by using [15N]glycine and [1-13C]leucine, *Am. J. Clin. Nutr.*, 50, 1395–1400, 1989.

25. Beaufrere, B., Fournier, V., Salle, B. et al., Leucine kinetics in fed low-birth-weight infants: importance of splanchnic tissues, *Am. J. Physiol.*, 263, E214–E220, 1992.

26. Mitton, S.G., Calder, A.G., and Garlick, P.J., Protein turnover rates in sick, premature neonates during the first few days of life, *Pediatr. Res.*, 30, 418–422, 1991.

27. Rivera, A., Jr., Bell, E.F., and Bier, D.M., Effect of intravenous amino acids on protein metabolism of preterm infants during the first three days of life, *Pediatr. Res.*, 33, 106–111, 1993.

28. Thureen, P.J., Anderson, A.H., Baron, K.A. et al., Protein balance in the first week of life in ventilated neonates receiving parenteral nutrition, *Am. J. Clin. Nutr.*, 68, 1128–1135, 1998.

29. Duffy, B. and Pencharz, P., The effects of surgery on the nitrogen metabolism of parenterally fed human neonates, *Pediatr. Res.*, 20, 32–35, 1996.

30. Poindexter, B.B., Karn, C.A., Leitch, C.A. et al., Amino acids do not suppress proteolysis in premature neonates, *Am. J. Physiol.*, 281, E472–E478, 2001.

31. Goldman, H.I., Freundenthal, R., Holland, B. et al., Clinical effects of two different levels of protein intake on low birth weight infants, *J. Pediatr.*, 74, 881–889, 1969.

32. Goldman, H.I., Liebman, O.B., Freundenthal, R. et al., Effects of early dietary protein intake on low-birth-weight infants: evaluation at 3 years of age, *J. Pediatr.*, 78, 126–129, 1971.

33. Tappy, L., Schwarz, J.-M., Schneiter, P. et al., Effects of isoenergetic glucose-based or lipid-based parenteral nutrition on glucose metabolism, *de novo* lipogenesis, and respiratory gas exchanges in critically ill patients, *Crit. Care Med.*, 26, 860–867, 1998.

34. Shew, S.B., Keshen, T.H., Jahoor, F. et al., The determinants of protein catabolism in neonates on extracorporeal membrane oxygenation, *J. Pediatr. Surg.*, 34, 1086–1090, 1999.

35. Forsyth, J.S., Murdock, N., and Crighton, A., Low birthweight infants and total parenteral nutrition immediately after birth. III. Randomised study of energy substrate utilization, nitrogen balance, and carbon dioxide production, *Arch. Dis. Child Fetal and Neonatal Ed.*, 73, F13–F16, 1995.

36. Jones, M.O., Pierro, A., Garlick, P.J. et al., Protein metabolism kinetics in neonates: effect of intravenous carbohydrate and fat, *J. Pediatr. Surg.*, 30, 458–462, 1995.

37. Jeenvanandam, M., Young, D.H., and Schiller, W.R., Nutritional impact on energy cost of fat fuel mobilization in polytrauma victims, *J. Trauma*, 30, 147–154, 1990.

38. Powis, M.R., Smith, K., Rennie, M. et al., Effect of major abdominal operations on energy and protein metabolism in infants and children, *J. Pediatr. Surg.*, 33, 49–53, 1998.

39. Paulsrud, J.R., Pensler, L., Whitten, C.F. et al., Essential fatty acid deficiency in infants induced by fat-free intravenous feeding, *Am. J. Clin. Nutr.*, 25, 897–904, 1972.

40. Friedman, Z., Danon, A., Stahlman, M.T. et al., Rapid onset of essential fatty acid deficiency in the newborn, *Pediatrics*, 58, 640–649, 1976.

41. Giovannini, M., Riva, E., and Agostoni, C., Fatty acids in pediatric nutrition, *Pediatr. Clin. N. Am.*, 42, 861–877, 1995.

42. Committee on Nutrition, European Society of Pediatric Gastroenterology and Nutrition, Comment on the content and composition of lipids in infant formulas, *Acta Paed. Scand.*, 80, 887–889, 1991.

43. Van Aerde, J.E., Sauer, P.J., Pencharz, P.B. et al., Metabolic consequences of increasing energy intake by adding lipid to parenteral nutrition in full-term infants, *Am. J. Clin. Nutr.*, 59, 659–662, 1994.

44. Cleary, T.G. and Pickering, L.K., Mechanisms of intralipid effect on polymorphonuclear leukocytes, *J. Clin. Lab. Immunol.*, 11, 21–26, 1983.

45. Perriera, G.R., Fox, W.W., Stanley, C.A. et al., Decreased oxygenation and hyperlipidemia during intravenous fat infusions in premature infants, *Pediatrics*, 66, 26–30, 1980.

46. Freeman, J., Goldmann, D.A., Smith, N.E. et al., Association of intravenous lipid emulsion and coagulase-negative staphylococcal bacteremia in neonatal intensive care units, *N. Engl. J. Med.*, 323, 301–308, 1990.

47. Blackburn, G.L., Bistrian, B.R., Mani, B.S. et al., Nutritional and metabolic assessment of the hospitalized patient, *J. Parenter. Enteral Nutr.*, 1, 11–22, 1977.

48. Jahoor, F., Desair, M., Herndon, D.N. et al., Dynamics of the protein metabolic response to burn injury, *Metabolism*, 37, 330–337, 1988.

49. Jones, M.O., Pierro, A., Hammond, P. et al., The metabolic response to operative stress in infants, *J. Pediatr. Surg.*, 28, 1258–1263, 1993.

50. Shew, S.B., Keshen, T.H., Glass, N.L. et al., Ligation of a patent ductus arteriosus under fentanyl anesthesia improves protein metabolism in premature neonates, *J. Pediatr. Surg.*, 35, 1277–1281, 2000.

51. Pierro, A., Carnielli, V., Filler, R.M. et al., Partition of energy metabolism in the surgical newborn, *J. Pediatr. Surg.*, 26, 581–586, 1991.

52. Jaksic, T., Shew, S.B., Keshen, T.H. et al., Do critically ill surgical neonates have elevated energy expenditure? *J. Pediatr. Surg.*, 36, 63–67, 2001.

53. Garza, J.J., Shew, S.B., Keshen, T.H. et al., Energy expenditure in ill premature neonates, *J. Pediatr. Surg.*, 37, 289–293, 2002.

54. Letton, R.W., Chwals, W.J., Jamie, A. et al., Early postoperative alterations in infant energy use increase the risk of overfeeding, *J. Pediatr. Surg.*, 30, 988–993, 1995.

55. Weinstein, M.R. and Oh, W., Oxygen consumption in infants with bronchopulmonary dysplasia, *J. Pediatr.*, 99, 958–961, 1981.
56. Briassoulis, G., Venkataraman, S., and Thompson, A.E., Energy expenditure in critically ill children, *Crit. Care Med.*, 28, 1166–1172, 2000.
57. Coss-Bu, J.A., Jefferson, L.S., Walding, D. et al., Resting energy expenditure in children in a pediatric intensive care unit: comparison of Harris-Benedict and Talbot predictions with indirect calorimetry values, *Am. J. Clin. Nutr.*, 67, 74–80, 1998.
58. Jensen, G.L., McGee, M., and Binkley, J., Nutrition in the elderly, *Gastroenterol. Clin. N. Am.*, 30, 313–333, 2001.
59. Kinney, J.M., Energy requirements of the surgical patient, in *Manual of surgical nutrition*, Ballinger, W.F., Collins, J.A., Druker, W.R. et al., Eds., W.B. Saunders, Philadelphia, 1975, pp. 223–235.
60. Blumberg, J., Nutrient requirements of the healthy elderly — should there be specific RDAs? *Nutr. Rev.*, 52, S15–S18, 1994.
61. Lau, H.C., Granick, M.S., Aisner, A.M., and Solomon, M.P., Wound care in the elderly patient, *Surg. Clin. N. Am.*, 74, 441–463, 1994.
62. Tellado, J.M., Garcia-Sabrido, J.L., Hanley, Ja., Shizgal, H.M., and Christou, N.V., Predicting mortality based on body composition analysis, *Ann. Surg.*, 208, 81–87, 1989.
63. Starling, R.D. and Poehlman, E.T., Assessment of energy requirements in elderly populations, *Eur. J. Clin. Nutr.*, 54, S104–S111, 2000.
64. Finch, S., Doyle, W., Lowe, C., Bates, C.J., Prentice, A., Smithers, G., and Clarke, P.C., National Diet and Nutrition Survey (NDNS) People Aged 65 Years and Over, Vol. 1, The Stationary Office, London, 1998.
65. Goran, M.I. and Poehlman, E.T., Total energy expenditure and energy requirements in healthy elderly persons, *Metabolism*, 41, 744–752, 1992.
66. Black, A.E., Coward, W.A., Cole, T.J., and Prentice, A.M., Human energy expenditure in affluent societies: an analysis of 574 doubly-labelled water measurements, *Eur. J. Clin. Nutr.*, 50, 772–792, 1996.
67. Mullen, J.L., Buzby, G.P., Matthews, D.C. et al., Reduction of operative morbidity and mortality by combined preoperative and postoperative nutritional support, *Ann. Surg.*, 192, 604–613, 1980.
68. Phillips, P., Protein turnover in the elderly: a comparison between ill patients and normal controls. Human Nutrition, *Clin. Nutr.*, 37, 339–344, 1983.
69. Mobarhan, S. and Trumbore, L.S., Nutritional problems of the elderly, *Clin. Geriatr. Med.*, 7, 191–213, 1991.
70. Borlase, B.C., Bell, S.J., Lewis, E.J. et al., Tolerance to enteral tube feeding diets in hypoalbuminemic critically ill, geriatric patients, *Surg. Gynecol. Obstet.*, 174, 181–188, 1992.
71. Ziegler, F., Ollivier, J.M., Cynober, L. et al., Efficiency of enteral nitrogen support in surgical patients: small peptides v non-degraded proteins, *Gut*, 31, 1277–1283, 1990.
72. Meredith, J.W., Ditesheim, J.A., and Zaloga, G.P., Visceral protein levels in trauma patients are greater with peptide diet than with intact protein diet, *J. Trauma*, 30, 825–829, 1990.
73. Feller, A., Rudman, D., and Caindec, N., Comparison of nutritional efficacy of Peptamin and Vivonex TEN elemental diets in elderly tube fed subjects, *J. Parent. Enteral Nutr.*, 13, 12S–18S, 1989.
74. Fischer, J.E., *Nutrition and Metabolism in the Surgical Patient*, Little, Brown, Boston, 1996.

75. Cederholm, T., Jagren, C., and Hellstrom, K., Outcome of protein-energy malnutrition in elderly medical patients, *JAMA*, 98, 67–74, 1995.

76. Pirlich, M. and Lochs, H., Nutrition in the elderly, *Best Pract. Res. Clin. Gastroenterol.*, 15, 869–884, 2001.

77. Bowman, V.A., Rosenberg, I.C.H., and Hohnson, M.A., Gastrointestinal function in the elderly, in *Nutrition for the Elderly, Nestle Nutrition Workshop Series*, Vol. 29, Munro, H.N. and Schief, G., Eds., Raven, New York, 1992, pp. 43–50.

78. Russell, R.M., Changes in gastrointestinal function attributed to ageing, *Am. J. Clin. Nutr.*, 55, 1203S–1207S, 1992.

79. Foote, J., Giuliano, A.R., and Harris, R.B., Older adults need guidance to meet nutritional recommendations, *J. Am. Coll. Nutr.*, 19, 628–640, 2000.

80. Levenson, S.M., Gruber, C.A., Rettura, G. et al., Supplemental vitamin A prevents the acute radiation-induced defect in wound healing, *Ann. Surg.*, 200, 494–512, 1984.

81. McCormack, P., Undernutrition in the elderly population living at home in the community: a review of the literature, *J. Adv. Nursing*, 26, 856–863, 1997.

82. Morley, J.E., Anorexia of aging: physiologic and pathologic, *Am. J. Clin. Nutr.*, 66, 760–773, 1997.

83. Baumgartner, R.N., Koehler, K.M., Gallagher, D., Romero, L., Heymsfield, S.B., Ross, R.R., Garry, P.J., and Lindeman, R.D., Epidemiology of sarcopenia among the elderly in New Mexico, *Am. J. Epidemiol.*, 147, 755–763, 1998.

84. Sturm, K., Parker, B., Wishart, J., Feinle-Bisset, C., Jones, K.L. et al., Energy intake and appetite are related to antral area in healthy young and older subjects, *Am. J. Clin. Nutr.*, 80, 656–667, 2004.

85. Sullivan, D.H. and Walls, R.C., The risk of life-threatening complications in a select population of geriatric patients: the impact of nutritional status, *J. Am. Coll. Nutr.*, 14, 29–36, 1995.

86. Chapuy, M.C., Arlot, M.E., Buoeuf, F. et al., Vitamin D_3 and calcium to prevent hip fracture in the elderly woman, *N. Engl. J. Med.*, 327, 1637–1642, 1992.

87. Ward, W. and Richardson, A., Effect of age on liver protein synthesis and degradation, *Hepatology*, 14, 935–948, 1991.

88. Williams, J.Z. and Barbul, A., Nutrition and wound healing, *Surg. Clin. N. Am.*, 83, 571–596, 2003.

89. Avenell, A. and Handoll, H.H., A systematic review of protein and energy supplementation for hip fracture aftercare in older people, *Eur. J. Clin. Nutr.*, 57, 895–903, 2003.

90. Ciocon, J.O., Silverstone, F.A., Graver, L.M. et al., Tube feedings in elderly patients: indications, benefits and complications, *Arch. Intern. Med.*, 148, 429–433, 1988.

91. Dawson-Hughes, B., Harris, S.S., Krall, E.A., and Dallal, G.E., Effect of calcium and vitamin D supplementation on bone density in men and women 65 years of age or older, *N. Engl. J. Med.*, 337, 670–676, 1997.

92. Woodcock, N.P., Zeigler, D., Palmer, M.D., Buckley, P., Mitchell, C.J., and MacFie, J., Enteral versus parenteral nutrition: a pragmatic study, *Nutrition*, 17, 53–55, 2001.

93. Garvin, G., Wound healing in pediatrics, *Nursing Clin. N. Am.*, 25, 181–192, 1990.

94. Hurwitz, S., Cutaneous diseases of the newborn, in *Neonatal Skin Structure and Function*, Maibach, H. and Boisits, E., Eds., Marcel Dekker, New York, 1992, pp. 239–263.

95. Eichenfield, L.F. and Hardaway, C.A., Neonatal dermatology, *Curr. Opin. Pediatr.*, 5, 471–475, 1999.

96. Solis, I., Krouskop, T., Trainer, N. et al., Supine interference pressure in children, *Arch. Phys. Med. Rehabil.*, 69, 524–526, 1988.

97. Harpin, V.A. and Rutter, N., Barrier properties of the newborn infant's skin, *J. Pediatr.*, 120, 419–425, 1983.
98. Mast, B.A., Diegelmann, R.F., Krummel, T.M., and Cohen, I.K., Scarless wound healing in the mammalian fetus, *Surg. Gynecol. Obstet.*, 5, 441–451, 1992.
99. Peacock, K.K., Madden, J.W., and Trier, W.C., Biological basis for the treatment of keloids and hypertrophic scars, *So. Med. J.*, 63, 755, 1970.
100. Albina, J.E., Nutrition and wound healing, *J. Parenter. Enteral Nutr.*, 18, 367–376, 1994.
101. Lansdown, A.B.G., Nutrition 2: a vital consideration in the management of skin wounds, *Br. J. Nursing*, 13, 1199–1210, 2004.
102. Meyer, N.A., Muller, M.J., and Herndon, D.N., Nutrient support of the healing wound, *New Horizons*, 2, 202–214, 1994.
103. Lifschitz, C.H., Carbohydrate needs in preterm and term newborn infants, in *Nutrition During Infancy*, Reginald, C.T. and Buford, L.N., Eds., Hanley and Belfus, Philadelphia, 1988, pp. 122–132.
104. The Veterans Affairs total parenteral nutrition cooperative study group, Perioperative total parenteral nutrition in surgical patients, *N. Engl. J. Med.*, 325, 525–532, 1991.
105. Mann, G.V., The impairment of transport of amino acid by monosaccharides, *Fed. Proc.*, 33, 221–226, 1974.
106. Wilson, P.W.F., Anderson, K.M., and Kannel, W.B., Epidemiology of diabetes mellitus in the elderly: the Framingham study, *Am. J. Med.*, 80, S3–S9, 1986.
107. Thomas, D.R., Goode, P.S., Tarquine, P.H., and Allman, R.M., Hospital-acquired pressure ulcers and risk of death, *J. Am. Geriatr. Soc.*, 44, 1435–1440, 1996.
108. Pinchkofsky-Devin, G.D. and Kaminski, M.V., Jr., Correlation of pressure sores and nutritional status, *J. Am. Geriatr. Soc.*, 34, 435–440, 1986.
109. Mechanick, J.I., Practical aspects of nutritional support for wound-healing patients, *Am. J. Surg.*, 188, 52S–56S, 2004.
110. Albina, J.E., Nutrition and wound healing, *J. Parenter. Enteral Nutr.*, 18, 367–376, 1994.
111. Hulsey, T.K., O'Neill, J.A., Neblett, W.R. et al., Experimental wound healing in essential fatty acid deficiency, *J. Pediatr. Surg.*, 15, 505–508, 1980.
112. Caffrey, B.B. and Jonnson, J.T., Jr., Role of essential fatty acids in wound healing in rats, *Prog. Lipid Res.*, 20, 641–647, 1981.
113. Nirgiotis, J.G., Hennessey, P.J., Black, C.T. et al., The effects of an arginine-free enteral diet on wound healing and immune function in the postsurgical rat, *J. Pediatr. Surg.*, 26, 936–941, 1991.
114. Albina, J.E., Abate, J.A., and Mastrofrancesco, B., Role of ornithine as a proline precursor in healing wounds, *J. Surg. Res.*, 55, 97–102, 1993.
115. Thomas, D.R., Improving outcomes of pressure ulcers with nutritional interventions: a review of the evidence, *Nutrition*, 17, 121–125, 2001.
116. Englard, S. and Seifter, E., The biochemical functions of ascorbic acid, *Annu. Rev. Nutr.*, 6, 365–406, 1986.
117. Henzel, J.H., DeWeese, M.S., and Lichti, E.L., Zinc concentrations within healing wounds. Significance of postoperative zincuria on availability and requirements during tissue repair, *Arch. Surg.*, 100, 349–357, 1970.
118. Prasad, A.S., Zinc deficiency in human subjects, *Prog. Clin. Biol. Res.*, 129, 1–33, 1983.
119. Liu, Z. and Barrett, E.J., Human protein metabolism: its measurement and regulation, *Am. J. Physiol.*, 238, E1105–E1112, 2002.
120. Takala, J., Ruokonen, E., Webster, N.R. et al., Increased mortality associated with growth hormone treatment in critically ill adults, *N. Engl. J. Med.*, 341, 785–792, 1999.

121. Yarwood, G.D., Ross, R.J., Medbak, S. et al., Administration of recombinant insulin-like growth factor-I in critically ill patients, *Crit. Care Med.*, 25, 1352–1361, 1997.

122. Demling, R.H. and Orgill, D.P., The anticatabolic and wound healing effects of the testosterone analog oxandrolone after severe burn injury, *J. Crit. Care*, 15, 12–17, 2000.

123. Denne, S.C., Liechty, E.A., Liu, Y.M. et al., Proteolysis in skeletal muscle and whole body in response to euglycemic hyperinsulinemia in normal adults, *Am. J. Physiol.*, 261, E809–E814, 1991.

124. Farrag, H.M., Nawrath, L.M., Healey, J.E. et al., Persistent glucose production and greater peripheral sensitivity to insulin in the neonate vs. the adult, *Am. J. Physiol.*, 272, E86–E93, 1997.

125. Sakurai, Y., Aarsland, A., Herndon, D.N. et al., Stimulation of muscle protein synthesis by long-term insulin infusion in severely burned patients, *Ann. Surg.*, 222, 283–297, 1995.

126. Thomas, S.J., Morimoto, K., Herndon, D.N. et al., The effect of prolonged euglycemic hyperinsulinemia on lean body mass after severe burn, *Surgery*, 132, 341–347, 2002.

127. Van den Berghe, G., Wouters, P., Weeks, F. et al., Intensive insulin therapy in critically ill patients, *N. Engl. J. Med.*, 345, 1359–1367, 2001.

128. Javid, P.J., Agus, M.S.D.A., Dzakovic, A. et al., Intravenous insulin improves protein breakdown in infants on extracorporeal membrane oxygenation (abstract), *J. Am. Coll. Surg.*, 2003, in press.

14 Pharmacologic Manipulation of the Healing Wound: The Role of Hormones

Robert H. Demling

CONTENTS

ROLE OF HORMONES IN NUTRITION AND WOUND HEALING

There is a very complex interrelationship between hormones, nutrition, and wound healing. Protein synthesis, with new tissue formation known as anabolism, requires the presence of anabolic hormones. Specific actions of the various anabolic hormones will be discussed in subsequent sections.

Good nutrition is essential for maintenance of lean body mass and for wound healing and hormones play a key role in nutrient utilization.[1–4] Protein energy malnutrition (PEM) caused, for example, by the catabolic stress hormone response to injury is characterized by a decrease in lean body mass.[5–9] Lean mass loss also occurs with the decrease in endogenous anabolic hormones seen with aging, malnutrition, and chronic illness.[10–14]

As shown in Table 14.1, morbidity, including impaired healing, is directly proportional to the degree of lean mass loss from "stress" or PEM.[13,15–17] Lean mass is the metabolically active body compartment containing all the protein plus water, in the body, as compared with the fat compartment, which is mainly an energy storage depot. Lean mass includes muscle, skin, and the immune system, all of which are composed of protein.

TABLE 14.1
Complications Relative to Loss of Lean Body Mass[a]

Lean Body Mass (% Loss of Total)	Complications (Related to Lost Lean Mass)	Associated Mortality (%)
10	Impaired immunity, increased infection	10
20	Decreased healing, weakness, infection	30
30	Too weak to sit, pressure sores, pneumonia, no healing	50
40	Death, usually from pneumonia	100

[a]Assuming no preexisting loss.

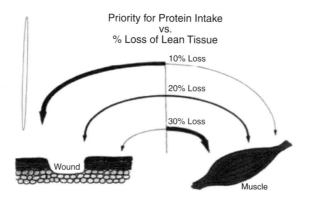

FIGURE 14.1 The wound takes priority for available nutrients as long as LBM loss does not exceed 10% of total. With increasing loss of lean body mass (LBM), more nutrients are used to restore lean mass while wound healing becomes markedly impaired until a portion of lost lean mass is restored.

Impaired Healing with Lean Mass Loss

Impaired healing is the result of the shunting of protein substrate away from the wound to be used instead for the restoration of lost lean mass. This process occurs with lean mass losses exceeding 15% of total[15–17] (Figure 14.1). This response is understandable, as the major risks for morbidity and mortality in moderate to severe protein energy malnutrition are complications caused by the loss of lean mass.[15–17]

Altered Nutrient Partitioning

There are two nutrient compartments, one for energy production and the second for protein synthesis or lean body mass. The metabolic response, to "stress" or to PEM, produces an alteration in normal nutrient partitioning. The result is the inappropriate use of protein for energy.

Normal metabolic pathways, which generate sufficient energy to meet daily demands and for new protein synthesis, are tightly regulated. The size of the lean mass compartment is genetically defined, with adaptation by environmental stimuli. Macronutrients in the form of fat and carbohydrates are channeled into production of energy, with excess being deposited as fat.[6–12]

Protein consumed is digested and absorbed as peptides and amino acids to be used for protein synthesis, restoring and maintaining the lean mass. Normally, only 5% of the protein is used for energy and 95% for protein synthesis. However, if normal anabolic activity decreases or catabolic hormone activity increases, there is an escape of protein from the protein synthesis compartment to the energy compartment.[7] This escape occurs when anabolic hormone levels are decreased, as in the elderly adult, and is the reason for the increased protein requirements in this population.[18,19] The same process occurs with activation of the stress response to injury,[7–9] where up to 25% of available protein substrate is burned for energy.[17–20] Anabolic hormone replacement can assist anabolic activity by directing protein substrate into

TABLE 14.2
Actions of Key Hormones in Metabolism

	Catechols	Cortisol	Insulin	Growth Hormone	Testosterone
Gluconeogenesis	↑	↑	↓	↑	—
Glycogen formation	↓	↓	↑	↓	—
Glycogenolysis	↑	↑	↓	↑	—
Lipogenesis	↓	↑	↑	↓	↓
Lipolysis	↑	↓	↓	↑	↑
Ketone production	↓	↓	↓	↑	—
Protein synthesis	↑	↓	↑	↑↑	↑
Proteolysis	↑	↑	↓	↓	↓

the protein synthesis pathway.[21,22] Resolution of the hypercatabolic state and restoration of anabolic hormone activity is needed to help restore and maintain activity of the protein synthesis pathway, which is necessary for wound healing.

HORMONAL RESPONSE TO WOUNDING

As shown in Table 14.2, there are a number of key hormones involved with energy production, catabolism, and anabolism, all directly or indirectly affecting wound healing.[6–9]

The stress response to injury activated by any significant body insult, especially a large wound, leads to a maladaptive hormone response, producing an increase in the catabolic hormones cortisol and epinephrine. A decrease in anabolic hormones, growth hormones, and testosterone, also occurs (Table 14.3).[6–9]

The altered hormonal environment can lead to both a significant increase in catabolism, or tissue breakdown, and a decrease in the overall anabolic activity

TABLE 14.3
Hormonal Response to Stress and Starvation

	Starvation	Stress
Catechols	↓	↑↑
Cortisol	↓	↑↑
Insulin	↓	↑
Glucagon	↓	↑
Growth hormone	↑↑	↓
Testosterone	↓	↓

Note: With starvation, an adaptive hormonal response is present, preserving lean mass and energy, while a maladaptive catabolic state occurs with the "stress response" activated by any wound.[12,31]

required to preserve lean mass and maintain the process of wound healing. Increasing anabolic activity using hormones can increase protein synthesis.[27–30]

In addition, the anabolic hormones, human growth hormone and the anabolic steroids, have been shown to have anticortisol activity. This effect decreases the catabolic response of cortisol but does not alter the protective anti-inflammatory response.

THE RATIONALE FOR HORMONAL MODIFICATION

It is now well recognized that the hormonal environment, so critical to wound healing, can be beneficially modified.[21–30] The specific aspects of each anabolic hormone will be described in depth in subsequent sections.

In general, restoration or improvement in net protein synthesis and, therefore, in wound healing, is the result of two processes. The first is an attenuation of the catabolic hormonal response, and the second is an increase in overall anabolic activity.

Attenuation of Catabolism

Any hormonal manipulation that decreases the rate of catabolism would appear to be beneficial for wound healing. The careful use of β-blockers to attenuate the stress-induced hyperadrenergic state has been shown to significantly decrease net catabolism in clinical studies on burn and trauma patients.[43–44] Blocking the cortisol response would seem to be intuitively beneficial, and as stated, growth hormone and testosterone analogs decrease the catabolic response to cortisol.[33–37]

However, any attempt to block the anti-inflammatory effects of cortisol will result in an increase in the acute destructive inflammatory response, further increasing morbidity.

Accentuation of Anabolic Activity

A number of clinical studies have demonstrated the ability of exogenous delivery of anabolic hormones to increase net nitrogen retention and overall protein synthesis.[35–42] Wound healing has been reported to be improved. However, it remains unclear as to how much of this response is the result of an overall systemic anabolic effect, or whether there is a direct effect on wound healing. Listed in Table 14.4 are the anabolic hormones for which there are available data (animal and clinical).

TABLE 14.4
Anabolic Hormone Studies

	Increased Anabolism	Direct Wound Effect
Insulin	Yes	Unclear
HGH	Yes	Unclear
IGF-1	Yes	Yes
Testosterone	Yes	No
Anabolic steroids	Yes	Yes

Note: HGH: human growth hormone; IGF-1: Insulin-like growth factor.

In summary, hormones in protein synthesis and new tissue growth are necessary for wound healing. In subsequent sections, individual anabolic hormones will be discussed, including human growth hormone, insulin-like growth factor, insulin, testosterone, and testosterone analogs, also known as anabolic steroids.

HUMAN GROWTH HORMONE (HGH)

ACTIONS

Human growth hormone (HGH) is a potent endogenous anabolic hormone produced by the pituitary gland in daily doses of 0.5 to 0.8 mg in children and young adults. Growth hormone is a large polypeptide, 191 amino acids long, that contains two receptor binding sites. There are a number of growth factor binding proteins (GHBP), and growth factor binding sites are found on a large variety of tissues, especially liver. Production decreases rapidly with increasing age. HGH levels are at their highest during the growth spurt. Starvation and intense exercise are two other potent stimuli, while acute or chronic injury or illness suppress HGH release, especially in the elderly.[45–48] The amino acids glutamine and arginine, when given in large doses, were also shown to increase HGH release.

HGH has a number of metabolic effects.[45–51] The most prominent is its anabolic effect. HGH increases the influx and decreases the efflux of amino acids into the cell. Cell proliferation is accentuated, as is overall protein synthesis and new tissue growth. HGH also stimulates insulin-like growth factor-1 (IGF1) production by the liver, and some of the anabolism seen with HGH is that produced by IGF-1, another anabolic agent. Other effects, listed in Table 14.5 and Table 14.6, include its effects on glucose and fat metabolism.

The effect on increasing fat metabolism is beneficial in that fat is preferentially used for energy production, and amino acids are preserved for use in protein synthesis (protein partitioning). Recent data indicate that insulin provides some of the anabolic effect of HGH therapy. At present, the issue as to the specific anabolic effects attributed to HGH versus that of IGF-1 and insulin remains unresolved.

TABLE 14.5
Anabolic Effects of Human Growth Hormone

Increases cell uptake of amino acids
Accelerates nucleic acid translation and transcription
Increases nitrogen retention
Increases protein synthesis
Decreases cortisol receptor activity
Increases releases of IGF-1
Increases insulin requirements

TABLE 14.6
Other Metabolic Effects of Human Growth Hormone

Increases hydrolysis of fat to fatty acids
Increases fat oxidation for fuel, decreasing fat stores
Increases metabolic rate (10 to 15%)
Produces insulin resistance, often leading to hyperglycemia
Causes some initial fluid retention

RESULTS OF EXOGENOUS HGH USE

Clinical studies have in large part focused on the systemic anabolic and anticatabolic actions of HGH.[52–54] Populations in which HGH has been shown to be beneficial include severe burn and trauma, HIV infection with wasting, and frail elderly adults (Table 14.7). In addition, HGH is being used to decrease the aging process. Increases in lean mass, muscle strength, and immune function have been documented in clinical use. HGH is approved only for use in children of short stature and is an orphan drug when used for improving protein synthesis. Increased anabolic activity requires implementation of a high-protein, high-energy diet.

WOUND HEALING EFFECT

As to its direct wound healing effects, skin is a target tissue for HGH, both directly through HGH receptors on the surface of epidermal cells and indirectly through the action of insulin-like growth factor IGF-1.[52–53] Exogenously administered HGH has been shown to increase skin thickness in normal humans.[46] Other effects on the wound include increased rate of re-epithelialization of skin graft donor sites in adults and children with severe burns or trauma[55–57] (Table 14.8). In addition, HGH has been shown to increase wound collagen content, granulation tissue and wound tensile strength, and the local production of IGF-1 by fibroblasts. These data are derived mainly from animal studies.[55–57]

TABLE 14.7
Clinical Uses of Human Growth Hormone

In the presence of severe catabolism from injury or illness
For malnourished patients with a superimposed catabolic illness
With an acute loss of > 15% lean body mass (muscle)
For treating large wounds (burns) or wounds with poor healing
For use in immunodeficiency states (AIDS), especially with weight loss
To decrease the rate of aging

TABLE 14.8
Wound Healing Effects of Human Growth Hormone

Increases re-epithelialization rate of donor sites
Increases wound collagen content
Increases granulation tissue
Increases wound tensile strength

COMPLICATIONS

Significant complications can occur with the use of HGH. The anti-insulin effects are problematic in that glucose is less efficiently used for fuel, and increased plasma glucose levels are known to be deleterious.

Increased insulin requirements occur. Complications are listed in Table 14.9.[58,59] It is important to also point out the findings of a multicenter European study of critically ill patients receiving HGH. In this study of critically ill postoperative cardiac patients, mortality was twofold greater in those treated with HGH compared to placebo.[58]

SUMMARY

In summary, use of HGH in conjunction with adequate nutrition and protein intake clearly results in increased anabolic activity and will positively impact wound healing by increasing protein synthesis in catabolic populations. There are some data that indicate that HGH can directly improve wound healing. However, the impact of IGF-1 and insulin on the effects of HGH remains undefined.

INSULIN-LIKE GROWTH FACTOR (IGF-1)

ACTIONS

Insulin-like growth factor-1 (IGF-1) is a large polypeptide that has hormone-like properties.[60–64] The IGF-1, also known as somatomedin-C, has metabolic and anabolic properties similar to insulin.

Although produced by a variety of wound cells, such as fibroblasts and platelets, the main source is the liver, where IGF synthesis is initiated by HGH. The IGF

TABLE 14.9
Potential Complications of Human Growth Hormone Therapy

Insulin resistance (hyperglycemia)
Fluid retention (usually self-limiting)
Hypercalcemia (uncommon with short-term use)
Modest increase in metabolic rate (10%)
Must be given parenterally

TABLE 14.10

Production by many cells, especially the liver
Production dependent on HGH
Production requires the presence of androgens
Actions much like insulin
Can produce hypoglycemia
Increases protein synthesis and anabolic activity
Levels decrease with severe trauma, infection
Attenuates stress-induced hypermetabolism

receptor is expressed in many different tissues, and the active peptide is bound in plasma by IGF binding proteins. IGF increases systemic nitrogen retention and protein synthesis. However, its anabolic activity is difficult to distinguish from that of HGH, as HGH needs to be present in order for IGF-1 to be produced and to have anabolic actions (Table 14.10). The combination of HGH and IGF-1 delivery results in a synergistic anabolic effect.[66]

The wound effects of HGH are also considered to be due in part to IGF-1.[66] IGF-1 production is also dependent on sufficient levels of circulating androgens.[62] Therefore, a close interrelationship exists between all of the anabolic hormones. IGF-1 levels are decreased with aging and also with a major bodily insult, such as trauma or sepsis, as are the other anabolic hormones. The decrease in IGF-1 levels increases the net nitrogen losses caused by wounding.

RESULTS OF EXOGENOUS IGF-1 USE

Properties of IGF-1 are summarized in Table 14.11. Metabolic properties include increased protein synthesis, a decrease in blood glucose, and an attenuation of stress-induced hypermetabolism, the latter two properties being quite different from HGH.[67–69] The attenuation of stress-induced hypermetabolism is a favorable property of IGF-1. The major complication is hypoglycemia. Clinical trials using an IGF-1 infusion have focused on demonstrating increased anabolic activity.[74–76] Increased protein synthesis and nitrogen retention has been reported in burns, head injury, and HIV-induced catabolic states.[74,75]

TABLE 14.11
Wound Healing and Insulin Growth Factor-1[a]

General wound healing stimulant
Increases cell replication
Increases epithelialization rate
Increases angiogenesis rate
Reverses both diabetes- and corticosteroid-induced impaired healing

[a]Animal studies.

WOUND HEALING EFFECT

The wound healing effects are described in Table 14.11.[74–78] IGF-1 is considered to be a wound healing stimulant, increasing cell proliferation and collagen synthesis. In addition, IGF-1 infusion has been shown to reverse the diabetes- and corticosteroid-induced impairment in wound healing. It is important to point out that these properties have largely been reported in animal studies. No direct effect on wound healing has been shown in man. However, increasing overall anabolism should benefit a wound.

COMPLICATIONS

The main complication is that of hypoglycemia. This agent, in general, appears to have fewer side effects than HGH.

INSULIN

ACTIONS

The hormone insulin is known to have anabolic activities in addition to its effect on glucose and fat metabolism.[79] In a catabolic state, exogenous insulin administration has been shown to decrease proteolysis in addition to increasing protein synthesis.[80–83] The anabolic activity appears to mainly affect the muscle and skin protein in the lean body mass compartment (Table 14.12). An increase in circulating amino acids produced by wound amino acid intake increases the anabolic and anticatabolic effect in both normal adults and populations in a catabolic state.[80–83]

RESULTS OF EXOGENOUS USE

A number of clinical trials, mainly in burn patients (Table 14.13) have demonstrated the stimulation of protein synthesis, decreased protein degradation, and a net nitrogen uptake, especially in skeletal muscle.[84–92] An increase in anabolic activity is also evident in diabetics who are provided more insulin. The positive insulin effect on protein synthesis decreases with aging.[89] This response is different from that found with the use of HGH and anabolic steroids, where age does not appear to blunt the anabolic response.

TABLE 14.12
Anabolic and Wound Healing Effects of Insulin

Increases cell amino acid influx
Decreases amino acid reflux
Increases muscle protein synthesis and decreases degradation
Increases skin wound protein content
Anabolic effect decreases with age
Increases rate of re-epithelialization and collagen synthesis in donor sites

---

TABLE 14.13
Clinical Studies on Insulin

Stimulates muscle protein synthesis in catabolic burn patients
Stimulates muscle protein synthesis in healthy humans
Decreases protein breakdown in catabolic patients
Increases re-epithelialization rate of donor sites in burn patients

---

WOUND HEALING EFFECT

Less data exist on the actions of insulin on wound healing over and above its systemic anabolic effect.[93–96] Increases in skin protein content have been demonstrated with a chronic insulin infusion. Increased re-epithelialization of skin graft donor sites was reported in one clinical trial in burn patients. Several animal studies have demonstrated increased collagen production with insulin and increasing the insulin administration to diabetic mice improved all phases of healing.[98] However, the effects of insulin on wound healing have not been well studied in man (Table 14.12).

COMPLICATIONS

The main complication is hypoglycemia. There does not appear to be any fluid retention or hypermetabolism with its use.

SUMMARY

In summary, hyperinsulinemia in catabolic patients and in normal adults increases net protein synthesis and decreases protein breakdown. An infusion of glucose is required to avoid hypoglycemia. In turn, inadequate insulin intake in diabetics leads to progressive lean mass loss, and hyperglycemia appears to accentuate the nitrogen loss. Although some positive data are present on insulin improving healing, data are limited.

TESTOSTERONE

ACTIONS

Testosterone, with a basic structure as a steroid ring, is the natural endogenous androgen.[97–99] Testosterone is synthesized primarily in the Leydig cells of the testes in males and by the ovaries and adrenal glands in females. Healthy adult men produce 3 to 10 mg/d, yielding plasma concentrations ranging from 300 to 1000 µg/dl.[93–95] Testosterone acts on the cell androgenic receptors found mainly in skin, muscle, and male sex glands. It has both androgenic or masculinizing properties and anabolic properties. Androgenic effects are present to some degree in all anabolic steroids. Androgenic affects include development of male sex glands, male hair growth pattern, increased libido, and assertiveness (Table 14.14). Most testosterone analogs or anabolic steroids have androgenic properties much lower than testosterone

TABLE 14.14
Testosterone Characteristics

Endogenous anabolic hormone
Produced mainly by the testes in males and the adrenal gland in females
Acts on androgenic receptors found mainly in muscle, skin, and sex glands
Has modest anabolic activity compared to its analogs
Androgenic activity includes male sex gland development, male pattern of hair, mood
Rapidly metabolized by the liver
Levels decrease with increasing age
Levels decrease with injury/infection
Decreased testosterone causes lean mass loss in healthy and injured man

itself.[97–99] The anabolic properties were defined in the 1930s. These included an increase in muscle size, synthesis, and strength. Increased skin thickness has also been noted with administration to hypogonadal men. The importance of testosterone is evidenced by the complications seen with low testosterone levels, which include sarcopenia or lost lean mass, increased rate of development of osteoporosis, anemia, thinning of skin, and weakness and impaired wound healing[98–100] (Table 14.15 and Table 14.16).

The native molecule was first used in the 1950s to correct a debilitated state, correct anemia, and increase calcium deposition in bone as well as to treat hypogonadal states.[93–96] The testosterone molecule is rapidly metabolized by the liver such that the half-life is only about 20 min. Adjustments were made to the molecule to increase its time of action, the most popular being testosterone enthanate.

Decreased production, leading to a hypogonadal state, occurs with increasing age as well as with injury or infection, especially severe trauma and chronic illness such as HIV infection and chronic wounds.

As seen in Table 14.16, a hypogonadal state is seen in many patient populations, including an acute severe injury state, infection, or more chronic states such as aging, chronic obstructive pulmonary disease (COPD), and other chronic illnesses.[96–99]

TABLE 14.15
Effect of Decreased Testosterone (The Hypogonadal State)

Lean mass loss
Thinning of skin
Increasing fat mass
Impaired wound healing
Decrease in physical and psychological masculinizing properties
Osteoporosis

TABLE 14.16
Populations at Risk for a Hypogonadal State

Elderly
Those with chronic illness
Those with chronic obstructive pulmonary disease
Those with autoimmune diseases
Those undergoing high-dose corticosteroid therapy
Those with severe acute injury or infection or who are critically ill

RESULTS OF EXOGENOUS USE

Testosterone administration is used mainly to correct a hypogonadal state, because testosterone analogs have much greater anabolic activity[100–104] (Table 14.16). Clinical studies have demonstrated a significant increase in net protein synthesis, especially in muscle and skin, with use of high doses of testosterone delivered parenterally.[105,106]

WOUND HEALING EFFECT

It is clear that testosterone is needed for the wound healing process, because decreased levels impede healing.[107–110] Adequate testosterone levels are required for IGF-1 production (IGF-1 being a wound healing agent). However, there are no reliable data that confirm that an increase in testosterone levels above normal improves wound healing. This is not the case with a number of anabolic steroids that have been shown to increase the rate of wound healing even in the absence of hypogonadism. These agents will be discussed next.

COMPLICATIONS

The major complications are the androgenic side effects. Some fluid retention has been reported with high doses. A decrease in high-density lipoproteins has also been reported with the use of large doses.

TABLE 14.17
Clinical Effects of Testosterone Administration

Correction of the androgenic/anabolic deficiency of a hypogonadal state
Increased anabolism and muscle synthesis in the elderly
Increased lean mass synthesis in healthy humans
Decreases bone loss
Androgenic side effects

SUMMARY

Testosterone is a necessary androgen for maintaining lean mass and wound healing. A deficiency leads to catabolism and impaired healing. The use of large doses exogenously has increased net protein synthesis, but a direct effect on wound healing has not yet been demonstrated.

ANABOLIC STEROIDS

ACTIONS

Anabolic steroids refer to the class of drugs produced by modification of testosterone.[22,24,108-110] These drugs were developed in order to take clinical advantage of the anabolic effects of testosterone while decreasing androgenic side effects of the naturally occurring molecule. Modifications in the steroid ring were made because of the short half-life of testosterone and its masculinizing properties. Modifications included a 17-α-methyl derivative for oral use and a 17-β-ester configuration for parenteral use. These changes markedly increased half-life and decreased androgenic properties (Table 14.18).

The mechanisms of action of testosterone analogs are also through activation of the androgenic receptors found in highest concentration in myocytes and skin fibroblasts. Some populations of epithelial cells also contain these receptors. Androgenic receptors were first isolated in the 1960s.[93-95,108-110]

Stimulation leads to a decrease in efflux of amino acids and an increase in influx into the cell. Activation of intracellular DNA and DNA polymerase also occurs with androgenic receptor stimulation. A decrease in fat mass is also seen due to the preferential use of fat for fuel. There are no metabolic effects on glucose production.

All anabolic steroids increase overall protein synthesis and new tissue formation, as evidenced by an increase in skin thickness and muscle formation.[110-114] All these agents also have anticatabolic activity, decreasing the protein degradation caused by cortisol and other catabolic stimuli.[114] In addition, all anabolic steroids have androgenic or masculinizing effects.

TABLE 14.18
Anabolic Steroids (History)

All are testosterone derivatives

Anabolic properties noted in the 1940s

Androgen receptors found in cytosol (1960s)

Attempt to increase anabolism (use of anabolic to androgenic ratio to judge new drugs; 1960 to present)

Derivatives

Oral are 17-α-methyl

Parenteral are 17-β-esters

Most cleared by the liver (concern for hepatotoxicity)

TABLE 14.19
Anabolic Activity of 17 Methyl Derivatives

Agent	Androgenic: Anabolic Activity	Indications	Hepatotoxicity
Testosterone	1:1	Hypogonadism	
Nandrolone	1:4	Anemia	Moderate to severe
Oxymetholone	1:3	Anemia	Severe
Oxandrolone[a]	1:3 to 1.13	Loss of body weight from injury or infection	Mild, rare

[a]The anabolic steroid oxandrolone is the only approved drug for restoration of lost body weight and lost lean mass.

The quality of a testosterone analog is determined by the ratio of androgenic to anabolic activity — the lower the better. A low value indicates very little masculinizing effects compared to a very potent anabolic effect (Table 14.19).

The anabolic steroid oxandrolone also happens to have the greatest anabolic and least androgenic side effects in the class of anabolic steroids.[112] Oxandrolone is the only steroid that has a carbon atom within the phenanthrene nucleus that has been replaced by another element, namely, oxygen. In addition, oxandrolone is cleared by the kidney and not the liver, so hepatotoxicity is rare.

CLINICAL USE OF ANABOLIC STEROIDS (EFFECT ON LEAN BODY MASS)

Most of the recent studies on anabolic steroids and lean body mass have used the anabolic steroid oxandrolone (Table 14.20).[112–121]

Oxandrolone is a 17-β-hydroxy-17-α-methyl ester of testosterone that is cleared primarily by the kidney. Hepatotoxicity is minimal, even at doses higher than the 20 mg/d recommended by the U.S. Food and Drug Administration (FDA). Oxandrolone has potent anabolic activity, being up to 13 times that of methyltestosterone. In addition, its androgenic effect is considerably less than testosterone, minimizing this complication common to other testosterone derivatives. The increased anabolic activity and decreased androgenic (masculinizing) activity markedly increase its

TABLE 14.20
Oxandrolone

Oral 17-α analog
Metabolized mainly by kidney
Not hepatotoxic
Readily absorbed by intestine with 99% bioavailability
Biologic life of 9 to 12 h
Highly anabolic
Minimal androgenic effects

TABLE 14.21
Clinical Effect of Anabolic Steroids

Attenuate the catabolic stimulus during the "stress response"
More rapid restoration of lost lean mass
Restore normal nutrient partitioning
Improved healing of chronic wounds with restoration of lost lean mass

clinical value. Oxandrolone is given orally, with 99% bioavailability. It is protein bound in plasma with a biologic life of 9 h.

The anabolic steroids, especially oxandrolone, have been successfully used in the trauma and burn patient population to both decrease lean mass loss in the acute phase of injury as well as more rapidly restore lost lean mass in the recovery phase.[37–41,117–121] A significant attenuation of catabolism and increase in lean mass, has also been reported with HIV infection, in the COPD population, and spinal cord injury population.[117–121] Demonstrated in several studies is an increase in the healing of chronic wounds. However, significant lean mass gains were also present.

It is important to point out that in all of the clinical trials where lean mass gains were reported, a high-protein diet was used. In most studies, a protein intake of 1.2 to 1.5 g/kg/d was used, 0.8 g/kg/day.

WOUND HEALING PROPERTIES

The effects of anabolic steroids on wound healing appear to be, in large part, due to a general stimulation of overall anabolic activity. However, there is increasing evidence of a direct stimulation of all phases of wound healing by these agents[122–128] (Table 14.22 and Table 14.23).

Falanga et al.[124] reported a stimulation of collagen synthesis with the anabolic steroid stanazol. Erlich et al.[125] reported a tenfold increase in the messenger RNA for collagen synthesis, in a human fibroblast culture with oxandrolone. Tenenbaum et al.[126] reported increased synthesis of bone, collagen, matrix, and epidermis in a wound of the oral cavity stimulated with oxandrolone. Demling[116] reported a marked increase in the healing of a cutaneous wound in the rat treated with oxandrolone compared to controls. A 50% increase in wound collagen was noted as well as a doubling of tensile strength at 3 weeks with oxandrolone. Histology also revealed

TABLE 14.22
Wound Healing Effects (*In Vitro* Human Fibroblasts)

Stimulation in messenger RNA for collagen synthesis
Stimulate collagen synthesis
Increases release of transforming growth factor-β (TGFβ)
Downregulation of expression of matrix metalloproteinase expression

---

TABLE 14.23
Wound Healing Effects (Animal Studies)

Increase in wound closure (contraction)
Increase in collagen deposition
Increased re-epithelialization
Increased angiogenesis
Increased wound tensile strength

TABLE 14.24
Treatment of Patient with Significant IWL, Protein Energy Malnutrition, or in a Catabolic State

Initiate optimum daily nutrition
35 calories/kg body weight
1.5 g protein/kg body weight
High potency multivitamin, multi-mineral per day
Vitamin C, 1 g
Water/1 ml per calorie

Initiate Oral Oxandrolone Therapy

10 mg/b.i.d.
Once nutrition is adequate
After prostate cancer has been ruled out with prostate-specific antigen (PSA)
After obtaining a normal PSA in patients over 50 yr of age
Until body weight is restored and catabolic state resolved

Monitor Liver Function Tests

Decrease or temporarily stop oxandrolone if AST or ALT increases by more than three times normal value

Monitor Prothrombin Time

If patient on coumadin
In order to adjust coumadin dose downward if necessary

Provide Insulin Only in Acute Care Setting

If hyperglycemia is present due to the increased caloric intake
Instead of decreasing calories

Provide Human Growth Hormone

Only if patient cannot take pills (oxandrolone)
In a dose of 5 to 10 mg sub q per day
Only if glucose levels can be carefully monitored

Provide Testosterone

If patient also has evidence of a hypogonadal state
Using testosterone enthanate 200 to 400 mg/IM every 2 weeks
Or using testosterone undercanoate 80 mg p.o./twice a day
After checking for prostate cancer

more densely packed collagen with more fibroblasts and mononuclear cells. Anabolic steroids have also been shown to release the growth factor TGF-β by human fibroblasts.[127] The mechanism of improved wound healing with the use of anabolic steroids is not yet defined. Stimulation of androgenic receptors on wound fibroblasts may well lead to a local release of growth factors.

SIDE EFFECTS

In addition to androgenic activity, a number of potential side effects exist for this drug class. Some fluid retention will occur initially but is usually transient.[109,112,113] Liver toxicity has been reported, ranging from a transient increase in aminotransferases to jaundice, liver failure, and, rarely, liver tumor.[128] The potential for liver change varies among anabolic steroids.[112] Oxandrolone appears to be the safest. A recent 1 year study in elderly men given oxandrolone demonstrated only transient increases in aminotransferases.

A change in the lipid profile has been reported.[129] Several studies have demonstrated a decrease in high-density lipoproteins, potentially increasing the risk of atherosclerosis. The lipid response differs among the drugs in this class.[130]

Anabolic steroids have been reported to increase the potency of coumadin, and coumadin dose often has to be decreased. Finally, this drug class is contraindicated in patients with prostate cancer, as this tumor is stimulated by androgenic receptors.[112,113]

CONCLUSION

Anabolic steroids are analogs of testosterone modified to increase anabolic and decrease androgenic side effects. All of these agents have been shown to increase lean body mass. In addition, there appears to be a direct wound healing effect. Side effects include liver dysfunction. Oxandrolone appears to be the most anabolic and safest anabolic steroid.

RECOMMENDATIONS FOR PHARMACOLOGIC MANIPULATION

Anabolic hormones are necessary to maintain the necessary protein synthesis required for maintaining lean body mass, including wound healing, assuming the presence of adequate protein intake. However, endogenous levels of these hormones are decreased in acute and chronic illness and with increasing age, especially in the presence of a large wound.

The corroborating data, for the use of anabolic hormones, are excellent for more rapidly restoring protein synthesis and lean mass with lean mass loss. A high-calorie, high-protein diet is required.

Because lost lean mass caused by the stress response, aging, and malnutrition, retards wound healing, the ideal use of these agents is to more effectively restore anabolic activity. All these agents can cause complications specific to the hormone used, which needs to be considered.

There are also data that indicate a direct wound healing stimulating effect for some of these hormones. However, more clinical data need to be obtained before a recommendation can be made to use anabolic hormones to increase the rate of wound healing in the absence of a catabolic state or an existing lean mass loss. Oxandrolone is the agent of choice unless contraindicated with the presence of prostate cancer.

FUTURE DIRECTIONS

Three areas of research and development are indicated at this point. The first area is to better define the effect of all of these anabolic hormones on the various stages of wound healing. This information is needed in order to determine the indications for the use of the available anabolic hormones. It is possible that combination therapy would be more beneficial if it is determined that these agents have different modes of action.

The second area is the development of analogs of the anabolic hormones, which appear to have the most beneficial wound healing effects. The analogs would be developed to maximize wound healing activity and minimize complications.

The third area would be the development of a topical form of the anabolic hormones that demonstrate the most beneficial wound healing effects. The topical form would provide a direct wound healing benefit without the potential complications of systemic use.

REFERENCES

1. Young, M., Malnutrition and wound healing, *Heart and Lung*, 17, 65–66, 1988.
2. Thomas, D., Role of nutrition in prevention and healing of pressure ulcers, *Clin. Geriatric Med.*, 13, 497–510, 1997.
3. Gilmore, S. and Rolumson, G., Clinical indications associated with unintentional weight loss and pressure ulcers in elderly residents of nursing facilities, *J. Am. Diet. Assoc.*, 95, 984–992, 1995.
4. Bergstrom, N., Lack of nutrition; in AHCPR preventive guidelines, *Decubitus*, 6, 4–6, 1993.
5. Bessey, Post traumatic skeletal muscle proteolysis; the role of the hormonal environment, *World J. Surg.*, 13, 465–470, 1989.
6. Wolfe, R., Relation of metabolic studies to clinical nutrition; the example of burn injury, *Am. J. Clin. Nutr.*, 64, 800–808, 1996.
7. Wolfe, R., An integrated analysis of glucose, fat and protein metabolism in severely traumatized patients, *Ann. Surg.*, 209, 63–72, 1989.
8. Streat, S. et al., Aggressive nutritional support does not prevent protein loss despite fat gain in septic intensive care patients, *J. Trauma*, 27, 262–266, 1987.
9. Wernerman, J., Brandt, R., and Strandell, T., The effect of stress hormones on the interorgan flux of amino acids and concentration of free amino acids in skeletal muscle, *Clin. Nutr.*, 4, 207–216, 1985.
10. Wallace, J., Schwartz, R. et al., Involuntary weight loss in older outpatients: incidences and clinical significance, *J. Am. Geriatric Soc.*, 43, 329–337, 1995.

11. Wallace, J.L., Involuntary weight loss in elderly outpatients: recognition, etiologies and treatment, *Clinics in Geriatr. Med.*, 13, 717–735, 1997.

12. Torun, B. and Cherv, F., Protein-energy malnutrition, in *Modern Nutrition in Health and Disease*, Shels. M., Ed., Lea & Felugan, Philadelphia, 1994, p. 950.

13. Roubenoff, R. and Kehajias, J., The meaning and measurement of lean body mass, *Nutr. Rev.*, 49, 163–175, 1991.

14. Moran, L., Custer, P., and Murphy, G., Nutritional assessment of lean body mass, *J. Pen.*, 4, 595, 1980.

15. Kotler, D., Magnitude of cell body mass depletion and timing of death from wasting in AIDS, *Am. J. Clin. Nutr.*, 50, 444–447, 1984.

16. Kimball, M.J. and Williams-Burgess, C., Failure to thrive: the silent epidemic of the elderly, *Arch. Psych. Nurs.*, 9, 99–105, 1995.

17. Woof, P., Hamill, R., and McDonald, J., Transient hypogonadism caused by critical illness, *J. Clin. Endocrinol. Metab.*, 60, 494–500, 1985.

18. Fiatarone, M., Lipsitz, L., and Evans, W., Exercise training and nutritional supplementation for physical frailty in very elderly people, *N. Engl. J. Med.*, 330, 1769–1775, 1994.

19. Heymsfield, S. and Wang, Z., Human body composition: advances in models and methods, *Ann. Rev. Nutr.*, 17, 527–558, 1997.

20. Jeveendra, M., Ramos, J., Shamos, R., and Shiller, R., Decreased growth hormone levels in the catabolic phase of severe injury, *Surgery*, 111, 495–502, 1992.

21. Ziegler, T. and Wilmore, D., Strategies for attenuating protein-catabolic responses in the critically ill, *Am. Rev. Med.*, 45, 459, 1994.

22. Forbes, G., The effect of anabolic steroids on lean body mass: the dose response curve, *Metabolism*, 34, 571–573, 1985.

23. Wray, C., Mammen, J., and Hasselgren, P., Catabolic response to stress and potential benefits of nutrition support, *Nutrition*, 18, 97, 2002.

24. Hasselgren, P. and Fischer, J., Muscle cachexia: current concepts of intracellular mechanisms and molecular regulation, *Am. Surg.*, 233, 9–17, 2001.

25. Hasselgren, P. and Fischer, J., Sepsis: stimulation of energy dependent protein breakdown resulting in protein loss in skeletal muscle, *World J. Surg.*, 22, 203–208, 1998.

26. Biols, G., Toigo, G., Ciocechi, B. et al., Metabolic response to injury and sepsis: changes in protein metabolism, *Nutrition*, 13, 52–57, 1997.

27. Krasner, D. and Belcher, Oxandroloen restores appetite. An increase in weight helps heal wounds, *Am. J. Nurs.*, 100, 53–57, 2000.

28. Demling, R. and Orgill, D., The anticatabolic and wound healing effects of the testosterone analog, oxandrolone, after severe burn injury, *J. Crit. Care Med.*, 15, 12–18.

29. Saito, H., Anabolic agents in trauma and sepsis reflecting body mass and function, *Nutrition*, 17, 554–556, 1998.

30. Fernando, A., Scheffield-Moore, M., Paddon-Jones, D. et al., Differential anabolic effects of testosterone and amino acid feeding in older men, *J. Clin. Endocrinol. Metab.*, 88, 358–362, 2003.

31. Cahill, G., Starvation in men, *N. Engl. J. Med.*, 282, 668–675, 1970.

32. Rico, R., Repamonti, R., Burns, A. et al., The effect of sepsis on wound healing, *J. Surg. Res.*, 102, 193–197, 2002.

33. Wolf, S., Nicolai, M., and Dazemis, G., Growth hormone treatment in catabolic states other than burns, *Growth Hormone IFG Res.*, 8, 117–119, 1998.

34. Woerman, H., Strack, R., de Boer, H. et al., Growth hormone secretion and administration in catabolic patients with emphasis on the critically ill patient, *Neth. J. Med.*, 41, 222–244, 1992.

35. Fleming, R., Rutan, R., Jahoor, F. et al., Effect of recombinant human growth hormone in catabolic hormones and free fatty acids following thermal injury, *J. Trauma*, 698, 703–707, 1992.
36. Hadley, J. and Hinds, C., Anabolic strategies in critical illness, *Curr. Open Pharmacol.*, 2, 700–707, 2002.
37. Demling, R. and DeSanti, L., The anabolic steroid oxandrolone reverses the wound healing impairment in corticosteroid dependent burn and wound patients, *Wounds*, 13, 203–208, 2001.
38. Demling, R. and DeSanti, L., The beneficial effects of the anabolic steroid oxandrolone in the geriatric burn population, *Wounds*, 15, 54–60, 2003.
39. Earthman, C., Reid, P., Harper, I. et al., Body cell mass repletion and improved quality of life in HIV infected individuals receiving oxandrolone, *JPEN*, 26, 357–365, 2002.
40. Hart, D., Wolf, S., Ramzy, P. et al., Anabolic effects of oxandrolone after severe burn, *Ann. Surg.*, 233, 556–564, 2001.
41. Nandi, J., Meguid, M., Inise, A. et al., Critical mechanisms involved with catabolism, *Curr. Open Clin. Nutr. Metab. Care*, 5, 407–408, 2002.
42. Kaiser, F., Silver, H., and Morley, The effect of recombinant human growth hormone on malnourished older individuals, *Am. Geriatric Soc.*, 39, 235–240, 1991.
43. Chrolero, R., Breitenstein, E., Thorin, D. et al., Effect of propranolol on resting metabolic rate after severe head injury, *Crit. Care Med.*, 17, 328–334, 1989.
44. Breitenstein, E., Chrolero, R., Jequier, E. et al., Effect of -blockade on energy metabolism following burns, *Burns*, 16, 259–264, 1990.
45. Hansen, T., Pharmacokinetics and acute lipolytic actions of growth hormone. Impact of age, body compensation, binding proteins and other hormones, *Growth Horm. IGF Res.*, 12, 372–378, 2002.
46. Vahl, N., Moller, N., Lauretzen, T. et al., Metabolic effects and pharmacokinetics of a growth hormone pulse in healthy adults: relation to age, sex and body composition, *J. Clin. Endocrinol. Metab.*, 82, 3612–3618, 1997.
47. Hansen, T., Granholt, C., Orskow, H. et al., Dose dependency of the pharmacokinetics and acute lipolytic actions of growth hormone, *J. Clin. Endocrinol. Metab.*, 87, 4691–4698, 2002.
48. Jackson, N., Carroll, P., Russell-Jones, D. et al., Effect of glutamine supplementation, GH and IGF-1 on glutamine metabolism in critically ill patients, *Am. J. Physiol. Endocrinol. Metab.*, 278, 226–233, 2002.
49. Suminski, R., Robertson, R., Goss, F. et al., Acute effect of amino acid ingestion and resistance exercise on plasma growth hormone concentration in young men, *Int. J. Sport Nutr.*, 7, 48–60, 1997.
50. Climmons, D. and Underwood, L., Role of insulin like growth factors and growth hormone in reversing catabolic states, *Horm. Res.*, 38, 37–40, 1992.
51. Bondanelli, M., Ambrosia, M., Margutti, A. et al., Evidence for integrity of the growth hormone/insulin like growth factor-1 axis in patients with severe head injury during recovery, *Metabolism*, 51, 1363–1369, 2002.
52. Lang, C. and Frost, R., Role of growth hormone, insulin-like growth factor-1 and insulin-like growth factor binding proteins in the catabolic response to injury and infection, *Curr. Opin. Clin. Nutr. Metab. Care*, 5, 271–279, 2002.
53. Ross, R., Bentham, J., and Coakley, J., The role of insulin, growth hormone and IGF-1 as anabolic agents in the critically ill, *Intensive Care Med.*, 19, 54–57, 1993.
54. Mulligan, K., Tai, V., and Schambelan, M., Use of growth hormone and other anabolic agents in AIDS wasting, *JPEN*, 23, 202–209, 1999.

55. Raschke, M., Kolbeck, S., and Bail, H., Homologous growth hormone accelerates healing of segmental bone defects, *Bone*, 4, 368–373, 2001.

56. Lal, S., Wolf, S., and Herndon, D., Growth hormone, burns and tissue healing, *Growth Horm. IGF Res.*, 10, 39–43, 2002.

57. Ghofrani, A., Holler, D., and Shulmann, K., The influence of systemic growth hormone administration on the healing time of skin graft donor sites in a pig model, *Plast. Reconstr. Surg.*, 104, 470–475, 1999.

58. Ruokonen, E. and Takala, J., Dangers of growth hormone therapy in critically ill patients, *Curr. Opin. Clin. Nutr. Care*, 5, 199–209, 2002.

59. Carroll, P. and Van den Berghe, C., Safety aspects of pharmacological GH therapy in adults, *Growth Horm. IGF Res.*, 11, 166–172, 2001.

60. Achmud, C., Insulin-like growth factors, *Cell Biol. Int.*, 19, 445–457, 1995.

61. Gore, D., Insulin-like growth factor-1 in hypercatabolic states, *Growth Horm. IGF Res.*, 8, 107–109, 1998.

62. Saito, N., Anabolic agents in trauma and sepsis: repleting body mass and function, *Nutrition*, 6, 554–556, 1998.

63. Boulivare, S., Tamborlane, D., Matthews, L. et al., Diverse effects of insulin-like growth factor-1 on glucose, lipid and amino acid metabolism, *Am. J. Physiol.*, 262, 130–133, 1992.

64. Dahn, M., Lange, M., and Jacobs, L., Insulin-like growth factor production is inhibited in human sepsis, *Arch. Surg.*, 123, 1409–1414, 1988.

65. Strock, L., Singh, H., Abdullah, A. et al., The effect of insulin-like growth factor on post burn hypermetabolism, *Surgery*, 108, 161–164, 1990.

66. Kupfer, S., Underwood, L., Baxter, R. et al., Enhancement of the anabolic effects of growth hormone and insulin-like growth factor-1 by use of both agents simultaneously, *J. Clin. Invest.*, 91, 391–393, 1993.

67. Guler, H., Zapf, J., and Froesch, E., Short term metabolic effects of recombinant human insulin-like growth factor-1 in healthy adults, *N. Engl. J. Med.*, 317, 137–140, 1987.

68. Wicke, C., Wagner, S., Trabold, O. et al., Age dependency of insulin-like growth factors, insulin-like growth factor binding proteins and acid labile subunit in plasma and wounds of surgical patients, *Wound Repair Regen.*, 10, 360–365, 2002.

69. Liu, Z. and Barrett, E., Human protein metabolism; its measurement and regulation, *Am. J. Physiol. Endocrinol. Metab.*, 283, 1105–1112, 2002.

70. Blumenfield, I., Saiiyi, S., and Lanir, Y., Enhancement of bone defect healing in old rats by TGF and IGF-1, *Exp. Gerontol.*, 37, 53–55, 2002.

71. Coerper, S., Wolf, S., and Thomas, S., Insulin-like growth factor accelerates gastric ulcer healings by stimulating cell proliferation and by inhibiting gastric and secretion, *Scand. J. Gastroenterol.*, 9, 921–927, 2001.

72. Betar, M., Insulin-like growth factor-1 reverscs diabetes induced wound healing impairment in rats, *Horm. Metab. Res.*, 8, 383–386, 1997.

73. Pierre, E., Perez-Polo, J., Mitchell, A. et al., Insulin-like growth factor-1 liposomal gene transfer and systemic growth hormone stimulate wound healing, *J. Burn Care Rehab.*, 4, 287–289, 1997.

74. Hatton, J., Rapp, R., Kudsk, K. et al., Intravenous insulin-like growth factor-1 in moderate to severe head injury: a phase II safety and efficacy trial, *Neurosurg. Focus*, 2, 1–17, 1997.

75. Lieberman, S., Bukar, J., and Chen, S., Effects of recombinant human insulin-like growth in cachectic patients with the acquired immunodeficiency syndrome, *J. Clin. Endocrinol. Metab.*, 78, 404–410, 1994.

76. Rooyackirs, O. and Nair, K., Hormonal regulation of human muscle protein metabolism, *Ann. Rev. Nutr.*, 17, 457–485, 1987.

77. Bhara, F., Dunkin, B., Batzri, S. et al., Effect of growth factors on cell proliferation and epithelialization in human skin, *J. Surg. Res.*, 59, 236–255, 1995.

78. Suh, D., Hunt, T., and Spencer, E., Insulin-like growth factor-1 reverses the impairment of wound healing induced by corticosteroid in rats, *Endocrinology*, 131, 2399–2403, 1992.

79. Biolo, G., Fleming, R., and Wolfe, R., Physiological hyperinsulinemia stimulates protein synthesis and enhances transport of selected amino acids in human skeletal muscle, *J. Clin. Invest.*, 95, 811–817, 1995.

80. Zhang, X., Chinkes, D., Irtun, O., and Wolfe, R., Anabolic action of insulin on skin wound protein is augmented by exogenesis amino acids, *Am. J. Physiol. Endocrinol. Metab.*, 282, 308–315, 2002.

81. Davis, T., Fiorotto, M., Burrin, D. et al., Stimulation of protein synthesis by both insulin and amino acids is unique to skeletal muscle in neonatal pigs, *Am. J. Physiol. Endocrinol. Metab.*, 282, 880–890, 2002.

82. Volpi, E., Mittendorfer, B., Rasmussen, B., and Wolfe, R., The response of muscle protein anabolism to combined hyperaminoacidemia and glucose induced hyperinsulinemia is impaired in the elderly, *J. Clin. Endocrinol. Metab.*, 85, 4481–4490, 2000.

83. Hadley, J. and Hinds, C., Anabolic strategies in critical illness, *Curr. Opin. Pharmacol.*, 2, 720–727, 2002.

84. Zhang, X., Chinkes, P., Irtien, O., and Wolfe, R., Insulin but not growth hormone stimulates protein anabolism in skin wound and muscle, *Am. J. Physiol.*, 276, 12–20, 1999.

85. Pierre, E., Barrow, R., Hawkins, H. et al., Effect of insulin on wound healing, *J. Trauma*, 44, 342–345, 1999.

86. Zhang, X., Chinkes, D., Wolf, S., and Wolfe, R., Insulin but not growth hormone stimulates protein anabolism in skin wound and muscle, *Am. J. Physiol. Endocrinol. Metab.*, 276, 712–720, 1999.

87. Phillips, T., Demircay, Z., and Sahu, M., Hormonal effects on skin aging, *Clin. Geriatr. Med.*, 17, 661–672, 2001.

88. Sakurai, Y., Aarsland, A., Herndon, D. et al., Stimulation of muscle protein synthesis by long term insulin infusion in severely burned patients, *Ann. Surg.*, 222, 283–287, 1995.

89. Zhang, X., Chinkes, P., Irtrin, O., and Wolfe, R., Anabolic action of insulin on skin wound protein is augmented by exogenous amino acids, *Am. J. Physiol. Endocrinol. Metab.*, 283, 1308–1315, 2002.

90. Ferrando, A., Chinkes, D., Wolf, S. et al., A submaximal dose of insulin promotes net skeletal muscle protein synthesis in patients with severe burns, *Ann. Surg.*, 229, 148, 1999.

91. Madibally, S., Solomon, V., Mitchell, R. et al., Influence of insulin therapy on burn wound healing in rats, *J. Surg. Res.*, 1099, 92–100, 2003.

92. Weringer, E., Kelso, J., Tamai, I., and Arquilla, E., Effects of insulin on wound healing in diabetic mice, *Acta Endocrinol.*, 99, 101–108, 1982.

93. Kuhn, C., Anabolic steroids, *Recent Prog. Horm. Res.*, 57, 411–434, 2002.

94. Christiana, J. and Frishman, W., Testosterone and other anabolic steroids as cardiovascular drugs, *Am. J. Ther.*, 6, 167–174, 1990.

95. Carson-Jurica, M. and Schrador, W., Steroid receptor family; structure and functions, *Endocrinol. Rev.*, 11, 201–220, 1990.

96. Phillips, T., Demircay, Z., and Sahu, M., Hormonal effects on skin aging, *Clin. Geriatr. Med.*, 17, 6610–6672, 2001.

97. Morley, J., Testosterone replacement in older men and women, *J. Ger. Specif. Med.*, 4, 49–53, 2001.

98. Matsumoto, A., Andropause: clinical implications of the decline in serum testosterone levels with aging in man, *J. Gerontol. Biol. Sci. Med. Sci.*, 57, 76–99, 2002.

99. Morley, J., Baumgartner, R., Roubenoff, R. et al., Sarcopenia, *J. Lab. Clin. Med.*, 127, 231–243, 2001.

100. Fernando, A., Sheffield, M., and Wolfe, R., Differential anabolic effects of testosterone and amino acid feeding in older man, *J. Clin. Endocrinol. Metab.*, 88, 358–362, 2003.

101. Janssens, H. and Vanderscheuren, D., Endocrinological aspects of aging in man; is hormone replacement of benefit? *Eur. J. Obstet. Gynecol. Reprod. Biol.*, 92, 9–12, 2000.

102. Bhasin, S., Storer, T., Berman, N. et al., The effects of supraphysiologic doses of testosterone on muscle strength and size in normal man, *N. Engl. J. Med.*, 335, 1–7, 1996.

103. Frankle, M. and Borrelli, J., The effects of testosterone proprionate and methenolane enthanate on the healing of humeral osteotomies in the Wistar rat, *J. Invest. Surg.*, 3, 93–113, 1990.

104. Ashcroft, G. and Mills, S., Androgen receptor mediated inhibitions of cutaneous wound healing, *J. Clin. Invest.*, 110, 615–624, 2002.

105. Thomas, P., Age related changes in wound healing, *Drugs Aging*, 18, 607–620, 2001.

106. Bolognia, J., Aging skin, *Am. J. Med.*, 98, 99–102, 1995.

107. Kopera, N., The history of anabolic steroids and a review of clinical experience with anabolic steroids, *Acta Endocrinol.*, 110, 11–18, 1985.

108. Hampt, N. and Raver, G., Anabolic steroids: a review of the literature, *Am. J. Sports Med.*, 12, 469–484, 1984.

109. Fox, M. and Minot, A., Oxandrolone, a potent anabolic steroid, *J. Clin. Endocrinol.*, 22, 921, 1962.

110. Sheffield, M., Wolfe, R. et al., The effect of short term oxandrolone treatment on peripheral amino acid metabolism, *J. Burn Care Rehab.*, 2, 127, 1999.

111. Lafferty, F., Spencer, G., and Pearson, O., Effect of androgens, estrogens and high calcium intakes on bone formation and resorption in osteoporosis, *Am. J. Med.*, 36, 514–528, 1969.

112. Karim, A., Ranney, E., Zagarella, B.A. et al., Oxandrolone disposition and metabolism in man, *Clin. Pharmacol. Ther.*, 14, 862–866, 1973.

113. Mendenhall, C.I., Anderson, S., Garcia-Pont, P. et al., A study of oral nutritional support with oxandrolone in malnourished patients with alcoholic hepatitis: results of a Department of Veterans Affairs Cooperative Study, *Hepatology*, 17, 564–570, 1993.

114. Hickson, R., Czerwinski, S., Falduta, M., and Young, A., Glucocorticoid antagonism by exercise and androgenic-anabolic steroids, *Med. Sci. Sports Exer.*, 22, 331–340, 1990.

115. Stanford, A., Barbieri, T., Van Loan, M. et al., Resistance exercise and supraphysiologic androgen therapy in eugonadal men with HIV related weight loss. A randomized placebo controlled trial, *JAMA*, 281, 1282–1290, 1999.

116. Demling, R.H., Oxandrolone, an anabolic steroid, enhances the healing of a cutaneous wound in the rat, *Wound Repair Regen.*, 8, 97–102, 2000.

117. Demling, R.H. and Orgill, D.P., The anticatabolic and wound healing effects of the testosterone analog oxandrolone after severe burn injury, *J. Crit. Care*, 15, 12–17, 2000.

118. Demling, R.H. and DeSanti, L., Involuntary weight loss and the nonhealing wound: the role of anabolic agents, *Adv. Wound Care*, 12, 1–14, 1999.

119. Demling, R.H., Comparison of the anabolic effects and complications of human growth hormone and the testosterone analog, oxandrolone, after severe burn injury, *Burns*, 25, 215–221, 1999.

120. Kim, C.S., Buchmiller, T.L., Fonkalsrud, E.W., and Phillips, J.D., The effect of anabolic steroids on ameliorating the adverse effects of chronic corticosteroids on intestinal anastomotic healing in rabbits, *Surg. Gynecol. Obstet.*, 176, 73–79, 1993.

121. Schols, A., Slangen, J., Voloiris, L., and Wauter, E., Weight loss is a reversible factor in the prognosis of chronic obstruction pulmonary disease, *Am. Rev. Resp. Dis.*, 157, 1791–1797, 1998.

122. Demling, R.H. and DeSanti, L., Closure of the "non-healing wound" corresponds with correction of weight loss using the anabolic agent oxandrolone, *Ostomy Wound Manage.*, 44, 58–62, 1998.

123. Beiner, J.M., Jokl, P., Cholewicki, J., and Panjabi, M.M., The effect of anabolic steroids and corticosteroids on healing of muscle contusion injury, *Am. J. Sports Med.*, 27, 2–9, 1999.

124. Falanga, V., Greenberg, A., Zhou, L. et al., Stimulation of collagen synthesis by the anabolic steroid Stanazol, *J. Invest. Dermatol.*, 11, 1193–1197, 1998.

125. Erlich, P., The influence of the anabolic steroid oxandrolone upon the expression of procollagen types I and II MRNA in human fibroblasts cultured in collagen or plastic, *Wounds*, 13, 66–72, 2001.

126. Tennenbaum, R. and Shkear, G., Effect of the anabolic steroid oxandrolone on wound healing, *Oral Surg.*, 30, 834–835, 1970.

127. Basaria, S., Wahlstrom, J., and Dobs, A., Anabolic-androgenic steroid therapy in the treatment of chronic diseases, *J. Clin. Endocrinol. Metab.*, 86, 5108–5117, 2001.

128. Sweeney, E. and Evans, D., Hepatic legions in patients treated with synthetic anabolic steroids, *J. Clin. Pathol.*, 29, 626–633, 1976.

129. Thompson, P., Cullinane, E., Sady, S. et al., Contrasting effects of testosterone and slanozolol on serum lipoprotein levels, *JAMA*, 261, 1165–1168, 1989.

130. Gherondacke, C., Dowling, W., and Pincus, G., Metabolic changes induced in elderly patients with an anabolic steroid oxandrolone, *Am. Geriatr. Soc.*, 47, 751–755, 1991.

Index

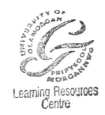